PSYCHOLOGY OF STRESS

NEW RESEARCH

PSYCHOLOGY OF EMOTIONS, MOTIVATIONS AND ACTIONS

Additional books in this series can be found on Nova's website under the Series tab.

Additional e-books in this series can be found on Nova's website under the e-book tab.

PSYCHOLOGY OF EMOTIONS, MOTIVATIONS AND ACTIONS

PSYCHOLOGY OF STRESS

NEW RESEARCH

LEANDRO CAVALCANTI
AND
SOFIA AZEVEDO
EDITORS

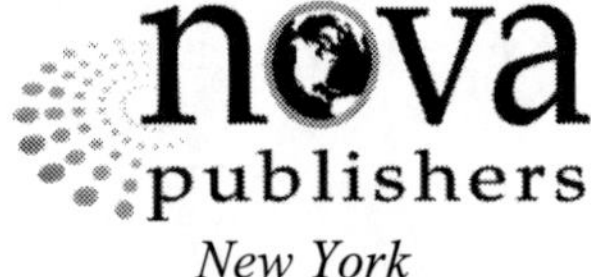

nova publishers

New York

NOTICE TO THE READER

Library of Congress Cataloging-in-Publication Data

Psychology of stress : new research / editors, Leandro Cavalcanti and Sofia Azevedo.
    p. cm.
  Includes index.
  ISBN: 978-1-62417-109-3 (hbk.)
  1. Stress (Psychology) I. Cavalcanti, Leandro. II. Azevedo, Sofia.
  RC455.4.S87P853 2013
  155.9'042--dc23
                        2012038756

Published by Nova Science Publishers, Inc. † New York

CONTENTS

PREFACE

In this book, the authors study the psychology of stress. Topics discussed include the integration of psychological factors and the metaphysical representation of the skin in cutaneous homeostasis under stress influence and its effect on skin wound healing; the use of the Dundee Stress State Questionnaire (DSSQ) in the investigation of task-induced stress; stress in adoptive parenthood; cognitive deficit and immune alterations after chronic stress exposure; stress and homosexuality; the psychological factors influencing inter-individual variation in carbon dioxide-induced stress response; and chronic psychosocial work stress in teachers.

Chapter 1 – Do animals, creatures phylogenetically less developed, present the same wound healing process as humans? Hypothetically yes, once many of these animals are used as experimental models for studies in wound healing.

The scientific literature is plentiful in researches on wound healing mechanisms. However, since in the year of 2000 it has also directed to the influence of psychological stress on it. There is an association between psychological stress and deficiency in wound healing in most of these studies. But there is a hyperproliferative disorder of the wound healing, whose maximum expression is the keloid, which results in excessive scar tissue; in other words, the correlation the greater stress the lower skin wound healing would not occur.

Keloid is a cicatricial and tumoral lesion that can be disfiguring. Usually this lesion presents pruritus and/or pain and causes significant loss on quality of life, self-esteem and even in the functional capacity, depending on the localization. However, keloid occurs only in humans. Why animals don´t develop keloid?

It was always precognized that immune and endocrine factors would be the main involved in an adequate wound healing. Currently, the neurogenic factor is focused, which would precede, during the wound healing, both factors cited above. It is because nerve endings are the first signaling structures injured. In a skin injure, a potential of action and a current of injury start immediately, that will be the healing process trigger. Only after this, the immune and endocrine factors act. When compared to the neurogenic factors performance, that slowness is due to the characteristics of cell signaling, less fast because it is cellular and serum, respectively. Afterwards, these three factors are intertwined and, from this interaction, the neuro-immune-endocrine modulation of the inflammatory phase of skin wound healing occurs.

The homeostatic status of the skin, which precedes and governs the wound healing process, is psycho-dependent. The limbic system, the center of emotions, formed by the amigdala and the hippocampus, connects directly to the *Locus Coeruleus*, the largest noradrenergic source of the Sympathetic Nervous System (SNS), and also to the conscious cortex, through the thalamus. The *Locus Coeruleus*, via hypothalamus and adenohypophysis, transmits the influence of the SNS to peripheral areas, by neurotransmitters, neuropeptides and hormones. Thus thoughts influence the skin and skin processes, because there is a way morpho-anatomical and functional from the conscious cortex to the skin. In addition, there is also the action of the spinothalamic tract in spinal cord dorsal ganglia, to produce more pro-inflammatory neuropeptides. Therefore, the homeostasis and the wound healing depend on the functioning of a Psychoneuroimmune and endocrine system. So, the amounts of studies on psychodermatology increases, which associate some forms of stress SNS to the exacerbation of skin diseases as psoriasis and dermatitis. Therefore, the skin is also a psycho-functional organ.

Humans have a single type of psyches in the animal kingdom and, therefore, the repercussions in their own, on skin homeostasis and wound healing. This chapter reviews the integration of psychological factors and the metaphysical representation of the skin in cutaneous homeostasis under stress influence and its effect on skin wound healing.

Chapter 2 – Task performance is frequently stressful, especially when the task imposes high cognitive demands. Research has shown that the subjective stress response to performance is multidimensional. Different types of task demand elicit different patterns of response. This chapter reviews the use of the Dundee Stress State Questionnaire in the investigation of task-induced stress. The DSSQ is based on a factor model that differentiates 11 primary state factors, which cohere around three higher-order dimensions of task engagement, distress and worry. Following a review of the psychometric evidence for this factorial structure, the chapter surveys evidence on the differing profiles of state change produced by a range of basic and applied performance tasks. It also reviews evidence that links stress states to cognitive appraisal and coping processes, consistent with the transactional model of stress. Data also show that the DSSQ factors predict objective performance. These findings may be understood in relation to the emerging cognitive neuroscience of attention. The final section of the chapter covers practical issues in using the DSSQ for assessment of stress in basic and applied contexts.

Chapter 3 – This chapter focuses on the stress that parents experience in raising adoptive children. Parenting stress is linked to the familiar functioning and to the children and adolescent psychological adjustment. Parenting stress is both condition and consequence of the family and psychological well being. On the one hand, for example, higher emotional or behavioral problems manifested by children affect parental stress. On the other hand, when parents face the task of rearing a child in a very stressful situation, it is more probable that child-rearing practices are affected. Through parental stress, it is possible to analyze bidirectional effects of individual and family processes involved.

Life in adoptive families is very similar to life in the non-adoptive ones. Nevertheless, they have to deal with challenges or tasks added by the fact of adoption. The authors are interested in learning how being an adoptive family affects parental stress. This chapter is based on the findings of the current empirical research with adoptive families, which counted on the participation of 260 adoptive families from Spain in the authors' own longitudinal research. The most widely used measures for parenting stress were applied. These measures are designed to identify parent/child or adolescent systems at-risk for dysfunctional parenting and problematic child adjustment.

When the analyzed adoptive families are not clinical but rather a representative sample of adoptive families, the picture they present is, broadly speaking, that of a good adjustment and a high satisfaction. Differences between families with adopted children and families with adopted adolescents are discussed. The authors identified several predictors of parenting stress. Consistent with the research findings on adoptive families, characteristics of the children, characteristics of the parents and context in which adoption takes place are significantly predictive scores for adoptive parenthood. So, for example, the parental stress is related to the age of arrival of the adopted children, to the parent educational levels, to the child-rearing practices and to the support and resources used regarding adoption.

This analysis allows us to focus the intervention into high stress areas and predicts children's future psychosocial adjustment. Important implications for the current and future adoptions are suggested. To sum up, identifying the most stressful aspects in the adoptive parenthood is useful to work in the pre-adoptive phases, but it is also necessary for organizing post-adoption services.

Chapter 4 – Stress is defined as any situation capable of perturbing the physiological or psychological homeostasis. While response to stress is a necessary survival mechanism, prolonged stress can have several repercussions affecting behavioral, endocrine and immunological parameters. Two genetically different inbred murine strains C57BL/6 and BALB/c, show distinct behavioral and immunological responses. In this chapter the authors show a comparative study on the effect of chronic mild stress upon learning and memory and immunity in BALB/c and C57BL/6 mice. Stressed BALB/c showed poor learning performance related to structural and neurochemical changes observed in the hippocampus, such as a decrease of neurogenesis, a decrease of neural nitric oxide synthase (nNOS) activity and an increase in reactive oxygen species (ROS) levels. These alterations were not found in C57BL/6 mice subjected to CMS. In vivo administration of a nNOS inhibitor induced behavioral alterations in both strains. Moreover, in vitro treatment with a nNOS inhibitor induced an increase in ROS levels. Respect to immune response, CMS BALB/c mice showed a decrease in the T-lymphocyte and an increase of B-lymphocyte mitogen-stimulated proliferation, and an imbalance towards Th2 cytokines. In addition, CMS BALB/c mice had poor antibody production after in vivo immunization with a T-cell depending antigen. On the contrary, CMS C57BL/6 animals showed an increase in the reactivity of T-lymphocytes without changes in the B-lymphocytes reactivity, no changes in humoral response after immunization and an imbalance towards Th1 cytokines. Concerning the participation of the classically stress-associated hormones (catecholamines and corticosterone) in the above mentioned findings, the results indicate that there was not a temporal coincidence between the increase of corticosterone and catecholamines and the behavioral and immune alterations. Taking into account, the authors' results suggest a different vulnerability to cognitive deficit and immune alterations after chronic stress exposure in BALB/c and C57BL/6 mice. These different responses could be related to a differential regulation of hippocampal NO production and peripheral Th1/Th2 cytokine balance. In addition, the relationship between these effects is also analyzed.

Chapter 5 – Homosexuals are one of the most stressed groups of individuals. The various stressful experiences which they face have been grouped under the term "minority stress". This model takes account of the excess amount of stress experienced by individuals belonging to these stigmatised social categories, in particular sexual minorities. Homosexuals are faced with numerous stressors such as family reactions, the attitudes of society and the revelation of their homosexuality. This revelation is often a stressful experience, and the stress is accentuated by the possibility that it may lead to rejection. At the same time, this announcement is a liberating experience conducive to the construction of identity and the improvement of quality of life.

The use or abuse of substances are coping strategies widely used by homosexuals to cope with the stress they are feeling. These strategies are particularly favoured in adolescence and early adulthood, as capacities to cope with stressful events are still being developed. Although adolescence is a period characterised by the presence of numerous stressors (emotional, physical, social, identity-related, affective...), young homosexuals are confronted with additional stressors (non-compliance with the norm, discrimination, revelation of their sexual orientation...). The ineffectiveness of coping strategies and the significant number of stressors are elements which may contribute to the suffering of young homosexuals amongst whom the incidences of consumption or abuse of substances, suicidal behaviour and psychiatric disorders are higher than amongst young heterosexuals.

According to the transactional stress model   it is the interpretation of the situation which generates stress, stress therefore depending on the cognitive evaluation made by the subject and the resources they think they have to cope with it. Based on this model, the authors have sought to evaluate the manner in which young homosexuals cope with the stress they feel when revealing their homosexuality. For this purpose, 400 young homosexuals replied to a questionnaire evaluating the risks encountered during this situation (primary evaluation), their options for action and the coping strategies which they had put in place (secondary evaluation). Two groups were created, the first being questioned on which revelation of their homosexuality had been the most stressful during their life (group 1), and the second on which situation during their life had been the most stressful for them (group 2); the authrs excluded those who replied the announcement of their homosexuality.

The authors' results demonstrate that the announcement of one's homosexuality is judged more "risky" than other stressful situations, the main fears being linked to the possibility of hurting someone as a result of this announcement. The respondents reported fewer possibilities for action during the revelation of their homosexuality than when faced with another stressful situation. During the announcement of their homosexuality, the most commonly used strategies related to personal growth and a positive re-evaluation of the situation. The announcement of one's homosexuality does not therefore necessarily constitute a negative stressor. This data supports the "stress-related growth" (SRG) model which argues that stressors do not systematically lead to negative consequences but that they can also induce positive changes. This data led to the creation of the term "coming-out growth" (COG), applying this model to the announcement of homosexuality.

Chapter 6 – People vary markedly in their response to the same stressor. Possibly, psychological factors hold promise in advancing the authors' understanding of this inter-individual variation in stress responsivity. Indeed, the psychology underlying stress reactivity is an active and important focus of extensive ongoing scientific investigation. Researchers interested in the psychology of stress have increasingly turned their attention towards laboratory stress provocation paradigms. This approach enables a controlled experimental environment in which to measure stress response before, during, and after the stressful provocation. It also affords the opportunity to manipulate putative causal factors implicated in individual stress response. Recently, use of 35% carbon dioxide (CO_2)-enriched air (the 35% CO_2 challenge) has emerged as a particularly promising laboratory stress provocation paradigm. The purpose of this chapter is to overview new findings about the psychology of stress that have been illuminated through 35% CO_2 provocation of the human stress response. The chapter focuses especially on the research conducted in the years since Zvolensky and Eifert (2001)'s seminal review of the psychology underlying the CO_2 response. Particular attention is spent on description of the psychological factors (e.g., anxiety sensitivity; Telch et al., 2011) that could aggravate stress responsivity. Emphasis is also placed on the need for research into factors promoting resilience in the face of the CO_2 stressor. Ultimately, clarifying how psychological factors influence individual differences in stress responsivity could yield targets for intervention in the treatment of extreme stress responses.

Chapter 7 – Recent evidence from epidemiological and prospective studies suggests that chronic work stress is a relevant risk factor for the progression and development of manifest disease such as cardiovascular disease, type 2 diabetes as well as psychiatric and psychosomatic conditions. Especially teaching has often been described as a highly demanding occupation, leaving many teachers with a general perception of being stressed and overworked. Here, the authors present an up-date on findings from the second part of the authors' Teacher Stress Study, in which the authorsinvestigated associations between work-related psychosocial stress in two independent samples of healthy school teachers and alterations in the regulation of different physiological systems. The goal of this project was to investigate the psychobiological pathways which link job stress to an increased risk for disease outcomes in order to increase the knowledge, which is necessary for the development of diagnostic tools that allow the early identification of potential risk factors. The authors' recent empirical results suggest an impact of chronic work stress in terms of effort-reward-imbalance and overcommitment on hypothalamus-pituitary-adrenal (HPA) axis stress responses and HPA axis feedback regulation, on stress responses of the blood coagulation system as well as on the regulation of the immune system. Furthermore, the authors found associations between exhaustion as a consequence of chronic work stress and stress reactivity of the blood coagulation system as well as HPA axis feedback regulation. To sum up, they observed subtle dysregulations in multiple stress sensitive, physiological systems even in apparently healthy, working school teachers. The authors' findings point to the need to protect employees from negative health outcomes, which are potentially associated with chronic work stress in the long run.

Chapter 1

PSYCHOLOGICAL STRESS AND SKIN WOUND HEALING: NEW HIGHLIGHTS

B. Hochman[1], F. Furtado[2], F. C. Isoldi[3],
M. A. Nishioka[4] and L. M. Ferreira[5]

[1]Plastic Surgery Division, Department of Surgery, Postgraduate Program in Plastic Surgery, Federal University of Sao Paulo (Unifesp), Sao Paulo-SP, Brazil
[2]Postgraduate Program in Plastic Surgery, Unifesp, Sao Paulo-SP, Brazil
[3]Improvement Program (*Latu sensu*), Plastic Surgery Division, Department of Surgery, Unifesp, Sao Paulo-SP, Brazil
[4]Postgraduate Program in Plastic Surgery, Unifesp, Sao Paulo-SP, Brazil
[5]Plastic Surgery Division, Department of Surgery, Postgraduate Program in Plastic Surgery, Unifesp, Sao Paulo-SP, Brazil

ABSTRACT

Do animals, creatures phylogenetically less developed, present the same wound healing process as humans? Hypothetically yes, once many of these animals are used as experimental models for studies in wound healing.

The scientific literature is plentiful in researches on wound healing mechanisms. However, since in the year of 2000 it has also directed to the influence of psychological stress on it. There is an association between psychological stress and deficiency in wound healing in most of these studies. But there is a hyperproliferative disorder of the wound healing, whose maximum expression is the keloid, which results in excessive scar tissue; in other words, the correlation the greater stress the lower skin wound healing would not occur.

Keloid is a cicatricial and tumoral lesion that can be disfiguring. Usually this lesion presents pruritus and/or pain and causes significant loss on quality of life, self-esteem and even in the functional capacity, depending on the localization. However, keloid occurs only in humans. Why animals don´t develop keloid?

It was always precognized that immune and endocrine factors would be the main involved in an adequate wound healing. Currently, the neurogenic factor is focused, which would precede, during the wound healing, both factors cited above. It is because nerve endings are the first signaling structures injured. In a skin injure, a potential of action and a current of injury start immediately, that will be the healing process trigger. Only after this, the immune and endocrine factors act. When compared to the neurogenic factors performance, that slowness is due to the characteristics of cell signaling, less fast because it is cellular and serum, respectively. Afterwards, these three factors are intertwined and, from this interaction, the neuro-immune-endocrine modulation of the inflammatory phase of skin wound healing occurs.

The homeostatic status of the skin, which precedes and governs the wound healing process, is psycho-dependent. The limbic system, the center of emotions, formed by the amigdala and the hippocampus, connects directly to the *Locus Coeruleus*, the largest noradrenergic source of the Sympathetic Nervous System (SNS), and also to the conscious cortex, through the thalamus. The *Locus Coeruleus*, via hypothalamus and adenohypophysis, transmits the influence of the SNS to peripheral areas, by neurotransmitters, neuropeptides and hormones. Thus thoughts influence the skin and skin processes, because there is a way morpho-anatomical and functional from the conscious cortex to the skin. In addition, there is also the action of the spinothalamic tract in spinal cord dorsal ganglia, to produce more pro-inflammatory neuropeptides. Therefore, the homeostasis and the wound healing depend on the functioning of a Psychoneuroimmune and endocrine system. So, the amounts of studies on psychodermatology increases, which associate some forms of stress SNS to the exacerbation of skin diseases as psoriasis and dermatitis. Therefore, the skin is also a psycho-functional organ.

Humans have a single type of psyches in the animal kingdom and, therefore, the repercussions in their own, on skin homeostasis and wound healing. This chapter reviews the integration of psychological factors and the metaphysical representation of the skin in cutaneous homeostasis under stress influence and its effect on skin wound healing.

1. GENERAL ASPECTS

The skin is a versatile organ that has many special features. It is the first contact interface between the body and the external environment. The skin is the second largest organ of the human body (about $1.8m^2$); however, it is the most visible because it is the outermost. Due to its visual range, the skin has an important social and interpersonal interaction function. In relation to the size, it is only surpassed by the endothelial tissue, but this one is in the intimacy of the blood vessels, thus not visible (GURTNER *et al.*, 2008).

Hypothetically, if no one had skin, everybody would have a similar appearance, presenting themselves as a mass of muscles, fascias, ligaments and tendons. This hypothesis demonstrates that the skin is our personal identifier. Therefore, under the psychic prism, analogously to the fingerprint that being unique identifies us as citizens, the skin would be the "fingerprint" of our personality.

Under the functional aspect, the skin is also a communication means and exchange with the environment. The skin presents itself as the first line of contact with the environment, protecting the body against toxic substances, solar radiation by ultraviolet rays (UVR), microorganisms, and mechanical trauma. It has a key role for the body hydroelectrolytic balance. It is involved in excretion and absorption of substances, and exercises a thermoregulatory function, immune and endocrine features activities, and others (HWA *et al.*, 2011).

2. ANATOMY OF THE SKIN AND STRESS LINKS

The skin is basically divided into two layers: the epidermis, which is the outermost and thus in contact with the external environment; and the dermis, located below the epidermis. The hypodermis or subcutaneous cellular tissue is not part of split skin and is located below the dermis. The epidermis and dermis can be studied together, because they have similar functions. The skin has different thicknesses in different regions of the body. The eyelid is the place where the skin is the thinnest, approximately 2 mm; on the soles and palms, 4 to 5 mm. The epidermis is only one tenth, on average, the total skin thickness (HWA *et al.*, 2011).

2.1. Epidermis

The epidermis consists of a keratinized squamous stratified epithelium and presents three major cell types: keratinocytes, melanocytes, and dendritic cells. It is divided into strata and deeply separated of the dermis by the basal membrane. It has no vascular system itself. Nutrients and oxygen arrives by diffusion from the blood vessels of the dermis. Regarding the nerve endings, only 5% of cutaneous nerve fibers are epidermal and the others are dermal. Some cutaneous annexes are originated from the epidermis, such as hair, nails, and sweat and sebaceous glands. Then, they migrate to deeper regions of the dermis according to its development (RINN *et al.*, 2008; KYPRIOTOU *et al.*, 2012)

2.1.1. Keratinocytes

The keratinocytes represent about 80% of all epidermal cells. The deeper stratum, which rests on the basement membrane, is the basal stratum or basal layer. In this stratum, the keratinocytes are under a "cuboid" shape. As these keratinocytes multiply and maturate in the basal layer, they start a migratory process, becoming superficial and forming the following strata. Thus, above the basal layer, is the stratum spinosum or spinous layer, called this way due to the development of cytoplasmic extensions resembling "thorns", by keratinocytes. In the sequence, they continue the differentiation, acquiring cytoplasmic granules and characterizing the next stratum in granny or granular layer. Superficially, the keratinocytes undergo apoptosis and form the stratum corneum or corneal layer, which is the outermost layer of the skin. On the palm of the hands and soles of feet, there is an intermediate layer before the corneal layer, called lucid layer. This cycle of transformation and cell superficialization, from the basal to the corneum stratum, in a young adult, takes about 70 days. This period can change to less or more days in the presence of some skin diseases or even in physiological processes. This time is reduced in psoriasis, characterizing classically scaly skin, whereas in elderly people the time is extended (DENDA *et al.*, 2007; DENDA & TSUTSUMI, 2011).

The keratinocytes are rich in cytoplasmic proteins composed mostly by keratin and kerato hyaline (or filaggrin). The keratin provides structural and tensile strength to the skin due to its provision in bands of fibers that extend between the cells. Surrounding keratinocytes themselves, there is a crossed network of these proteins, in a cornified way, which protects the cell and serves as an anchor for the keratin (HENRY *et al.*, 2012).

2.1.1.1. Keratinocytes under Stress

These cells have another important function in the skin immune regulation, by the secretion of inflammatory mediators. They are also closely related to melanocytes, regulate their own proliferation, have enzymatic function, express membrane proteins and release growth factors - such as Neural Growth Factor (NGF) (PINCELLI *et al.*, 1994; STEFANATO *et al.*, 2003; CIRULLI & ALLEVA, 2009), one of the main central and peripheral marker of stress, which are precursors of proinflammatory neuropeptide of the skin , Substance P (SP), and Calcitonin Gene-Related Peptide (CGRP), which will be detailed below. Keratinocytes are involved in the melanogenesis and dendritogenesis of melanocytes (DI MARCO *et al.*, 1991; YAAR *et al.*, 1991). Its expression is up-regulated by UVR, suggesting yet another paracrine influence of keratinocytes on melanocytes with possible relevance to the tanning response (DI MARCO *et al.*, 1993).

2.1.2. Melanocytes

Melanocytes represent about 19% in the amount of epidermal cells. They are also supported in the basal membrane between the basal cells. Embryologically, melanocytes derive from neural crest cells. During embryonic development, these cells migrate to the basal layer of the epidermis (YAAR & PARK, 2012). Thus, because of its neuroectodermal origin, as such Perypheral Nervous System (PNS) and Central Nervous System (CNS) cells, the melanocyte is considered a "skin neuron", presenting, as it is in fact, cell body, axons, dendrites, and synapses, by means of neurotransmitters (KAWAKAMI & FISHER, 2011; YAAR & PARK, 2012). And, as it is known in the field of phylogeny, neurons have evolved to exercise command, control, and integration activities. This way, the skin melanocyte acts commanding trophic functions and homeostasis of the skin, including the wound healing. Without approaching details about melanocyte nature, Navarro asserts that by the fact that the embryological origin of the epidermis occurs in the ectoderm, from where also is the CNS, it could be recognized as an "external brain" (NAVARRO, 1991). He continues his line of reasoning by stating that in the skin is contained the "Self", therefore, chronic disorders of the skin would be responses to a malfunction of the "Self".

The melanocyte commands on average 36 keratinocytes, by means of neurotransmitters. This is the "thinking" unit of the skin (SLOMINSKI *et al.*, 2004). The melanin, a pigment produced by the melanocytes, is the final product of dopamine from tyrosine transformation, an essential amino acid. Dopamine is also an adrenaline and noradrenaline precursor. Therefore, the bioavailability of melanin is neurotransmitter-dependent, a typical nerve cell event.

Neurons and myocardial cells do not multiply because they are highly specialized, except in very precise circumstances. Melanocytes, however, still preserve this ability and perform cellular multiplication (COSTIN & HEARING, 2007). Another difference between CNS neurons and melanocytes is related to its disposal in the body. The neurons maintain their cell bodies located in the encephalon and spinal cord and also in dorsal root ganglia, distributing nerve fibers throughout the whole body; melanocytes are completely inserted in the epidermis.

2.1.2.1. Melanocytes under Stress

Increased circulating levels of Pro-Opiomelanocortin-derived peptides (POMC), such as alpha-Melanocyte-Stimulating Hormone (α-MSH) and Adrenocorticotropic Hormone

(ACTH) in horses and humans exposed to sunlight stimulate the production and secretion of ACTH, α-MSH (SCHAUER *et al.*, 1994) and Corticotropin-Releasing Hormone (CRH) (SLOMINSKI *et al.*, 1996) in cultured melanocytes and keratinocytes. Therefore, activation of the local cutaneous neuronal axis could contribute to the systemic response to stress (SLOMINSKI *et al,.* 1993; SLOMINSKI & MIHM, 1996;). Moreover, melanocytes respond to CRH and ACTH with an enhanced production of cortisol/corticosterone (SLOMINSKI *et al.*, 2005b). In normal melanocytes, production of CRH peptide could be stimulated with Ultraviolet Radiation B (UVB; wavelength 290–320 nm) (ZBYTEK *et al.*, 2006); normal human skin, α-MSH was found in epidermal melanocytes and Langerhans cells, and ACTH was found in differentiating keratinocytes (WAKAMATSU *et al.*, 1997).

2.1.3. Dendritic Cells

Dendritic cells (Langerhans cells) are about 1% of epidermal cells. However, despite its name and format suggesting that also would include nerve cells, they are only cells of mesenchymal origin, derived from macrophages. They have immunological function with the surface antigens identification, in other words, dendritic cells are the main activators and regulators of diverse immune responses, which determine responses of immediate and late hypersensitivity by antigen-antibody binding. Its subtypes can be distinguished by the location in the tissue, by the phenotype and function in the homeostasis of normal skin, and in the cutaneous inflammatory response, influenced by the extracellular microenvironment to which they belong (TEUNISSEN *et al.*, 2012).

2.1.3.1. Dendritic Cells under Stress

Dendritic cells are a potent initiators of skin immune responses (VALLADEAU & SAELAND, 2005), providing the first line of defense against invading pathogens and sensitizing substances. They are very close connected with epidermis nerve fibers (HOSOI *et al.*, 1993) and they express receptors for many neuropeptides and neurohormones (MISERY, 1998; SEIFFERT *et al.*, 2002; KODALI *et al.*, 2003; KODALI *et al.*, 2004). Their modulation pay special emphasis on mediators of the Sympathetic Nervous System (SNS). Glucocorticoids applied to human skin *in vivo*, for instance, lead to a reduction of dendritic cell number (ASHWORTH *et al.,* 1988) and can induce their apoptosis *in situ*. Thus, catecholamines appear to decrease epidermal immune reactions by inhibiting antigen presentation by dendritic cell. This corroborates with a worsening of the cutaneous cellular immunity in stressful situations.

2.2. Dermis

Various cell types are found in the dermis, but only fibroblasts has dermal origin; in other words, fibroblast is the unique autochthonous cell of the dermis and the main cell type. Other important cells present in the dermis, but of migratory character, appearing as needed, are leukocytes (or white blood cells), and monocytes, mast cells and neutrophils, which are inflammatory cells and also have a key role in wound healing (RINN *et al.*, 2008; KYPRIOTOU *et al.*, 2012).

Other important structures located in the dermis are the cutaneous annexes: sweat glands, sebaceous glands with their hair (pilo-sebaceous unit), and nerve endings, which are sensorial and belonging to the SNS.

2.2.1. Fibroblasts

Fibroblasts function is the synthesis of Extracellular Matrix (ECM) proteins, mainly collagen. Twenty-eight types of collagens have been identified, and the characterization of the nature and functions of several collagens have been well established. The common structural feature of collagens is the presence of a triple helix composed by aminoacids hidroxiprolin, hidroxilisin and glicin. Collagens are the major fibrous proteins in ECM of the skin, bone or ligaments and other organs. In the skin, collagen fibrils are composed mainly of collagen type I (80–85%), collagen type III (10–15%) and smaller amounts of collagen type V (ONO *et al.*, 2000; RICARD-BLUM, 2011).

In practice, fibroblasts are identified by their spindle-shaped morphology with diverse appearances depending on their location and activity. The main function of fibroblasts is to maintain the structural integrity of connective tissues by continuously secreting precursors of the ECM. The composition of the ECM determines the physical properties of connective tissues (HULMES, 2002).

Also, fibroblasts play an important role in wound healing. Following tissue injury, they migrate to the site of damage, where they deposit new collagen and facilitate the healing process. This occurs mainly at the proliferative phase of wound healing, in which there are fibroblasts proliferation and an active angiogenesis, creating new capillaries and allowing nutrient delivery to the wound site. Then, fibroblasts compose the granulation tissue which are activated and acquire a smooth muscle cell-like phenotype, then being referred to as myofibroblasts, which synthesize and deposit ECM components that replace the provisional matrix. They also have contractile properties mediated by alpha-smooth muscle actin organized in microfilament bundles or stress fibers (MYLLYHARJU & KIVIRIKKO, 2001).

Some neuropeptides have a proliferative effect on fibroblasts and may cause disturbances of wound healing. One of them, SP, has the ability to induce synthesis and proliferation of keratinocytes and human dermal fibroblasts through arachidonic acid metabolites, and has been linked to cutaneous immune reactions. SP is a potent chemoattractant for human fibroblasts *in vitro*, triggering a concentration-dependent migratory response. The ability of SP to promote chemotaxis in human fibroblasts, which extends to the fibroplasia phase of wound healing, is another proinflammatory activity of this neuropeptide (HOFFMANN *et al.*, 2010).

2.2.1.1. Fibroblasts under Stress

Increased levels of circulating glucocorticoids can down-regulate local tissue levels of insulinlike growth factor-1 and lead to impaired fibroblast function (BITAR, 2000). In addition, glucocorticoids can impact upon angiogenesis by inhibiting Vascular Endothelial Growth Factor (VEGF), VEGF expression, and impaired matrix deposition by down-regulating Transforming Growth Factor-beta (TGF-β) receptor levels (NAUCK *et al.*, 1998; ROY, 2000). TGF-β modulates wound contraction and myofibroblast differentiation (HINZ *et al.*, 2001; MONTESANO & ORCI, 1988; REED *et al.*, 1994). Gene expression of TGF-β was dramatically altered in a model of glucocorticoid-impaired wound healing (FRANK *et al.*, 1996). Evidence demonstrates that chronic psychological stress enhance endogenous glucocorticoids modulating the expression of TGF-β2 and TGF-β3 during normal healing, which resulted in alterations in fibroblast migration, proliferation, and differentiation within the wound granulation tissue (GROSE *et al.*, 2002; CAMPANER *et al*, 2006). Thus, altered expression of TGF-β delays fibroblast migration, proliferation, and differentiation. That is, stress adversely affects wound closure by significantly impairing wound contraction (HORAN *et al.*, 2005; VILEIKYTE, 2007).

2.2.2. Inflammatory Cells

Although there are various types and subtypes of inflammatory cells, this sub-section will report only those important and directly linked to the skin wound healing, such as mast cells, monocytes/macrophages and neutrophils.

2.2.2.1. Mast Cells

Mast cells contain many granules rich in histamine and heparin. Although their role in allergy and anaphylaxis, they play an important function in the skin wound healing and defense against pathogens. Nevertheless, mast cells are originated from bone marrow precursors; circulate in an immature form, and only maturing once in a tissue site. They are present in most tissues of the body characteristically surrounding blood vessels and nerves, and are especially prominent in the skin, playing a key role in the inflammatory process. When activated, a mast cell rapidly releases its granules and various hormonal mediators into the interstitium. This event, degranulation, can be started by direct injury, cross-linking of Immunoglobulin E (IgE) receptors, or by activated complement proteins (KASHIWAKURA *et al.*, 2011; JAMUR & OLIVER, 2011).

2.2.2.1.1. Mast Cells under Stress

Mast cells are powerful inflammatory cells which are in close functional and anatomical association with sensory nerves in the skin. Mast cell activation is a characteristic feature of chronic inflammation, a condition that may lead to fibrosis as a result of increased collagen synthesis by fibroblasts (CAIRNS & WALLS, 1997). During psychological stress the peripheral sensory nerves are activated leading to release of many mediators, such as neuropeptides, neurotrophins and hormones, which are capable of activating mast cells. On the other hand, mast cell mediators released, such as histamine, tryptase and NGF can in turn excite and stimulate surrounding neuropeptide-containing C-fibers, for example SP (HARVIMA & NILSSON, 2012), possibly resulting in feedforward loop and potentiation of neurogenic inflammation. In these mechanisms, proinflammatory cytokines and chemokines are released from mast cells. In chronic skin diseases the contacts between tryptase-positive mast cells and sensory nerves are increased in number, which provides the morphological basis for increased mast cell - sensory nerve interaction in chronically inflamed skin (PETERS *et al.*, 2005; HARVIMA *et al.*, 2010).

Thus, it is clear that any stress could affect the dermal nerves and mast cells immediately. Moreover, stress could be retained in "memory" over a long period of time and may be invoked when some factor affects the skin. Mast cells compute activation signals received via both systemic and locally generated stress messengers such as CRH, NGF and SP. Upon activation, mast cells release a multitude of factors. The close level of mast cell integration into neuroendocrine-immune networks is probably most easily examined and best documented in the skin (ARCK & PAUS, 2006).

2.2.2.2. Monocytes

Monocytes are a type of white blood cell and part of the innate immune system. They play multiple roles in immune function in response to inflammation signals, moving quickly to the site of infection where they differentiate into macrophages and dendritic cells to elicit an immune response. Therefore, monocytes circulate in the bloodstream for about one to three days and then typically move into tissues throughout the body, where they mature into macrophages in response to a skin injury, for instance. Macrophages are responsible for protecting tissues from foreign substances by phagocytosis, antigen presentation, and cytokine production (MAHDAVIAN *et al.*, 2011).

2.2.2.2.1. Monocytes under Stress

Stress, like severe sleep disruption, can impair healing, altering proinflammatory cytokine profiles as well as Growth Hormone (GH) secretion (LEPROULT *et al.*, 1997; VGONTZAS *et al.*, 1999; IRWIN, 2002). GH enhances healing through several functions including stimulating monocyte migration, enhancing macrophage activation, and amplifying bacterial killing by macrophages (ZWILLING & HILBURGER, 1994). Because the majority of GH release occurs during sleep (VELDHUIS & IRANMANESH, 1996), stress can substantially affect GH production by altering sleep architecture, and impairing immune system directly and wound healing indirectly (CHRISTIAN *et al.*, 2006). Interestingly, it has also been demonstrated that various aspects of the immune response, such as cytokine production, antibody production, chemotaxis of monocytes and neutrophils, can be affected by glucocorticoids as well as peptides such as ACTH, endorphins, SP, and somatostatin (BLALOCK, 1989; YANG & GLASER, 2002).

2.2.2.3. Neutrophils

Neutrophils are the most abundant type of white blood cells are an essential part of the innate immune system. In general, they are referred to as either neutrophils or polymorphonuclear neutrophils, and are subdivided into segmented and banded neutrophils. Neutrophils are normally found in the blood stream. During the acute phase of inflammation, neutrophils are one of the first-responders of inflammatory cells to migrate towards the site of inflammation. They migrate from the blood vessels to the tissue, following chemical signals within minutes. The average lifespan of the neutrophils are about 5 days (PILLAY *et al.*, 2010).

2.2.2.3.1. Neutrophils under Stress

Adults with higher perceived stress scores had elevated levels of salivary cortisol and decreased concentrations of the inflammatory cytokines Tumor Necrosis Factor-alpha (TNFα), Interleukin (IL), such as IL-1α, IL-6 and IL-8 at wound sites. Moreover, this state of stress was associated with a temporary dysregulation in the balance of Th1-Th2, consistent with suppression of neutrophil activity. (GODBOUT & GLASER, 2006). Besides, neutrophil function appears compromised as bacterial counts in the wound increase in stress state (ROJAS *et al.*, 2002). Impaired neutrophil functioning is likely due to reduced oxygen availability, as alpha-adrenergic activation causes peripheral vasoconstriction and thus reduces oxygen and nutrients to the wound (AHLQUIST, 1976). The responses of macrophages and neutrophils, both important players in wound healing, can be altered by adrenergic agonists (BARNES, 1999; EIJKELKAMP *et al.*, 2007).

2.2.3. Sweat Glands

The sweat glands are numerous and found throughout the body surface, except in some regions such as the glans and lips. Its secretory apparatus is considered merocrine because its cells are not destroyed in the process of secretion. The substance produced and secreted by these glands, the sweat, is diluted and contains, in general, inorganic substances such as sodium, potassium, urea and ammonia, and organic substances as some proteins. The cells that compose their ducts are rich in mitochondria, and this is a characteristic of ions and water carrying cells. They can be classified according to their mode and place of secretion as eccrine, apocrine and apoecrine (WILKE *et al.*, 2007). The eccrine glands have their excretory canal opened directly into the pores of the skin surface. They are generally small and start functioning since birth. Their secretion is clear, colorless and odorless, similar to an aqueous fluid. Its composition varies depending on the rate of secretion, the transit time within the secretive duct, the aldosterone activity, the individual's physical activity and acclimatization phase, and the ambient temperature. The apocrine glands are present in the armpits, in the urogenital area, on the nipples, and in some male face areas. In the skin, these glands release their content along the hair follicle. The sweat secreted is more viscous because it contains a larger amount of lipids and proteins. They begin to function in the puberty period, because of the high sex hormonal activity, and are also stimulated in moments of stress and sexual excitement. The third glandular type, apoecrine, presents some characteristics of both previous glandular types. It is found in the armpits and responds rapidly to stressful factors, contributing to the characteristic high transpiration (SATO *et al.*, 1987; NOËL *et al.*, 2012).

The cutaneous transpiration function is mainly related to a reduction in body temperature. It is generally stimulated by the environment temperature elevation or by physical activity, for example. Another related situation, which has its mechanism still poorly understood, is the transpiration caused by emotional stress and by spicy foods consumption.

The sweat glands activity is directly controlled by the CNS. The hypothalamus is the main thermoregulatory center. This center not only responds to variations in body temperature, but also to hormones, endogenous pyrogenic factors, physical activity, and emotions. The rate of sweat secretion is also affected by the local thermal elevation of the skin, caused by increased secretion of neurotransmitters, and by the increased sensitivity of the sweat glands themselves to neurotransmitters, during the increased temperature period.. Constitutional and environmental factors such as gender, level of daily physical activity, menstrual cycle period, circadian cycle, humidity of air, among others, also contribute to the rate of excretion (OGAWA & SUGENOYA, 1993; HÖLZLE, 2002; DIPASQUALE *et al.*, 2003).

2.2.3.1. Sweat Glands under Stress

Emotional sweating is a physical reaction to emotional stimuli such as stress, fear, anxiety or pain, and occurs throughout the body surface, more evident on the palms, soles and armpits (EISENACH *et al.,* 2005). Unlike thermoregulation, the emotional transpiration occurs regardless of environmental characteristics, and decrease during relaxation and sleep. In general, emotional sweating involves the eccrine glands, typically activated by cholinergic fibers from SNS under adrenergic stimulation (WARNDORFF, 1972; SATO *et al.,* 1987; NAKAZATO *et al.,* 2004). The emotional transpiration central via is not completely understood yet, however, the amygdala, a constituent part of the limbic system, is probably involved in it (TRANEL & DAMASIO, 1994; ASAHINA *et al.*, 2003).

2.2.4. Pilosebaceous Unit

The pilosebaceous unit consists of the hair follicle associated with the corresponding sebaceous gland. It is morpho-functionally independent, with its own nutrition and vascular innervation. Sebocytes are the major component cells of it. Those cells are located in the dermis and are considered holocrine glands. In other words, unlike sweat glands, the glandular secretion of these is composed of the mature sebocytes that underwent apoptosis and its lipid content. These glands can be found in all terrestrial mammals, distinguishing between species by their cell density in different parts of the body, and by the composition of produced sebum. In adults, the sebaceous gland can be divided in three distinct zones, which contain sebocytes in different stages of differentiation. The peripheral zone consists of young cells mitotically active and small. As these cells mature, they lose their mitotic activity and migrate more toward the center of the gland, where they accumulate lipid droplets, composing the maturation zone. In the central region of the gland, these cells complete their differentiation into mature sebocytes, undergo cell death and release their internal lipid content through holocrine secretion via. This continuous cell differentiation via is controlled by hormonal mechanisms and neural mediators, which act on different receptors expressed on the cell membrane of sebocytes. In the follicular bulge, a specialized region of sebaceous gland, are located mesenchymal stem cells, which are also responsible for the hair growth and assist in wound healing (ZOUBOULIS, 2009a; SCHNEIDER *et al.,* 2009; SCHNEIDER & PAUS, 2010).

Sebum is mainly composed by neutral lipids, with a relative amount of triglyceride, free fatty acids, wax esters, cholesterol, and squalene. Among these, squalene and wax esters are unique and typical components of the sebum. Its presence in skin plays important roles in cutaneous functional barrier. It acts in the physicochemical barrier composition of the skin and contributes to the antimicrobial activity (WILLE &, KYDONIEUS, 2003; SMITH & THIBOUTOT, 2008).

2.2.4.1. Pilosebaceous Unit under Stress

The sebocytes are also involved in the regulation of immune function and inflammatory processes. They are able to produce different cytokines and lipid-derived inflammatory mediators, mostly proinflammatory (ALESTAS *et al.*, 2006; NAGY *et al.*, 2006). They are still able to produce several hormones also secreted by the hypothalamus, anterior pituitary, and peripheral organs, such as CRH, α-MSH, which are basically considered hormones of stress, SP, and others (SLOMINSKI & WORTSMAN, 2000; SLOMINSKI *et al.*, 2008; ZOUBOULIS, 2009b).

There is increasing evidence that the sebaceous gland expresses receptors for several neuropeptides and is involved in responses to stress. (KRAUSE *et al.*, 2007)

Culture of sebocytes provides a new insight into the participation of neuropeptides, notably SP, in the pathophysiology of acne. Acne is a complex, chronic and common skin disorder of pilosebaceous units, and its exacerbation results from emotional stress. Dermal nerves around the sebaceous glands of acne patients express SP (BÖHM *et al.*, 2002; BODÓ *et al.*, 2004; LEE *et al.*, 2008).

2.2.5. Nerve Endings

The skin has a somatic postganglionic sympathetic and parasympathetic sensory innervations (BOULAIS & MISERY, 2008). These nerve fibers are of various types, which differ as to size, degree of myelination, conduction speed and sensory specificity. They are categorized into three fiber groups: Aβ, Aδ and C. The top two groups of nerve fibers are covered with myelin. Nerve fibers C-type have no myelin being, therefore, considered unmyelinated. The fiber diameter is related to the nerve conduction speed of the electrical impulse transmitted. The higher the fiber diameter, the higher the speed of impulse transmission. In descending order, the Aβ-fiber has the largest diameter, followed by the Aδ-fiber, and finally by the C-fiber. Regarding the transmitted stimulus type, nerve fibers Aβ-type are responsible for conducting the tactile sensation; and Aδ- and C-fibers are thermoceptive and nociceptive, while C-fibers is related to inflammation (LAWSON, 2002).

The endings of these nerve fibers have sensory receptors, currently classified as mechanoreceptors (tactile, deep vibrational, pressure), thermoceptors (hot and cold temperature) and nociceptors (pain). There are some fibers that have their endings in the skin freely, without receptors. The thermoceptors and nociceptors are primarily involved in the mechanism of wound healing, as it will be detailed further ahead.

Interestingly, these nervous fibers form a complex neural network that, in an animal study, the sciatic nerve was severed in one leg and the other leg was treated with capsaicin (a C-fiber neuropeptides depletory), and skin wound healing was evaluated. There was no difference between the two research groups, concluding that it is difficult to knock out all cutaneous sensory innervation. Thirty per cent of C-fibre innervation seems enough to ensure a normal wound healing (WALLENGREN *et al.,* 1999).

2.2.5.1. Nerve Endings under Stress

Emotional stress can affect, reveal or exacerbate many skin disorders (psoriasis, atopic dermatitis, pruritus and others). There is increasing evidence that stress contributes to the skin inflammation through modulating hypothalamic-pituitary-adrenal axis and releasing neuropeptides, neurotrophins, citokynes and other chemical mediators from nerve endings and dermal cells. The central role in cellular skin reactivity may be attributed to dermal mast cells, as they show close connections with sensory nerve endings and may release a huge number of proinflammatory mediators (REICH *et al.,* 2010; PETERS, 2012).

2.3. Multisystem Functional Complexity of the Skin

Once understood the skin anatomy and some of their interrelations with the neural network and stress, it becomes easier to understand why the skin is currently considered an organ of psychoneuroimmuneendocrinefunctional interaction (MISERY, 1997; ZMIJEWSKI & SLOMINSKI, 2011).

Currently, studies on Psychoendoneuroimmunology are already possible. They are more and more employed (LOTTI *et al.,* 1995) in the holistic understanding about mind-body relationship and its influences on the skin (KOO & LEBWOHL, 2001; CHOI *et al.,* 2005; CONSOLI *et al.,* 2006; SAMPOGNA *et al.,* 2007; GRIFFITHS & BARKER, 2007). These studies also try to clarify the pathophysiological pathways of cutaneous lesions, by means of the integration of body systems (AZAMBUJA, 2000). So it is possible to understand how a mental event, which would be a stressful event, could turn into a skin disorder or disease on the skin (AZAMBUJA, 2000). Studies proposing the understanding of this mechanism also propose strategies of focal intervention about stress and about facing the disease.

It is classically preconized that, in the process of skin wound healing, the immune and endocrine factors are vitally important for proper tissue healing. Little is said about the neural factor involved. Currently, more importance has been given to this last factor, because in the cutaneous wound, the first signalizing structure of the injury caused is the nervous structure, triggering the initial electrical stimulus of the whole healing process. Then, later, immune and endocrine factors act, which are cellular and serum. Consequently, the modulation wound healing is reached by the interaction of all the following factors: nervous, immune, and endocrine.

To a better comprehension about the complexity of the skin, the holistic view will be addressed in a Cartesian way: in the next topics, the skin will be dismembered, in a didactical manner, and the relation to stress will be mentioned where appropriate.

3. SKIN AS A NEUROFUNCTIONAL ORGAN

Due to the common neuroectodermal origin of the skin with the CNS, there is a growing scientific attention to the brain-skin connections over the past decade. This is reflected by the skin's innervation related to numerous neurotransmitters, neuropeptides, neurotrophins or neurohormones present locally and acting both as major targets and effector messengers of the stress response (ARCK *et al.*, 2006)

3.1. Cutaneous Nervous System

In the skin, dermal-epidermal nerve fibers in conjunction with melanocytes are referred to as "cutaneous nervous system" or "cutaneous neurosensory system" (TOYODA *et al.*, 1999; LUGER, 2002; ROOSTERMAN *et al.*, 2006). This neural network, in addition to having primary activities on the skin itself, such as the participation in inflammation, immunity, functional regulation of its annexes, thermoregulation, and modulation of its homeostasis, is also part of healing (SLOMINSKI *et al.*, 1993; BESNÉ *et al.*, 2002; LIANG *et al.*, 2004; JUNIOR ESTEVES *et al.*, 2004). In other words, the neurological part of the skin acts in conjunction with the immune and endocrine systems of the skin to perform local physiological processes, such as the healing process (OAKLANDER & SIEGEL, 2005; ROOSTERMAN *et al.*, 2006; FERREIRA *et al.*, 2009). Furthermore, by its electrical nature, the cutaneous neurological system would respond faster to stimuli triggered on the skin than the other two systems, which act as cellular and humoral; moreover, another way of executing this system is by releasing neuropeptides which, like the CNS cells, act as neurotransmitters, but with some peculiarities to be discriminated below.

The CNS is directly (via efferent nerves or CNS-derived mediators) or indirectly (via the adrenal glands or immune cells) connected to skin function. In the skin, cutaneous nerve fibers are principally sensory, with an additional complement of autonomic nerve fibers

(BREATHNACH, 1977; MUNGER & IDE, 1988). Both C and Aδ fibers respond to a variable range of stimuli such as physical as well as chemical agents (STEINHOFF *et al.*, 2003). Thus mediators derived from sensory or autonomic nerves may play an important regulatory role in the skin under many physiological and pathophysiological conditions. Upon direct stimulation by physical stimuli (thermal, ultraviolet light, mechanical, electrical), chemical, or indirect stimuli such as allergens, haptens, microbiological agents, trauma, or inflammation, a significant increase of regulatory neuropeptides, neurotrophins, neurotransmitters, or reactive oxygen products such as nitric oxide can be detected in vitro and in vivo. Thus the skin "talks" to the brain via primary afferents thereby revealing information about the status of peripherally derived pain, pruritus, and local inflammation. (ROOSTERMAN *et al.*, 2006; ARCK *et al.*, 2006; ZOUMAKIS *et al., 2007*)

3.1.1. Cutaneous Nervous System under Stress

It is known that the skin has an electrical potential difference called "skin battery", as an electric or galvanic cell, where at the level of the stratum corneum is located the negative pole, and at the level of the vascular subdermal plexus the positive pole (BARKER *et al.*, 1982; JAFFE & VANABLE, 1984). These skin bioelectrical properties also define that the greatest impedance or electrical resistance factor occurs in the stratum corneum; and the higher conductance or electrical conductivity occurs at subdermal layer. Therefore, in patients with increased stress and SNS cholinergic function exaltation, with the increase of secretion in sebaceous and sudoriparous glands, there is, respectively, an increase of impedance and electrical conductance of the skin (ARCK *et al.*, 2006; ZOUMAKIS *et al., 2007*). This phenomenon will reflect directly in both neurogenic inflammation and skin wound healing process, as explained below.

3.1.2. Neurogenic Inflammation

Inflammatory events and initiators of the wound healing result from direct stimulation of tissue nerve fibers, and in the skin, it is generally known as neurogenic inflammation. As a nerve fiber has potentially two intrinsic functions, electric activity and transport of neurotransmitters and neuropeptides, the neurogenic inflammation can be didactically divided into two components, in chronological sequence, the neuroelectric component and the neuropeptidergic component (the latter also called neuroendocrine or neurohormonal).

3.1.3. Neuroelectric Component of Neurogenic Inflammation

The primary actuation of a nerve fiber, even when it is injured, occurs with successive phenomena of despolarization and electric repolarization, sequentially, this fiber will be stimulated to secrete neurotransmitters and neuropeptides. Therefore, currently, the neuroelectric component of neurogenic inflammation should be considered as the first trigger of skin wound healing, and the neuropeptidergic component the second. For a better understanding of the neuroelectric component, it will be didactically divided into the following sub-chapters.

3.1.3.1. Skin Battery and Cell Galvanotaxis

The movement of ions from outside to inside the cells, and vice-versa, produces potential differences through the cell membrane, and thus the formation of an endogenous electric field (SZATKOWSKI *et al.*, 2000; AL-BAZZAZ & GAILEY, 2001; BORBA *et al.*, 2011). This endogenous electric field play a significant role in major biological processes such as embryogenesis, wound healing and tissue regeneration (NUCCITELLI, 1988). Nerves and muscles are electrically excitable tissues and are major sources of action potentials. The perpetuation of these action potentials in nerve fibers, by the conduction of electrical impulses, generates an electric field at the body surface (SUSSMAN & BYL, 2001). The electrical activity is essential and necessary for maintaining cutaneous homeostasis. This fact becomes relevant because the life on this planet have started with an electrical discharge; also because the human body requires electricity to keep its various vital functions activated and, therefore, without electricity there would be no life. Thereby, due to continuous depolarization and repolarization of skin Aδ and C fibers axions (BESNE *et al.*, 2002), the undamaged skin has a difference in electrical potential called "skin battery". No correlation was found between skin battery voltage and age or sex, but consistent anatomical variations were observed and the influence of sweating (FOULDS & BARKER, 1983). Voltage measures were made in animal models in which ~0.5–10 mV across hairy skin and 30–100 mV across glabrous regions of skin (BARKER *et al.*, 1982). In human, the skin battery voltages were ranging from 10 mV to ~60 mV depending on the region measured (FOULDS & BARKER, 1983).

The cutaneous battery is able to attract or repel cells and proteins, according to its polarities (BARKER *et al.*, 1982). This phenomenon is called galvanotaxis (*galvano* derived from a Latin word, which means: the type of electrical current; and *taxis*, which means: the electrical attraction or repulsion handling). A major cellular effect of electric fields is galvanotaxis, which is directional movement towards the cathode (negative pole) or the anode (positive pole) (MYCIELSKA & DJAMGOZ, 2004). In most cells studied, galvanotaxis is thought to depend on changes in intracellular Ca2+ concentration, that possible change the intracellular milieu, and thus induce galvanotaxis (ONUMA & HUI, 1988). The endogenous electric field might also affect other voltage-gated conductance, such as the voltage-gated Na+ channel (MYCIELSKA & DJAMGOZ, 2004).

In summary, cells possess a surface charge owing to the presence of charged substances in the cell membrane and/or to free ions. Interestingly, surface charge can be changed with the pathophysiological state of the cell, and this could affect galvanotaxis (MYCIELSKA & DJAMGOZ, 2004). Indeed, increased negative surface charge is known to be associated with malignant cancer cells (ABERCROMBIE & AMBROSE, 1962; CARTER & COFFEY, 1988; CARTER *et al.*, 1989; PRICE *et al.*, 1987).

Other mechanisms have also been implicated in galvanotaxis are the chemoattractants, which involves protein kinases (NUCCITELLI *et al.*, 1993; ZHAO *et al.*, 2002; MCBAIN *et al.*, 2003) and growth factors and their receptors, especially Epidermal Growth Factor (EGF), Fibroblast Growth Factor (FGF), TGFβ (ZHAO, 1996; ZHAO *et al.*, 2002) and VEGF (ZHAO *et al.*, 2004).

When there is a skin wound, the endogenous electric field immediately undergoes a short circuit, generating a current of injury. In this sense, there are changes in the local electrical patterns of injury, which induce the cellular migration to start the wound healing process (TAI *et al.*, 2009; BORBA *et al.*, 2011). To migrate effectively to the wound site, the cells must know not only when to migrate but, in which direction (ZHAO, 2009). The endogenous electric field at wounds have also been proposed as an orientation that directs the cells to migrate in wound healing (JAFFE & NUCCITELLI, 1977; BORGENS *et al.*, 1979; JAFFE, 1981; JAFFE & VANABLE, 1984). It is important to state that not all cells will respond to an electric field by undergoing migration and for those that do, they will not all migrate in the same direction. Precisely why certain cells migrate to the negative pole while others migrate to the positive pole is not known, even when cells are of the same lineage (ZHAO *et al.*, 2004; BROWN & DRANSFIELD, 2008).

3.1.3.2. Current of Injury

When the skin is damage, immediately is generated a current of injury due to a short-circuit created in the skin battery (BECKER & MURRAY, 1967, BARKER *et al.*, 1982; NUCCITELLI, 2003; BROWN & DRANSFIELD, 2008; ZHAO, 2009). The potential at the wound drops, becoming more negative in relation to the potential underneath the unwounded epidermis. This potential gradient drives the current of injury towards the more negative site. This electric current is orientated towards the wound from the surrounding tissues and then out from the wound, returning underneath the stratum corneum (NUCCITELLI, 1992; BORBA *et al.*, 2011). Cells away from the wound keep transporting ions to maintain the skin battery. Those cells keep driving the electric currents until the wound heals and the cutaneous barrier restored (ZHAO, 2009), pela reepitelização. While there is the solution of continuity of skin, a temporary polarity inversion of this field occurs; and the status will return to normality when the epithelization is finished. This change of polarity is responsible for the first electrotaxis phenomena of the elements needed for wound healing; in other words, while the charge on the surface of the wound is negative, a natural electrical atraction of elements required for defense and for the beginning of granulation will occur, such as leukocytes, macrophages and endothelial cells. In the epithelization, which occurs in humans about five days after injury, the created polarity is inverted, returning to the status of basal skin battery and, thus, the negativity on the surface attracts electrically positive cells, such as fibroblasts for the production of the collagen matrix (BORGENS, 1988a; BORGENS, 1988b) (Figure 1).

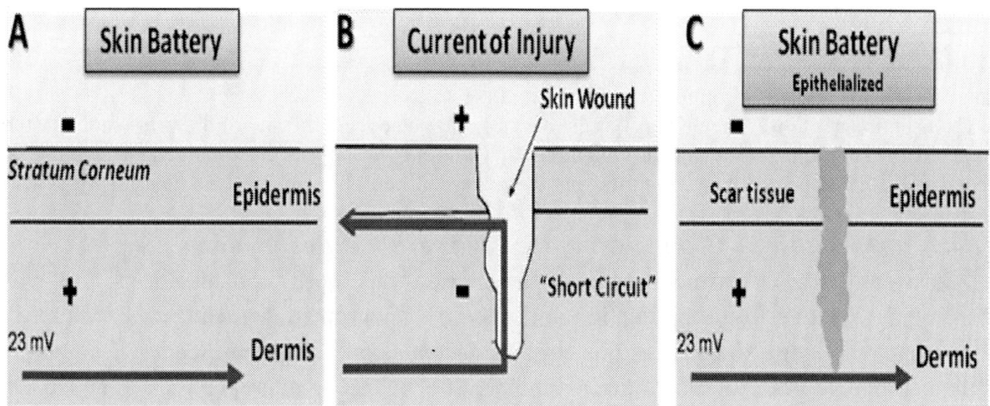

Figure 1. Model of the skin battery and current of injurty.
A: Model of skin battery; B: Current of injury originated after a skin wound. There is a polarity inversion due to the " short cut"; C:When the wound is epithelialized the skin battery returns to its normal polarity state.

That way, the generation of an electrical current, immediately to the cutaneous lesion occurrence, would be the first trigger of tissue wound healing (BECKER, 1960). At first, the affected area has a resistance greater than the tissue near the lesion. The electrical flow decrease, in the injured area, reduces the cellular capacitance. This could be one of the reasons for inflammatory reactions. Pain, warmth, swelling and redness are characteristics of inflamed tissues. Electricity flows faster through these inflamed fluids (WINDSOR *et al.*, 1993).

At the same time that the skin lesion disturbs the local bioelectric environment, generating a current of injury, part of this stimulus triggers a dromic electrical impulse; in other words, following by cutaneous nerve fibers to the dorsal root ganglion of the spinal cord. A part of this impulse is transmitted to the cerebral cortex, in order to "alert" the injury occurrence, and the other part returns to the dorsal root ganglion of the spinal cord, in the opposite direction, anti-dromic, carrying neurotransmitters and neuropeptides back to the skin, at the wound site, as explanation further ahead. This second part is the second trigger of healing (Figure 2).

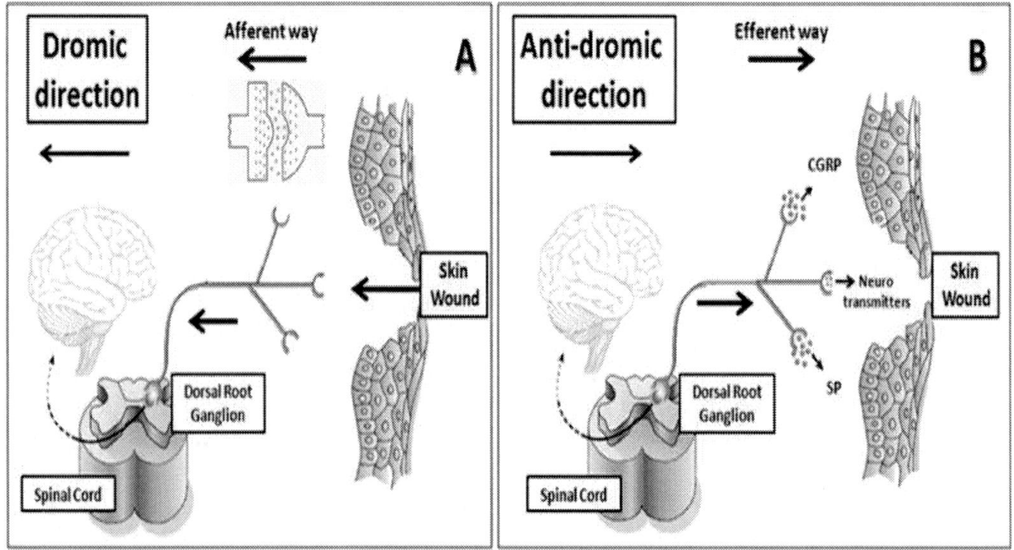

Figure 2. Dromic and anti-dromic nerve fiber stimuli.
A, The dromic direction (afferent way) of the electrical impulse from the site of the skin wound to the Dorsal Root Ganglion. B: The anti-dromic direction (efferent way) of the electrical response to the skin wound site from de Dorsal Root Ganglion and the release of neurotransmitters and neuropeptides.

3.1.4. Neuropeptidergic Component of the Neurogenic Inflammation

Classically, the term neurogenic inflammation has been considered as the whole phenomenon relative to the production and release of neuropeptides. But, it is preferred, in the current knowledge, to consider this classic concept as only the neuropepdergic component of the neurogenic inflammation, and it is the result of releasing neuropeptides (LYNN, 1988; BARNES *et al.*, 1990; LOTTI *et al.*, 1995; FELTEN, 2000).

3.1.4.1. Neuropeptides

Neuropeptides, which are special neurotransmitters, are released by exocytosis from peptidergic cutaneous C-fibers, and in smaller amounts by A-delta fibers (PETERSEN *et al.*, 1997; WEIDNER *et al.*, 2000; TOYODA & MOROHASHI, 2003). These neuropeptides are synthesized mainly in sensory neurons of the dorsal root ganglion (HOLZER, 1998; ROSSI

& JOHANSSON, 1998; WATSON *et al.*, 2002) and cause pain and inflammation (HOLZER, 1998; SAUERSTEIN *et al.*, 2000). This phenomenon has been reported to affect several organs, including the skin (SAUERSTEIN *et al.*, 2000; AKAISHI *et al.*, 2008; HOCHMAN *et al.*, 2008; FERREIRA *et al.*, 2009).

In the skin, there are about 20 kinds of neuropeptides, which vary in quantity, actions, and functions. Some examples are CGRP (the most abundant and the most potent vasodilator known), tachykinins (SP is the main representative), Neurokinin A (NKA), Vasoactive Intestinal Peptide (VIP), somatostatin, and many others, such as NGF which is precursor of some neuropeptides (EEDY, 1993; LOTTI *et al.*, 1995; PETERS *et al.*, 2006). Usually, nerve endings deep in the dermis contain increased quantities of CGRP, SP, VIP and NKA, while those that penetrate the epidermis contain only SP, CGRP and NKA (LOTTI *et al.*, 1995; HAGNER *et al.*, 2002; KALIL-GASPAR, 2003). The cutaneous concentration of neuropeptides changes according to the anatomic location.

Neuropeptides are also called neurotrophins or neurohormones and are released in much smaller amounts than common small-molecule neurotransmitters, such as catecholamines. However, neuropeptides are usually 1000 times more potent than neurotransmitters and act on their target cells by paracrine, juxtacrine or endocrine signaling (STEINHOFF *et al.*, 2003). Their action is slow and has prolonged effects that may last for days, months or years. Therefore, neuropeptides promote long-lasting changes in the mechanism of cellular metabolism by activating or deactivating specific genes (STEINHOFF *et al.*, 2003).

Neuropeptides are involved in the transmission of signals not only between nerve cells but also between nerve cells and immune system cells. They are predominantly expressed in neurons and gland cells derived from embryologic precursors of nerve tissue. Thus, neuropeptides represent a class of extremely potent substances acting on a variety of target cells by binding to specific receptors. Their regulatory influence are as components of the autonomic nervous system, acting locally at peripheral sites; as brain peptides, acting on central regulatory centers; and as neurohormones, reaching their target organs by way of the hypophysial portal vessels, or by way of the general circulation.

Since 1990's, cutaneous neurogenic inflammation has been studied more extensively (LOTTI *et al.*, 1995). Sympathetically dependent, it triggers a strong arteriolar vasodilator effect that modulates the amount of inflammatory mediators such as histamine, arachidonic acid, bradykinin, and prostaglandins, and the recruitment of immune-inflammatory cells, which together activate the inflammatory phase of wound healing (BALUK, 1997; HOLZER, 1998; ROSSI & JOHANSSON, 1998; SAUERSTEIN *et al.*, 2000). Also, the biodisponibility of neuropeptides modulating the neurogenic inflammation can be influenced by nutrients (FERREIRA *et al.*, 2010) Then, as a direct consequence, the neurogenic inflammation promotes the release of cytokines and growth factors, inducing ECM synthesis by fibroblasts on the proliferative phase (AKAISHI *et al.*, 2008; HOCHMAN *et al.*, 2008; FERREIRA *et al.*, 2009).

3.1.4.1.1. Neuropeptides under Stress

There are few studies relating CGRP and stress. An acute experimental social stress is associated with a reduction in frequency (HOSOI *et al.*, 1998; RUIZ *et al.*, 2003) and altered morphology (KAWAGUCHI *et al.*, 1997; HOSOI *et al.*, 1998) of epidermal dendritic cells, accompanied by reduction of cutaneous CGRP (Kleyn CE *et al.*, 2008). In addition, CGRP expression was up-regulated in the peripheral nerves of the upper dermis and lower epidermis (SEIKE *et al.*, 2002).

SP is a mediator of the systemic stress response (ARCK & PAUS, 2006). There are evidence that changes in SP content occur in brain areas known to be implicated in processing emotions and stress reactions in response to aversive situations (HERPFER & LIEB, 2005; EBNER & SINGEWALD, 2006). On the basis of these findings, SP and its preferred eceptor, NK1R, pathways have been proposed to be involved in the physiopathology of a number of stress-related diseases such as depression and anxiety disorders (HERPFER & LIEB, 2005; MCLEAN, 2005). Since the lateral septum, a key brain structure implicated in stress, anxiety, and depression (SHEEHAN *et al.*, 2004), contains one of the densest SP innervations (LJUNGDAHL *et al.*, 1978; SAKANAKA *et al*, 1982; GALL & MOORE, 1984; SZEIDEMANN *et al*, 1995; HÖKFELT *et al*, 2004), and has been suggested to be involved in the modulation of emotional processes and stress reactions (CULMAN & UNGER, 1995; RUPNIAK, 2002; EBNER & SINGEWALD, 2006).

Stress also exacerbates skin dermatitis via SP-dependent cutaneous neurogenic inflammation and subsequent local cytokine shifting (PAVLOVIC et al., 2008). And, in psoriasis, pruritus has been correlated to the severity of stress and secretion of SP (REMRÖD et al., 2007). Both physical and psychological stress significantly enhanced the degranulation of dermal mast cells and increased the number of SP-positive nerve fibers in the skin (KAWANA et al., 2006).

The presence and release of CGRP and SP is directly controlled by the availability of NGF. Likewise, SP and CGRP may induce an increase in the NGF concentration in the skin, indicating the probable existence of a mutual trophic communication whose importance (WALLENGREN, 1997) supports the concept of the brain-skin axis. Also, SP and CGRP are frequently present in the same nerve fiber and they are released in response to physical or chemical factors in the skin (WALLENGREN & HÅKANSON, 1987). The release of SP may induce the co-release of CGRP, which in turn may enhance the action of SP, although CGRP may have long-lasting effects (WALLENGREN & HÅKANSON, 1987; SCHOLZEN *et al.*, 1998; OLERUD *et al.*, 1999; WU *et al.*, 2007). Clinically, CGRP potentiates SP-induced edema in rat skin (NEWBOLD & BRAIN, 1993). Together, they play a significant role as modulators of neurogenic inflammation by cytokines and chemokins production and cell proliferation (OLERUD *et al.*, 1999; ZEGARSKA *et al.*, 2006).

NGF is recognized as an important parameter in stress responses (ALOE *et al.*, 2002), besides the classical stress-related neurohormones like CRH, ACTH, prolactin and glucocorticoids (AMARA *et al.*, 1982; ROSENFELD *et al.*, 1983; AMARA *et al.*, 1984). Recent findings indicate that circulating levels of NGF undergo significant variations after exposure to stressful events (AMARA *et al.*, 1982; ROSENFELD *et al.*, 1983), like sun exposure. It is now generally accepted that the activation of the SNS and the release of NGF and SP during stress response trigger an intense inflammatory response in the skin, whereas a systemic inflammatory response generally is suppressed (ROSENFELD *et al.*, 1983; Hagner *et al.*, 2002; JOHANSSON *et al.*, 2002; TOYODA & MOROHASHI, 2003; BRAIN & GRANT, 2004; ARCK & PAUS, 2006; PETERS *et al.*, 2010; LIEZMANN *et al.*, 2011). Also, stress enhances neurogenic inflammation in a peripheral inflammatory disease by epidermal hyperplasia, vascular activation or infiltration by eosinophils depended on SP and NGF (PAVLOVIC *et al.*, 2008; PETERS *et al.*, 2004).

Therefore, psychological stress activates a defined, hierarchically organized cascade of events in which NGF, SP and mast cells play key roles. Indeed, NGF directly stimulates activation of mast cells via functional neurotrophin receptors (MARSHALL *et al.*, 1999), thus aggravating cutaneous neurogenic inflammation. Furthermore, in response to stress, mast cells secrete proteinases which may subsequently trigger additional cytokine release, cell migration, recruitment of leukocytes and endothelial-cell activation (STEINHOFF *et al.*, 2000). These mechanisms probably act synergistically with NGF and SP to upregulate the neurogenic inflammation cascade (ARCK, 2006). NGF-dependent neurons are essential for the establishment of neural networks for interoception (sensitivity to stimuli originating inside of the body) and homeostasis, and play crucial roles in brain-immune-endocrine interactions and inflammation (INDO, 2010).

3.1.4.2. Neurotransmitters

On the other hand, approximately, a hundred different neurotransmitters exist. Each neuron produces and releases only one or a few types of neurotransmitters, but can carry receptors on its surface for several types of neurotransmitters. Neurotransmitters act as a pool in a rapid, massive transient manner on target cells. They are released into and diffuse across the synaptic cleft, where they bind to specific receptors in the membrane on the postsynaptic side (ELIAS & SAUCIER, 2005). Release of neurotransmitters usually follows arrival of an action potential at the synapse, but may also follow graded electrical potentials. In general, they are classified as either excitatory or inhibitory activity. They can be also classified into its composition as amino acids, peptides, monoamines and others.

3.1.4.2.1. Neurotransmitters under Stress

Serotonin (5HT), for instance, is an amine that acts in a wide variety of sites in the CNS and PNS (SLOMINSKI *et al.*, 2005). Functionally, its dysregulation may lead to sleep disorders, anxiety, depression, and aggressiveness. 5HT is also important for basic cell functions such as proliferation, differentiation, maturation, and migration. Besides its presence in the CNS and PNS, it is also released from platelets and mast cells (in animal models) after tissue injury. 5HT in the skin causes pro-edema, vasodilatation, proinflammatory and is pruritogenic (SLOMINSKI *et al.*, 2003; LONNE-RAHM *et al.*,2008). Stress involves different neuromediators including the SP (MANTYH, 2002) and the serotonergic system. 5HT blood level is considered as a marker of severity of stress. Mental stress resulted in an increase in platelet responses and to 5HT and catecholamine, and significant effect on platelet aggregation (PIETRASZEK *et al.*, 1991). And, in turn, each platelet aggregated is a power plant supplier of Platelet-Derived Growth Factor (PDGF), which is a growth factor essential for the production of ECM and collagen fibers (TAKEHARA, 2000).

4. SKIN AS AN IMMUNOFUNCTIONAL ORGAN

The skin is also considered an imunofuncional organ because its direct contact with the outside world, presenting itself as the first line of defense. In it, as mentioned above, there are resident cells (dendritic cells) and migratory cells (leukocytes and macrophages), which make up the cutaneous immune system. These cells produce several factors and inflammatory cytokines, as needed in the event of an aggression on the skin. Furthermore, each of the cells and skin appendages is also capable to produce these same inflammation mediators, which are mostly proinflammatory. In other words, the skin has a power plant its own, with the capacity to produce locally all these factors related to inflammation, even without the presence of these circulating immune cells. This fact causes an increase in the cutaneous immunoinflammatory potencial at the time of the wound healing process, especially under circumstances of exacerbation of the SNS as stress (Figure 3).

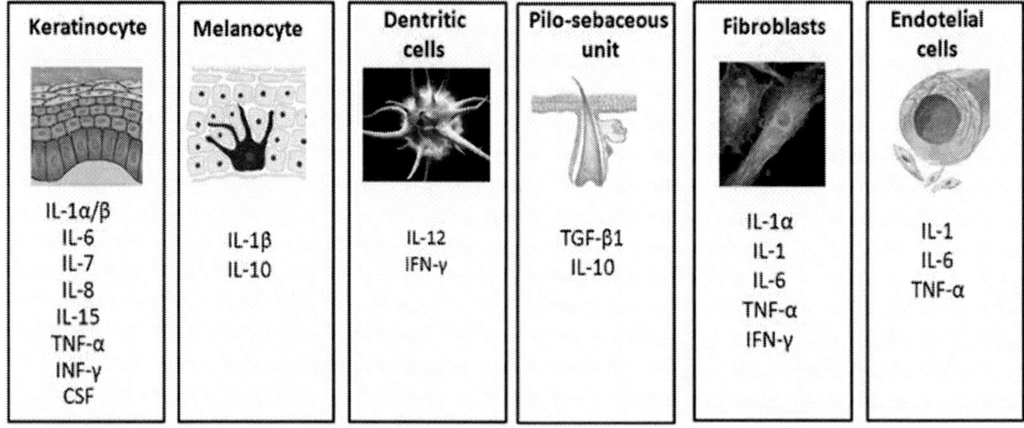

Figure 3. Cytokines and growth factors produced by skin cells involved with the immunecutaneous system.
IL: Interleukins; TNF-α: Tumor Necrosis Factor –alpha: IFN-γ: Interferon-gama;CSF: Granulocyte-Macrophage Colony –Stimulating Factor.

Recently, the concept of an immunocutaneous system complementary to the neurosensorial cutaneous axis is emerging. This has provided new forms to interpret the physiopathologic response of skin to a nociceptive stress, particularly the modulation of inflammation and immunity (FRAITURE *et al.*, 1998). The close anatomical and physiological link between skin, immunity and the nervous system supports the existence of a unified system (MISERY, 2000). This connections between nerve fibers and immune cells have been demonstrated, by their production of neurotransmitters (acetylcholine, catecholamines and endorphins) and neuropeptides (SP and CGRP), which allow them to modulate cutaneous function through membrane receptors (WEIDERMANN, 1987; MISERY, 1997). In addition, certain areas of primary and secondary lymphoid organs, such as lymph nodes and the spleen, are innervated with noradrenergic sympathetic neuronal fibers (O'SULLIVAN *et al.*, 1998). In skin epidermis, dendritic cells (MISERY, 1998) express neurotrophic factors and neuropeptide receptors giving further support to the theory that there is a functional relationship between the immune and the nervous systems (TSUCHIYA *et al.*, 1996; TORII *et al.*, 1997). This relationship is also based on the fact that hypertrophic scars, which contains a great number of nerve fibers and neuropetides than normal scars (PARKHOUSE *et al.*, 1992; CROWE *et al.*, 1994), also presenting an increased number of dendritic cells (NIESSEN *et al.*, 2004). These neuropeptides modulate bidirectional communication between the nervous and the immune systems (BLALOCK, 1989; REICHLIN, 1993) and provide firm evidence for a mind-body connection in the skin (O'SULLIVAN *et al.*, 1998).

4.1. Immunocutaneous System under Stress

Using an animal model, β-Endorphin, which is a neurotransmitter, was produced by macrophages, lymphocytes in response to the stress. This model suggests that immune cells may actually initiate or modify the perception of pain (O'SULLIVAN *et al.,* 1998). It is possible that the immune system might constitute a sixth sense by converting stimuli from environmental factors into "biochemical information in the form of neurotransmitters, hormones, and cytokines (BLALOCK, 1994). Finally, lymphocytes and macrophages express a wide range of hormone, neuropeptide, and steroid receptors (LOTTI *et al.,* 1995). The discovery of such concrete pathways of neuroimmune modulation dovetails with the observation that chronic or repetitive mental stress seems to alter immune response (MANUCK *et al.*, 1991). Stress effects on delayed-type hypersensitivity responses, including modification of delayed-type hypersensitivity responses (HICKIE *et al.*, 1993). In the skin, a stressful life may exacerbate psoriasis, acne and contact dermatitis (FARBER *et al.,* 1968; FARBER & NALL, 1974; GUPTA et *al.*, 1994). During the course of skin disorders, the neuroimmunocutaneous system is destabilized, and it can also be responsible for the induction and maintenance of the inflammatory process (MISERY, 1997).

In addition, the stress-induced up-regulation of glucocorticoids suppresses many proinflammatory factors such as TNFα and IL-6. This state, as observed in chronic stress, leukocytes can mount a counter regulatory response and down-regulate the expression and function of receptors for glucocorticoid hormones, and the immune system's sensitivity to cortisol declines, thereby leading to excessive inflammation (VILEIKYTE, 2007).

5. SKIN AS AN ENDOCRINOFUNCTIONAL ORGAN

Hormones are specific chemical substances which act as biomarkers. In general, they are secreted in small amounts, acting at the cellular and tissue levels, over short or long distances through the bloodstream. Thus, they play a regulatory role (inhibitor or inductive) in target organs. They have, in general, a slow-acting and long lasting, and they regulate growth, development, reproduction and metabolic processes of the body.

The several stimuli suffered by the skin from the external environment, generate responses to the body, in an effort to deal with and defend itself of these aggressions. The signaling pathways activation and regulation, especially the hormonal, from the CNS, is one of the ways to keep the integrity of the organism. The hormones produced and secreted activate other hormones and signaling pathways, in a "signaling cascade", until they reach the periphery of the body or the target organ, in order to effect and modulate the effects of aggression suffered, as well as to start processes of defense.

5.1. Endocrinofunctional Approach under Stress

The major neuroendocrine pathway known, responsible for the adaptive response to systemic stress, is the hypothalamic-pituitary-adrenal axis. However, other secondary routes related to the reception, transmission, interpretation, and stress response have been described as the sympathetic pathway of the Autonomic Nervous System. In this sense, recently, the skin itself has been investigated by presenting some similarities to the CNS itself, as well as regarding the production and secretion of neurohormones.

5.2. Hypothalamic-Pituitary-Adrenal Axis

The hypothalamus is the major center of monitoring information received from the periphery and coordinates responses releasing neurotransmitters, neuropeptides and hormones. All type of information from the organs of sense and emotional situations are focused to the hypothalamus which alerts and prepare the whole body to emergences and environmental hazards. From this integrative center, the brain controls an axis which releases many hormones to target tissues in a cascade. This is the hypothalamic-pituitary-adrenal axis (HPA) which is the mainly way involved in the neurobiology of mood disorders and functional illnesses (SPENCER & HUTCHINSON, 1999). It is activated in response to systemic stress (SLOMINSK *et al.*, 1998; PRUESSNER *et al.,* 1999; PADGETT & GLASER, 2003) involving the production and releasing of CRH, followed by production and secretion of ACTH, by the anterior pituitary gland. ACTH induces production and secretion of the cortisol, by the cortex of the adrenal gland, which by negative feedback terminates the stress response and attenuates CRH and ACTH production. This physiological function is triggered in response to any acute stressors in an attempt to the CNS to return to the homeostatic state (McEWEN, 1998; JUSTER *et al.*, 2010). Dysregulations in this mechanism may be an etiological link between stress and the subsequent development of many pathologies.

5.2.1. Hypothalamic-Pituitary-Adrenal Axis under Stress

Cortisol is a glucocorticoid responsible to alter the function of tissues in order to mobilize or store energy to meet the demands of the stress challenge (DE KLOET *et al.*, 2006). Release of cortisol in response to certain stressors may be adaptive in the short term situation, as it leads to behavioral and physical changes to deal with the acute threat (CHROUSOS, 1995). Prolonged exposure to cortisol from exaggerated, extended, or repeated activation of the HPA axis, however, may be maladaptive (ZOCCOLA & DICKERSON, 2012), leading to losses in many normal body functions. A defective HPA-axis response can mimic the glucocorticoid-deficient state and thus cause resistance to infections and neoplasms, but increased susceptibility to autoimmune or inflammatory disease (CHROUSOS, 1995). Conversely, an excessive HPA axis response to inflammation can mimic the state of stress or hypercortisolemia and thus increase susceptibility to infectious agents and tumors, but enhance resistance to autoimmune or inflammatory disease (CHROUSOS, 1995).

Stress-induced cortisol production has been associated with delayed wound healing (EBRECHT *et al.*, 2004). Furthermore, exogenous administration of glucocorticoid slowed wound healing as well (PADGETT & GLASER, 2003). Besides, two other hypothalamic peptides, oxytocin and vasopressin, modulated physiological stress responses and social work processes. Individuals who had more positive interactions with their partner during a social support task had higher plasma oxytocin levels. Higher circulating oxytocin levels were in turn associated with faster healing. Furthermore, in women, but not in men, greater plasma vasopressin levels were related to faster healing (GOUIN *et al.*, 2010). Exogenous oxytocin administration attenuated the stress-induced corticosterone production, in animal models, and impairment in wound healing (SARAIYA, 2003; DETILLION *et al.*, 2004; VITALO *et al.*, 2009).

Prolactin is likely to be involved as a mediator in the "brain–skin axis" (PAUS, 1991; SLOMINSKI & WORTSMAN, 2000; ARCK *et al.*, 2006; PAUS *et al.*, 2006a; PAUS *et al.*, 2006b). Strikingly, prolactin is also expressed in mammalian skin, where it is transcripts and protein are most prominently found in the hair follicle, in both mice (CRAVEN *et al.*, 2001; FOITZIK *et al.*, 2003) and humans (FOITZIK *et al.*, 2006). Therefore, it has been now joined the ranks of other intracutaneously expressed pituitary hormones. Elevation of serum prolactin levels has been demonstrated after thermal injury and hemorrhage after trauma (BRIZIO-MOLTENI *et al.*, 1984). Given that psychoemotional stress can retard wound healing (FLORIN *et al.*, 2006), a process that requires appropriate responses. These observations suggest that PRL may be involved in the stress-induced impairment of wound healing (FOITZIK *et al.*, 2009). On the other hand, hyperinsulinemia because of obesity with intrinsic systemic inflammatory response, associated with physical and psychological trauma could contribute to the stimulation of prolactin secretion and sustained hyperprolactinemia. This state, in turn, may cause hypertrophic scars not readily amenable to preventive and conservative therapeutic treatment methods (SARAIYA, 2003).

5.3. Sympathetic-Adrenal-Medullary Axis

The activation of the SAM is parallel and secondary the HPA axis activation, and releases neurohormones as catecholamines, norepinephrine and epinephrine (PADGETT & GLASER, 2003).

It is known that catecholamines also participate and modulate many immune functions, including cell proliferation, cytokine and antibody production and cell trafficking (SANDERS & KOHM, 2002; MADDEN, 2003). When the levels of cortisol are elevated due to activation of the HPA axis it results in catecholamine production and secretion from the adrenal medulla (CARRASCO & VAN DE KAR, 2003).

5.3.1. Sympathetic-Adrenal-Medullary Axis under Stress

Norepinephrine is released from sympathetic nerve fibers in direct approximation with target tissues when the organism faces an immediate threat, providing a first line of alert, known as "fight or flight" reaction, in which there is an increased heart rate and increased blood flow to skeletal muscles.

Catecholamines mediate their effect on target tissues through adrenergic receptors. These receptors can be divided into two subgroups, the α and β-adrenergic receptors (GILMAN, 1987; MADDEN, 2003). Since stress induces elevated levels of plasma catecholamines, events related to wound healing could be negatively affect like fibroblast growth and proliferation (SAITO *et al.*, 1997); the responses of macrophages and neutrophils (BARNES, 1999); the α and β-adrenergic receptor blockade in dermal healing (EIJKELKAMP *et al.*, 2007); reduce the keratinocyte motility and migration in vitro (SIVAMANI *et al.*, 2009). If the SAM axis is chronically activated, the secretion of excessive catecholamines can dysregulate immune function, supported by the observations that noradrenergic sympathetic nerve fibers run from the CNS to lymphoid organs (FELTEN *et al.*, 1992).

5.4. Endocrinocutaneus System

The HPA axis has intrinsically three stations. According to the hierarchy, the first station is located in the hypothalamus, which produces corticotrophin, among these the CRH (ACTH precursor). The second station is located in the anterior pituitary gland or adenohypophysis, where trophic hormones are produced, which act in target organs (for example, the ACTH and Thyrotropin - TSH). The second station is located in the anterior pituitary gland or adenohypophysis, where trophic hormones are produced, which will act in target organs (for example, the ACTH and TSH). And the third station, located in the periphery, in some target organ, wherein the trophic hormone previously produced and released, that will produce and release the final hormone, will act. In this sense, CRH stimulates the production and release of ACTH, which stimulates the adrenal gland to produce and release cortisol; TSH also stimulates the production and release of thyroxin by the thyroid gland. Therefore, the skin contains an endocrine power plant of such magnitude that in itself contains and performs functions, or most of them, relating to the three stations of HPA axis mentioned (ZIEGLER CG *et al.*, 2007) The skin has the ability to produce CRH, ACTH and cortisol, for example. In other words, the three stations of the HPA axis are contained in the cutaneousendocrine system (SKOBOWIAT *et al.*, 2011) (Figure 4).

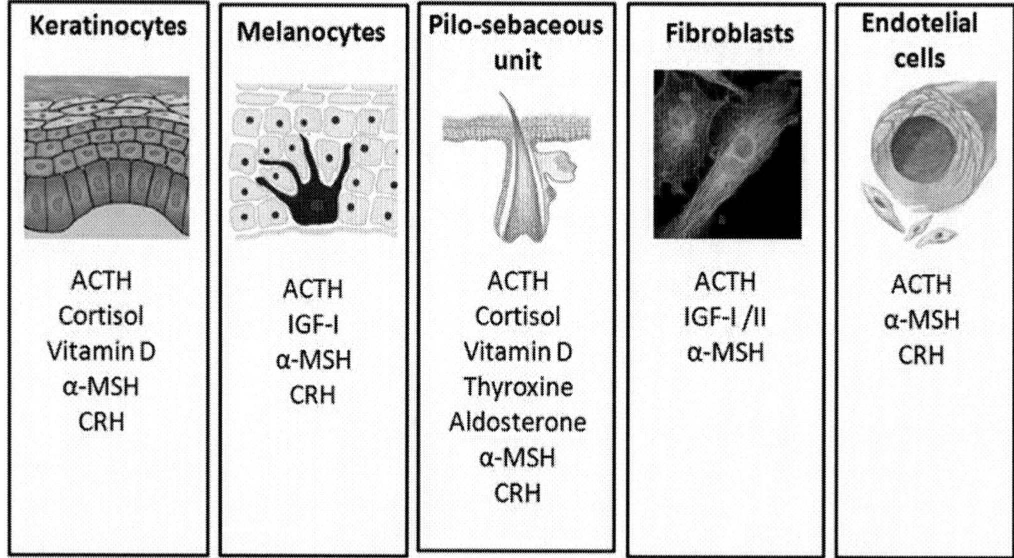

Figure 4. Hormones produced by skin cells involved with the endocrimecutaneous system. ACTH: Adrenocortictropic Hormone; α-MSH: Alpha Melanocyte-Stimulating Hormone; CRH: Corticotropin-Releasing Hormone; IGF-1 and 2: Insulin-Like Growth Factor Binding Protein 1 and 2.

5.4.1. Endocrinocutaneus System under Stress

In melanocytes and skin fibroblasts, the stimulation of its CRH receptors hyper-regulate the expression and production of systemic ACTH. Thus, they respond with a higher cortisol production. In vitro, cells of pilosebaceous unit also have a functional endocrine axis equivalent to the HPA axis, including the synthesis and secretion of cortisol which, by negative feedback, acts by reducing the expression of central CRH. Thus, the production of all of these hormones by the skin cells, mimicking the main central endocrine axis, supports the existence of a cutaneous system of stress response (SLOMINSKI *et al.*, 1999). When the skin is subjected to environmental stresses, stimuli are transmitted to the CNS by afferent peripheral neural signaling. Then, the sebaceous glands release CRH (SLOMINSKI *et al.*, 2006; KRAUSE *et al.*, 2007), which through an endocrine pathway, combines with the hypothalamic CRH and, consequently increasing the release of POMC-derived peptides, also known as "stress hormones" (ACTH, MSH and prolactin) (GRÜTZKAU *et al.*, 2000, KONO *et al.* 2001, SLOMINSKI *et al.*, 2004). Conversely, the same stimuli synergistically activate the SNS by stimulating the SAM axis (DHABHAR & McEWEN, 1999).

6. SKIN AS A PSYCHOFUNCTIONAL ORGAN

The skin is also a psychofunctional organ. Stress is a source of homeostasis disturbance, and stress factors may be exogenous (external) and endogenous (internal). Currently, among the exogenous factors, the UVR (sunlight) has been most studied, due to the strong disfunction of the skin homeostasis caused by them. Among the endogenous factors, the most damaging to the skin is the psychological stress, which is the subject of this chapter. In general, psychological stress is triggered by structures belonging to the emotional regulation center, the limbic system. For this reason, it grows more and more a new branch of biomedical science, called Psychodermatology. According to this, currently it is already known that at least 70% of skin diseases have psychogenic origin (JAFFERANY, 2007; FERM *et al.*, 2010). In this sense, the most studied cutaneous diseases are acne and psoriasis, in which the proinflammatory neuropeptide influence has already been proved (TOYODA & MOROHASHI, 2003; SARACENO *et al.*, 2006). Currently, it was found that the keloid, maximum expression of pathological scarring, also presentes, in its pathogenesis, psycho-neuro-phisiological disorders, including increased in innervation and neuropeptides (PARKHOUSE *et al.*, 1992; BARROS, BARROS, 1996; FURTADO *et al.*, 2009). Thus, to better understand the mind-skin relationships – expression more and more used in Psychodermatology and Psychobiology –, it is needed to review aspects regarding the functional neuroanatomy.

The Limbic System consists of brainstem and brain areas (telencephalon and diencephalon). The cortical portion is composed by the cingulate gyrus, parahippocampal gyrus and hippocampus. The subcortical region is formed by the amygdaloid body, septal area, mammillary nuclei, anterior nuclei of the thalamus, and habenular nuclei (MACHADO, 2006).

It is perhaps more important to understand the connections than describe structures that make up the Limbic System. Therefore, basically, there are the intrinsic and extrinsic connections. Regarding the first category, the various components of the limbic system keep each other numerous and complex intercommunications, known as the Papez circuit. Most of the extrinsic afferent connections that bring visual, auditory, somesthesic or olfactory information, has access to the Limbic System, make this indirectly. On the other hand, the information related to visceral sensitivity have access directly through the links of the solitary tract nucleus to the amygdaloid body or, indirectly, via hypothalamus. It should be noted here the numerous serotonergic, noradrenergic, and dopaminergic projections, originating from the reticular formation, which exert modulatory function on neuronal activity of this System. The extrinsic efferent connections are important because they mediate the participation in the effector mechanisms of emotions in the peripheral component, controlling the Autonomic Nervous System activity. These functions are performed through the connections that the Limbic System maintains with the reticular formation of the mesencephalon and the hypothalamus. The hypothalamus is the main arm of implementation of the Limbic System (MACHADO, 2006).

6.1. The Limbic System, Under Stress, in the Hypothalamic-Pituitary-Adrenal Axis (HPA)

The acute stress stimulates the release of CRH from neurons of cortical-limbic areas. The main effector branch of the Limbic System to the Hypothalamus is through the medial forebrain bundle (mesencephalon). The hypothalamic CRH stimulates the production of ACTH in the anterior pituitary which, in its turn, stimulates the cortex of the adrenal glands to synthesize glycocorticoids. The HPA axis activation, by the acute stress, produces a transient increase in plasma cortisol and a partial resistance to it, caused by the decreased sensitivity and by the amount of cortisol receptors in the brain (for example, hippocampus). Then, the cortisol concentration decreases, associated with the reduction of CRH, by negative feedback, normalizing the density of receptors (LEONARD, 2005).

When compared to acute stress, the chronic stress evolves with lower plasma levels of ACTH and cortisol. However, the chronic stress also results in hypersecretion of cortisol and sustained activation of the central and peripheral sympathetic system. These changes occur due to the desensitization function of central cortisol receptors and the resistance to negative feedback, as described above. The increase in plasma cortisol concentration is still raised by arginine vasopressin from the hypothalamus and by proinflammatory cytokines (IL-1, IL-6, TNF and interferon), commonly associated with cutaneous inflammatory diseases (LEONARD, 2005) (Figure 5-A).

6.2. The Limbic System, under Stress, in the Autonomic Nervous System

The hypothalamus and the reticular formation have direct connections with preganglionic neurons of the Autonomic Nervous System (MACHADO, 2006). Thus the Limbic System, regulatory center of emotions, because of their connections with these structures, is also involved in autonomic control. Therefore, any organ or tissue that has sympathetic or parasympathetic effector innervation, including the skin, can be influenced by the emotions. The peripheral reactions, such as the sweat and sebaceous secretion increase are one of the ways that emotion is expressed in skin (ZOUBOULIS, 2004; WILKE *et al.*, 2007)

The main noradrenergic nucleus of the body is the Locus Coeruleus (Locus Coeruleus-norepinephrine system), consequently, the stress nucleus of CNS. This way, there is communication through the conscious cortex until the thalamus, and from this to the hypothalamus until the skin, as will be described below; so, good and bad thoughts can influence the skin and cutaneous processes, because there is an anatomic morpho-functional pathway from the thinking cortex to the skin, made up nervous system of the skin (TOYODA & MOROHASHI, 2003; FURTADO *et al.*, 2009).

The *Locus Coeruleus* is located in the pons and reflects its fibers to the cortex, cerebellum, hypothalamus, hippocampus and spinal cord (AMARAL & SINNAMON, 1977) (Figure 5-B).

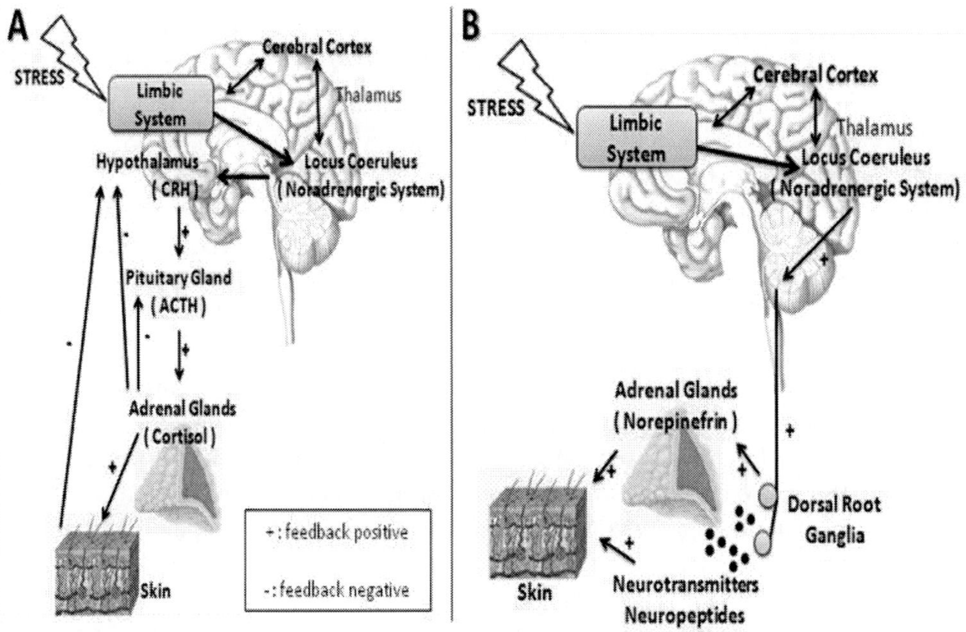

Figure 5. The Limbic System under stress, endocrine and nervous pathways to the skin.
A: Stress stimulating the Hypothalamus-Pituitary-Adrenal axis; B: Stress stimulating the Sympathetic Adrenal-Medulary axis.

6.3. The Limbic System, under Stress, in the Spinal Pathways of Pain

The Aδ and C fine fibers are responsible for conducting nociceptive stimuli from the periphery to the jelly-like substance, found in the posterior column of the spinal cord. In general, C fibers release neuropeptides, such as substance P and CGRP, while Aδ fibers release glutamate. These fibers conduct impulses in both directions, as described in previous items: from the periphery to the dorsal root ganglion (dromic direction) or vice-versa (anti-dromic direction). By the large Neoespinal-thalamic and Paleoespinal-thalamic afferent pathways, painful information reach the thalamus (posterolateral ventral nucleus - which is part of the lateral portion of the thalamus; and intralaminar nuclei – which are part of the medial portion of the thalamus –, respectively) and to the reticular formation of brainstem (periaqueductal gray matter). Projections depart from thalamus to the primary sensory cortex. This last one predominantly process the sensory components, to the cingulate gyrus (part of the Limbic System) responsible for the painful affective qualities, and projections also depart from thalamus to the prefrontal cortex (part of the Limbic System), responsible for cognitive and affective elements.

It is important to highlight that pain is a complex phenomenon, which presents several neurophysiological components, including sensitive, (burning, cramps, sharp pain) affective (torturous, terrifying) and cognitive evaluative (unbearable), among others (MELZACK, 1975). The set of all these neurophysiological components is called "painful experience"; for all these reasons, the pain is always subjective.

Brainstem areas and the Locus Coeruleus are responsible for sending descending fibers to the spinal cord, with inhibitory functions on the spinal pain circuits (FIELDS & BASBAUM, 1978, WILLIS & WESTLUND, 1997). These areas of the trunk, that include the magnus raphe nucleus and the magnocellular reticular nucleus, are rich in 5HT and SP and receive excitatory afferents from the periaqueductal gray matter, which also sends afferent fibers to the spinal cord. Efferent fibers originating in the raphe magnus nucleus and magnocellular reticular nucleus, through the dorsolateral funiculus, control nociceptive impulses of the gelatinous substance.

Fibers originating from the brainstem, such as 5HT and SP, are responsible for neurotransmitters and neuropeptides release, which activate interneurons located in the dorsal root ganglion. When activated, these interneurons release opioid neurotransmitters, such as enkephalin, β-endorphin and dynorphin. Therefore, the same neuropeptides that primarily work as excitatory nociceptive stimulation, in a descending inhibitory mechanism, work in analgesia. When activated, these interneurons release opioid neurotransmitters, such as enkephalin, β-endorphin and dynorphin. Therefore, the same neuropeptides that primarily work as excitatory nociceptive stimulation, in a descending inhibitory mechanism, work in analgesia.

Chronic pain is due to the continuous stimulation of nociceptive receptors. An example is the chronic pain resulting from tissue damages caused by tumor compression or chronic inflammation, as observed in keloid. The activity of nociceptors results in primary hyperalgesia, excessive sensitivity to stimuli in the injured tissue, with decreased pain threshold (LUNDY-EKMAN, 2008).

Similarly, the interaction of stress with chronic pain is also described (MELZACK, 1998); for this purpose, afferent fibers originating from the limbic system, in the dorsal raphe nucleus, are relevant (KIERNAN, 2004). In addition to the painful stimulus, the chronic stress, via CRH, induces the dorsal raphe nucleus activation, causing changes in the serotonergic system, such as the increase and decrease, respectively, of serotonin 5-HT2A and 5-HT1A receptors. Mastocytes are also activated by the CRH. They contribute to increase the concentration of proinflammatory cytokines, which are already well established in inflammatory skin diseases.

The phenomena described above contribute to the onset of anxiety and depression symptoms (LEONARD, 2005). Recently, the melanogenesis was induced by serotonin, through 5-HT2A receptor (LIAO *et al.*, 2012) e 1A (LEE *et al.*, 2011). Therefore, because of these anatomical relationships, the complex interrelationships of the binomial "chronic pain of somatic origin" and "chronic pain of psychic origin" are highlighted, by noradrenergic and serotonergic pathways, respectively. Thus, ultimately, it is consolidated the binomial concept "psychophysiologic disorder" versus "homeostasis/skin healing" or, in other words, the mind-skin relationship.

7. ADQUIRED KNOWLEDGE AND PERSPECTIVES

This chapter has dealt with the skin from its most basic concept, by means of descriptive anatomy, its functioning, histology and physiology of cellular and adnexial components, and their relationships and interactions, both regional and systemic, through signaling pathways and axles of the following levels: neural, immune, endocrine, and, with greater focus, the psychological level. Accordingly, the understanding about the skin should not be limited only as the first line of defense against external aggression and penetration of micro-organisms, the first barrier that separates the internal of the external environment, the body covering waterproof, the thermal regulation mechanism, or even the Hydro Salt balance maintainer. The skin, because of its own mixed cutaneous nervous system, with dermal nerve endings arising from neurons of the posterior horn of spinal cord, and functional epidermal neurons, which are melanocytes, henceforth should have a focus essentially *neuropsychophysiological*; even more taking into consideration that this cutaneous nervous system acts synergistically and in feedback with SNS and HPA axis; so it is implicit that the skin may act as important and as similar to the CNS.

In this context, Navarro and other researchers (NAVARRO, 1991; ZOUMAKIS *et al.,* 2007; CHAPMAN & MOYNIHAN, 2009) have already inserted the skin as our "external brain", according to Reichian view. In a morphofunctional definition, the "thinking" element is the melano-epidermic unit, in which a melanocyte controls about 36 keratinocytes, which interact with NHS and HPA axis, by means of their own melanocytes, keratinocytes, neurotransmitters and NGF secretion, also on interaction with dermal nerve endings (REICH *et al.,* 2010).

Thus, skin disorders should be interpreted in a holistic way; in other words, evaluating the individual as a whole, under a neuro-psycho-immune-endocrine-functional perspective. Since most, or perhaps all, of cutaneous somatization, that have been long neglected, now becomes the target of researches in which the psychogenic part has gained prominence because there is no dermatosis in which the psychological factor is not involved (JAFFERANY, 2007).

The skin wound healing of is a vitally important event for the organism, because it remains vulnerable until the full recovery of cutaneous integrity. It presents several complex mechanisms which, in harmony and synchronism one another, result in normal scar of the skin. As reported previously, the trigger wound healing depends on neurogenic, electrical and neurosecretory factors that, in its turn, are also premodulated by psychological factors. Once the neurogenic trigger is activated, it stimulates the wound healing immune and endocrine factors and, then, these three factors (nervous, immune and endocrine), along with the psychic, interact and inter-modulate. Any change in this quadruple circuit may interfere in the normal formation of a scar, resulting since hyperproliferative healing (hypertrophic scars and keloid) until wound healing deficit (atrophic scars and ulcerations).

Under some conditions, stress can suppress cell-mediated immune function, whereas under other conditions stress can enhance cell-mediated immunity *in vivo*. Substantial evidence from animal and humans studies indicate that chronic psychological stress can retard the initial inflammatory phase of wound healing. Glucocorticoids seem to hind the wound healing process, causing a decreasing in cellular proliferation, in neovascularization, and in matrix production. Occurs a delay in the afflux of macrophages, neutrophils, fibroblasts and proinflammatory cytokines and growth factors. It is owned that corticosteroids reduce the inflammatory phase of wound healing. The chronical state (or chronic use) of corticoids may influence negatively reepithelization, neovascularization, and collagen synthesis[3] and can result in an impaired wound healing (GLASER & KIECOLT-GLASER, 2005; GOUINA & KIECOLT-GLASER, 2011; ALBERTI *et al.*, 2012). It has been suggested that a stress-induced suppression of immune function may be evolutionarily adaptive because immunosuppression may conserve energy which is required to deal with the immediate demands imposed by the stressor (MAIER *et al.*, 1994).

Acute stress causes a significant enhancement of skin delayed type hypersensitivity and results in a rapid, significant, and rapidly reversible decrease in absolute numbers of leukocytes (T cells, B cells, NK cells and monocytes) in the blood. This represents a redistribution of leukocytes from the blood to organs such as the skin (DHABHAR *et al.* 1996; DHABHAR & MCEWEN, 1997), which ends up being a positive modulatory factor for wound healing.

Keloid is the hyperproliferative disorder of maximum expression in the healing process and only occurs in humans, in which the psychological chronic stress component is already demonstrated (HOCHMAN *et al.*, 2005; FURTADO *et al.*, 2012a), including an increase in salivary cortisol. However how can we explain the fact that patients with Keloid present exacerbated inflammatory response? During inflammation, cytokines from the periphery activate the CNS through multiple routes. This results in stimulation of the HPA axis which, in turn through the immunosuppressive effects of the glucocorticoids, generally inhibits inflammation. Recent studies indicate that physiological levels of glucocorticoids are immunomodulatory rather than solely immunosuppressive. Interruptions of this loop at any level and through multiple mechanisms can render an inflammatory resistant host susceptible to inflammatory disease, including increased resistance of glucocorticoid receptors (STERNBERG, 2001; AVITSUR *et al.*, 2001).

The healing process undergoes a multiplicity of influences of factors that go beyond the organic component, and the psychological/emotional stress being vital importance. This fact can be corroborated when the body-mind connection is broken. Patients operated on for reduction mammaplasty and subjected to hypnosis in the postoperative period presented, according to the author, better healing (GINANDES *et al.*, 2003). In fact, hypnosis has a long history in the treatment of skin disorders, chronic spontaneous urticaria is a common disorder that causes a great deal of suffering and often responds poorly to antihistamine drugs, necessitating recourse to a variety of drugs, some of which have significant side effects and may be ineffective (SHERTZER & LOOKINGBILL, 1987; BROOM, 2010).

However, experimental models of wound healing in animals such as rats and pigs, which are submitted to several types of physical and psychological stress, show similar results to those occurring in humans; in other words, animals submitted to chronic stress show a delayed healing of the skin, and when they are submitted to acute stress, they have a positive stimulus in the wound healing. Then, why does keloid occur only in humans? What characteristic animals (phylogenetically lower than men) have that protect them from this condition? Or, perhaps, what is a needed characteristic for the keloid appearance, that animals do not possess; and would be it intrinsic to human beings?

From a metaphysical approach, if the skin is the outermost of human organs, so the body has a social nature and a more social responsibility. This statement corresponds to the truth as the skin is the organ that gives physical identity to each individual, or the organ that strongly marks the personality of each one, according to the earlier description in this chapter. The skin is our individual frontier within the social sphere. Consequently, each time this frontier is pervaded by an external cause (injury or surgery) or opened by an internal cause (acne, chickenpox or other skin rash), the exposure of the individual essence or soul can take several stereotypes, as status or psychological stability that preceded the moment of the frontier rupture. Following the universal law of physics, according to which for every action there is always a reaction of equal magnitude and in an opposite direction, it can be said that the reaction to the social frontier disruption (skin) will be directly proportional to the intensity of mental disharmonies (revolts, frustration, social shame or inferiority complex) that the individual keeps within himself, in a secret way, but conscious. The somatic form to express this reaction is the resulting scar.

Therefore, through a holistic and metaphysical view, stressed patients undergoing adaptive physiological changes to time and social context, exacerbating the SNS, cause a basal inflammatory metabolic activity on the individual skin (frontier), which enhances the neurogenic inflammation phase during the healing process. In other words, the people bring themselves inflammation, when sweat excessively facing a situation that exalts them, whose fury lets them with "the nerves on edge". This psychosocial situation, which is more common in adolescents, coincides with the appearance of keloid, which is the maximum expression of a pathological scar, resulting from a reaction to a preexisting social aversion (revolt, frustration, or shame). In a more simplistic way, the projection of the "Self" of a person with keloid means: "this horrible scar produced by myself is a consequence of an aggression suffered in the social environment, and shows how much I'm angry and I want you to stay away from me because of the appearance of my scars". What would be implicit in the projection of this person which presents a keloid is: "I'm enjoying that I already had a not assumed inferiority complex, even before forming the scar, and with the distance between us I feel safer because I am not inserted in the social context". For this reason, as I am socially closeted in my inferiority complex, I also take advantage of the horrible keloids as an excuse for not being among you; so, I don't go to the beach, I don't take the shirt, I don't expose myself or I am ashamed to expose myself in the intimacy... ". And as for the keloid symptoms, the meaning of the "Self" would be: "the sudden quickness of the lesions, the redness and swelling, the pruritis, irritation and burning, and the (at times) extreme scratching all (in the symbolic and psychodynamic view) suggestively parallel the human experience of affect on the anger spectrum (anger, rage, irritation, frustration, resentment)" (BROOM, 2010; FURTADO *et al.*, 2012b).

Internal attitudes trigger psychological mechanisms and are among the main causes of organic ills. Thus, healing, as a global manner, such as the normal skin wound healing, is influenced by factors (body condition, personal attitudes and relationships) that facilitate or hinder the process. Positive attitudes facilitate healing, and negative ones impede healing. Positive attitudes include a strong will to feel better; a sense of purpose; acceptance; patience; hope and a willingness to work. Negative attitudes thought to be detrimental to healing include many destructive attitudes and feelings (GLAISTER, 2001). And in this context, a negative attitude of the "Self", and strictly social, which directly affects the health of the skin and, therefore, its healing process, is the ostentatious vanity. Unlike deprived vanity, in which the individual auto-sustain himself (he guarantees himself) in the social context he lives (for example, a person uses an expensive pen in his pocket just because he likes to use this pen), in the ostentatious vanity, in which the person, having inferiority complex and, therefore, does not sustaining himself (not guarantee) in its context he seeks to other ways to feel inserted in social life, and thus compensates his complex (for example, one uses an expensive pen in his pocket to make him feel better seen and admired by others). This ostentatious attitude creates a continuous level of attention that, in its turn, is reflected in a social stress which keeps the SNS exalted. This tensional condition changes the normal physiology of the skin and provides a pathological formation of scar tissue, as described in the subchapter "Cutaneous Nervous System."

Animals do not have vanity ostentatious. They use tricks related to beauty for other purposes, such as camouflage and courtship, both with the purpose of maintenance and survival of the species, respectively. Then, because they don't live in a continuous social tension state in its habitat (except occasionally, in the presence of predators), the physiology of the skin and wound healing of animals is not influenced by this desire in social life; obviously, in experimental laboratory conditions, under stress effect (and never of vanity), changes occur in physiology and wound healing of the skin of animals, though keloid never occurs.

The present chapter reviews the psychoneuroimmunendocrine physiology of the skin responsible for its multiple functions and the extreme disturbances of the healing process. It was seen the excess of the extracellular matrix deposition, such as in keloid and hyperthophic scar; however, there is the other side of the coin, which represents the deficiency of the extracellular matrix deposition, that is atrophic scars and skin ulcerations.

However, even for the latter, the metaphysical reasoning does not change, but its projection. The patient with healing disability presents the psychological profile similar to patients with keloid, described above, but when its frontier (skin) is disrupted, by failing to guarantee himself, he clings to the fear and does not react, keeping its frontier open (ulceration) or weakly closed (atrophic scar). Similarly, in patients with hypertrophic scar, the frontier is more closed than it should, and in patients with keloid the frontier is overly closed. However, in spite of all literature evidences, despite the clinical experience and the metaphysical approach detailed above, more studies should be directed, with this focus on the research of the skin healing in the body-mind connection, because of the importance it holds.

There comes a time when the understanding of the cutaneous healing process becomes essential due to the need for a precocious tissue repair to reduce the physical, social, and psychological morbidity. In wound healing, the "body-mind" connection, or the holistic healing which encompasses the Body, Emotions, Mind, and Spirit? Metaphysical diagnosis takes into account many signs and symptoms, which are then interpreted according to life details that only you can provide. "If the eyes are the mirror of the soul, the skin is the mirror of the mind" - Bernardo Hochman, 2009.

REFERENCES

Abercrombie M, Ambrose EJ. The surface properties of cancer cells: a review. *Cancer Res.* 1962 Jun;22:525-48.

Ahlquist RP. Present state of alpha and beta adrenergic drugs. II. The adrenergic blocking agents. *Am Heart J.* 1976 Dec;92(6):804-7.

Akaishi S, Ogawa R, Hyakusoku H. Keloid and hypertrophic scar: neurogenic inflammation hypotheses. *Med Hypotheses* 2008; 71: 32-8.

Al-Bazzaz FJ, Gailey C. Ion transport by sheep distal airways in a miniature chamber. *Am J Physiol Lung Cell Mol Physiol.* 2001 Oct;281(4):L1028-34.

Alberti LR, Vasconcellos Lde S, Petroianu A. Influence of local or systemic corticosteroids on skin wound healing resistance. *Acta Cir Bras.* 2012 Apr;27(4):295-9.

Alestas T, Ganceviciene R, Fimmel S, Müller-Decker K, Zouboulis CC. Enzymes involved in the biosynthesis of leukotriene B4 and prostaglandin E2 are active in sebaceous glands. *J Mol Med* (Berl). 2006 Jan;84(1):75-87.

Aloe L, Alleva E, Fiore M. Stress and nerve growth factor: findings in animal models and humans. *Pharmacol Biochem Behav.* 2002;73:159–66.

Amara SG, Evans RM, Rosenfeld MG. Calcitonin/calcitonin gene-related peptide transcription unit: tissue-specific expression involves selective use of alternative polyadenylation sites. *Mol Cell Biol* 1984; 4: 2151-60.

Amara SG, Jonas V, Rosenfeld MG, Ong ES, Evans RM. Alternative RNA processing in calcitonin gene expression generates mRNAs encoding different polypeptide products. *Nature.* 1982;298:240-4.

Amaral DG, Sinnamon HM. The locus coeruleus: neurobiology of a central noradrenergic nucleus. *Prog Neurobiol.* 1977;9(3):147-96.

Arck P, Paus R. From the brain-skin connection: the neuroendocrine-immune misalliance of stress and itch. *Neuroimmunomodulation.* 2006;13(5-6):347-56.

Arck PC, Slominski A, Theoharides TC, Peters EM, Paus R. Neuroimmunology of stress: skin takes center stage. *J Invest Dermatol.* 2006 Aug;126(8):1697-704.

Asahina M, Suzuki A, Mori M, Kanesaka T, Hattori T. Emotional sweating response in a patient with bilateral amygdala damage. *Int J Psychophysiol.* 2003 Jan;47(1):87-93.

Ashworth J, Booker J, Breathnach SM. Effects of topical corticosteroid therapy on Langerhans cell antigen presenting function in human skin. *Br J Dermatol.* 1988 Apr;118(4):457-69.

Avitsur R, Stark JL, Sheridan JF. Social stress induces glucocorticoid resistance in subordinate animals. *Horm Behav.* 2001 Jun;39(4):247-57.

Azambuja RD. Dermatologia integrativa: a pele em novo contexto. *An Bras Dermatol.* 2000 Jul-Ago;75(4):393-420.

Barker AT, Jaffe LF, Vanable JW. The glabrous epidermis of cavies contains a powerful battery. *Am J Physiol.* 1982;242:358.

Barnes PJ. Effect of beta-agonists on inflammatory cells. *J Allergy Clin Immunol.* 1999 Aug;104(2 Pt 2):S10-7.

Barnes PJ, Belvisi MG, Rogers DF. Modulation of neurogenic inflammation: novel approaches to inflammatory disease. *Trends Pharmacol Sci.* 1990 May;11(5):185-9.

Barros J, Barros M. Cicatrizes hipertróficas y homeopatía. *Gac Homeop Caracas.* 1996 Jun;4(2): 73-8.

Becker RO. The bioelectric field pattern in the salamander and its simulation by an electronic analog. *IRE Trans Med Electron.* 1960 Jul;ME-7:202-7.

Becker RO, Murray DG. A method for producing cellular dedifferentiation by means of very small electrical currents. *Trans N Y Acad Sci.* 1967 Mar;29(5):606-15.

Besné I, Descombes C, Breton I. Effect of age and anatomical site on density of sensory innervation in human epidermis. *Arch Dermatol.* 2002; 138(11):1445-50.

Bitar MS. Insulin and glucocorticoid-dependent suppression of the IGF-I system in diabetic wounds. *Surgery.* 2000 Jun;127(6):687-95.

Blalock JE. A molecular basis for bidirectional communication between the immune and neuroendocrine systems. *Physiol Rev.* 1989 Jan;69(1):1-32.

Blalock JE. The syntax of immune neuroendocrine communication. *Immunol Today.* 1994 Nov;15(11):504-11.

Bodó E, Kovács I, Telek A, Varga A, Paus R, Kovács L, Bíró T. Vanilloid receptor-1 (VR1) is widely expressed on various epithelial and mesenchymal cell types of human skin. *J Invest Dermatol.* 2004 Aug;123(2):410-3.

Böhm M, Schiller M, Ständer S, Seltmann H, Li Z, Brzoska T, Metze D, Schiöth HB, Skottner A, Seiffert K, Zouboulis CC, Luger TA. Evidence for expression of melanocortin-1 receptor in human sebocytes in vitro and in situ. *J Invest Dermatol.* 2002 Mar;118(3):533-9.

Borba GC, Hochman B, Liebano RE, Enokihara MM, Ferreira LM. Does preoperative electrical stimulation of the skin alter the healing process? *J Surg Res.* 2011 Apr;166(2):324-9.

Borgens RB. Stimulation of neuronal regeneration and development by steady electrical fields. *Adv Neurol.* 1988a;47:547-64.

Borgens RB. Voltage gradients and ionic currents in injured and regenerating axons. *Adv Neurol.* 1988b;47:51-66.

Borgens RB, Vanable JW, Jaffe LF. Role of subdermal current shunts in the failure of frogs to regenerate. *J Exp Zool.* 1979;209:49-56.

Boulais N, Misery L. The epidermis: a sensory tissue. *Eur J Dermatol.* 2008 Mar-Apr;18(2):119-27.

Brain SD, Grant AD. Vascular actions of calcitonin gene-related peptide and adrenomedullin. *Physiol Rev* 2004; 84: 903–34.

Breathnach AS. Electron microscopy of cutaneous nerves and receptors. J Invest Dermatol. 1977;69:8–26.

Brizio-Molteni L, Molteni A, Warpeha RL, Angelats J, Lewis N, Fors EM. Prolactin, corticotropin, and gonadotropin concentrations following thermal injury in adults. *J Trauma.* 1984;24:1–7.

Broom BC. A reappraisal of the role of 'mindbody' factors in chronic urticaria. *Postgrad Med J.* 2010 Jun;86(1016):365-70.

Brown SB, Dransfield I. Electric fields and inflammation: may the force be with you. *ScientificWorldJournal.* 2008 Dec 25;8:1280-94.

Cairns JA, Walls AF. Mast cell tryptase stimulates the synthesis of type I collagen in human lung fibroblasts. *J Clin Invest.* 1997 Mar 15;99(6):1313-21.

Campaner AB, Ferreira LM, Gragnani A, Bruder JM, Cusick JL, Morgan JR. Upregulation of TGF-beta1 expression may be necessary but is not sufficient for excessive scarring. *J Invest Dermatol.* 2006 May;126:1168–76.

Carrasco GA, Van de Kar LD. Neuroendocrine pharmacology of stress. *Eur. J. Pharmacol.* 2003;463:235–72.

Carter HB, Coffey DS. Cell surface charge in predicting metastatic potential of aspirated cells from the Dunning rat prostatic adenocarcinoma model. *J Urol.* 1988 Jul;140(1):173-5.

Carter HB, Partin AW, Coffey DS. Prediction of metastatic potential in an animal model of prostate cancer: flow cytometric quantification of cell surface charge. *J. Urol.* 1989;142:1338-41.

Chapman BP, Moynihan J. The brain-skin connection: role of psychosocial factors and neuropeptides in psoriasis. *Expert Rev Clin Immunol.* 2009 Nov;5(6):623-7.

Choi EH, Brown BE, Crumrine D, Chang S, Man MQ, Elias PM, Feingold KR. Mechanisms by which psychologic stress alters cutaneous permeability barrier homeostasis and stratum corneum integrity. *J Invest Dermatol.* 2005 Mar;124(3):587-95.

Christian LM, Graham JE, Padgett DA, Glaser R, Kiecolt-Glaser JK. Stress and wound healing. *Neuroimmunomodulation.* 2006;13(5-6):337-46.

Chrousos GP. The hypothalamic-pituitary-adrenal axis and immune-mediated inflammation. *N Engl J Med.* 1995 May 18;332(20):1351-62

Cirulli F, Alleva E. The NGF saga: from animal models of psychosocial stress to stress-related psychopathology. *Front Neuroendocrinol.* 2009 Aug;30(3):379-95.

Consoli SM, Rolhion S, Martin C, Ruel K, Cambazard F, Pellet J, Misery L. Low levels of emotional awareness predict a better response to dermatological treatment in patients with psoriasis. *Dermatology.* 2006;212(2):128-36.

Costin GE, Hearing VJ. Human skin pigmentation: melanocytes modulate skin color in response to stress. *FASEB J.* 2007 Apr;21(4):976-94.

Craven A, Ormandy C, Robertson F, Kelly P, Nixon A, Pearson A. Prolactin signalling influences the timing mechanism of the hair follicle: analysis of hair growth cycles in prolactin receptor knockout mice. *Endocrinology.* 2001;142:2533–9.

Crowe R, Parkhouse N, McGrouther D, Burnstock G. Neuropeptide-containing nerves in painful hypertrophic human scar tissue. *Br J Dermatol.* 1994 Apr;130(4):444-52.

Culman J, Unger T. Central tachykinins: mediators of defence reaction and stress reactions. *Can J Physiol Pharmacol.* 1995;73:885–91.

De Kloet CS, Vermetten E, Geuze E, Kavelaars A, Heijnen CJ, Westenberg HG. Assessment of HPA-axis function in posttraumatic stress disorder: pharmacological and non-pharmacological challenge tests, a review. *J Psychiatr Res.* 2006 Sep;40(6):550-67.

Denda M, Nakatani M, Ikeyama K, Tsutsumi M, Denda S. Epidermal keratinocytes as the forefront of the sensory system. *Exp Dermatol.* 2007 Mar;16(3):157-61.

Denda M, Tsutsumi M. Roles of transient receptor potential proteins (TRPs) in epidermal keratinocytes. *Adv Exp Med Biol.* 2011;704:847-60.

Detillion CE, Craft TK, Glasper ER, Prendergast BJ, DeVries AC. Social facilitation of wound healing. *Psychoneuroendocrinology.* 2004 Sep;29(8):1004-11.

Dhabhar FS, McEwen BS. Acute stress enhances while chronic stress suppresses cell-mediated immunity in vivo: a potential role for leukocyte trafficking. *Brain Behav Immun.* 1997 Dec;11(4):286-306.

Dhabhar FS, McEwen BS. Enhancing versus suppressive effects of stress hormones on skin immune function. *Proc Natl Acad Sci U S A.* 1999 Feb 2;96(3):1059-64.

Dhabhar FS, Miller AH, McEwen BS, Spencer RL. Stress-induced changes in blood leukocyte distribution. Role of adrenal steroid hormones. *J Immunol.* 1996 Aug 15;157(4):1638-44.

Di Marco E, Marchisio PC, Bondanza S, Franzi AT, Cancedda R, De Luca M. Growth-regulated synthesis and secretion of biologically active nerve growth factor by human keratinocytes. *J Biol Chem.* 1991;266:21718–22.

Di Marco E, Mathor M, Bondanza S, Cutuli N, Marchisio PC, Cancedda R et al. Nerve growth factor binds to normal human keratinocytes through high and low affinity receptors and stimulates their growth by a novel autocrine loop. *J Biol Chem.* 1993;268:22838–46.

DiPasquale DM, Buono MJ, Kolkhorst FW. Effect of skin temperature on the cholinergic sensitivity of the human eccrine sweat gland. *Jpn J Physiol.* 2003 Dec;53(6):427-30.

Ebner K, Singewald N. The role of substance P in stress and anxiety responses. *Amino Acids.* 2006;31:251–72.

Ebrecht M, Hextall J, Kirtley LG, Taylor A, Dyson M, Weinman J. Perceived stress and cortisol levels predict speed of wound healing in healthy male adults. *Psychoneuroendocrinology.* 2004 Jul;29(6):798-809.

Eedy DJ. Neuropeptides in skin. *Br J Dermatol.* 1993 Jun;128(6):597-605

Eijkelkamp N, Engeland CG, Gajendrareddy PK, Marucha PT. Restraint stress impairs early wound healing in mice via alpha-adrenergic but not beta-adrenergic receptors. *Brain Behav Immun.* 2007 May;21(4):409-12.

Eisenach JH, Atkinson JL, Fealey RD. Hyperhidrosis: evolving therapies for a well-established phenomenon. *Mayo Clin Proc.* 2005 May;80(5):657-66.

Elias LJ, Saucier DM. *Neuropsychology: Clinical and Experimental Foundations.* Boston: Pearson; 2005.

Esteves Junior I, Ferreira LM, Liebano RE. Peptídeo relacionado ao gene da calcitonina por iontoforese na viabilidade de retalho cutâneo randômico em ratos. *Acta Cir Bras.* 2004;19(6):626-9.

Farber EM, Bright RD, Nall ML. Psoriasis: a questionnaire of 2144 patients. *Arch Dermatol.* 1968 Sep;98(3):248-59.

Farber EM, Nall ML. The natural history of psoriasis in 5,600 patients. *Dermatologica.* 1974;148(1):1-18.

Felten DL. Neural influence on immune responses: underlying suppositions and basic principles of neural-immune signaling. *Prog Brain Res.* 2000;122:381-9.

Felten SY, Felten DL, Bellinger DL, Olschowka JA. Noradrenergic and peptidergic innervation of lymphoid organs. *Chem. Immunol.* 1992;52:25–48.

Ferm I, Sterner M, Wallengren J. Somatic and psychiatric comorbidity in patients with chronic pruritus. *Acta Derm Venereol.* 2010 Jul;90(4):395-400.

Ferreira AC, Hochman B, Furtado F, Bonatti S, Ferreira LM. Keloids: a new challenge for nutrition. *Nutr Rev.* 2010 Jul;68(7):409-17.

Ferreira LM, Gragnani A, Furtado F, Hochman B. Control of the skin scarring response. *An Acad Bras Cienc.* 2009 Sep;81(3):623-9.

Fields HL, Basbaum AI. Brainstem control of spinal pain-transmission neurons. *Annu Rev Physiol.* 1978;40:217-48.

Florin L, Knebel J, Zigrino P, Vonderstrass B, Mauch C, Schorpp-Kistner M *et al.* Delayed wound healing and epidermal hyperproliferation in mice lacking JunB in the skin. *J Invest Dermatol.* 2006;126:902–11.

Foitzik K, Krause K, Conrad F, Nakamura M, Funk W, Paus R. Human scalp hair follicles are both a target and a source of prolactin, which serves as an autocrine and/or paracrine promoter of apoptosis-driven hair follicle regression. *Am J Pathol.* 2006;168:748–56.

Foitzik K, Krause K, Nixon AJ, Ford CA, Ohnemus U, Pearson AJ *et al.* (2003) Prolactin and its receptor are expressed in murine hair follicle epithelium, show hair cycle-dependent expression, and induce catagen. *Am J Pathol.* 2003;162:1611–21.

Foitzik K, Langan EA, Paus R. Prolactin and the skin: a dermatological perspective on an ancient pleiotropic peptide hormone. *J Invest Dermatol.* 2009 May;129(5):1071-87.

Foulds IS, Barker AT. Human skin battery potentials and their possible role in wound healing. *Br J Dermatol.* 1983;109:515–22.

Fraiture AL, Piérard-Franchimont C, Piérard GE. The cutaneous neurosensory axis and the neuro-immuno-cutaneous system. *Rev Med Liege.* 1998 Nov;53(11):676-9.

Frank R, Adelmann-Grill BC, Herrmann K, Haustein UF, Petri JB, Heckmann M. Transforming growth factor-beta controls cell-matrix interaction of microvascular dermal endothelial cells by downregulation of integrin expression. *J Invest Dermatol.* 1996 Jan;106(1):36-41.

Furtado F, Hochman B, Farber PL, Muller MC, Hayashi LF, Ferreira LM. Psychological stress as a risk factor for postoperative keloid recurrence. *J Psychosom Res.* 2012a Apr;72(4):282-7

Furtado F, Hochman B, Ferrara SF, Dini GM, Nunes JM, Juliano Y, Ferreira LM. What factors affect the quality of life of patients wih keloid? *Rev Assoc Med Bras.* 2009;55(6):700-4.

Furtado F, Hochman B, Ferreira LM. Evaluating keloid recurrence after surgical excision with prospective longitudinal scar assessment scales. *J Plast Reconstr Aesthet Surg.* 2012b Jul;65(7):e175-81.

Gall C, Moore RY. Distribution of enkephalin, substance P, tyrosine hydroxylase, and 5-hydroxytryptamine immunoreactivity in the septal region of the rat. *J Comp Neurol.* 1984;225:212–27.

Glaister JA. Healing: analysis of the concept. *Int J Nurs Pract.* 2001 Apr;7(2):63-8.

Glaser R, Kiecolt-Glaser JK. Stress-induced immune dysfunction: implications for health. *Nat Rev Immunol.* 2005 Mar;5(3):243-51.

Gilman AG. G proteins: transducers of receptor-generated signals. *Annu. Rev. Biochem.* 1987;56:615–49.

Ginandes C, Brooks P, Sando W, Jones C, Aker J. Can medical hypnosis accelerate post-surgical wound healing? Results of a clinical trial. *Am J Clin Hypn.* 2003 Apr;45(4):333-51.

Godbout JP, Glaser R. Stress-induced immune dysregulation: implications for wound healing, infectious disease and cancer. *J Neuroimmune Pharmacol.* 2006 Dec;1(4):421-7.

Gouin JP, Carter CS, Pournajafi-Nazarloo H, et al. Marital behavior, oxytocin, vasopressin, and wound healing. *Psychoneuroendocrinology.* 2010 August;35(7):1082–90.

Gouin JP, Kiecolt-Glaser JK. The impact of psychological stress on wound healing: methods and mechanisms. *Immunol Allergy Clin North Am.* 2011 Feb;31(1):81-93.

Griffiths CE, Barker JN. Pathogenesis and clinical features of psoriasis. *Lancet.* 2007 Jul 21;370(9583):263-71

Grose R, Werner S, Kessler D, Tuckermann J, Huggel K, Durka S, Reichardt HM, Werner S. A role for endogenous glucocorticoids in wound repair. *EMBO Rep.* 2002 Jun;3(6):575-82.

Grützkau A, Henz BM, Kirchhof L, Luger T, Artuc M. alpha-Melanocyte stimulating hormone acts as a selective inducer of secretory functions in human mast cells. *Biochem Biophys Res Commun.* 2000 Nov 11;278(1):14-9.

Gurtner GC, Werner S, Barrandon Y, Longaker MT. Wound repair and regeneration. *Nature.* 2008 May 15;453(7193):314-21.

Gupta MA, Gupta AK, Schork NJ, Ellis CN. Depression modulates pruritus perception: a study of pruritis in psoriasis, atopic dermatitis, and chronic idiopathic urticaria. *Psychosom Med.* 1994 Jan-Feb;56(1):36-40.

Hagner S, Haberberger RV, Overkamp D, Hoffmann R, Voigt KH, McGregor GP. Expression and distribution of calcitonin receptor-like receptor in human hairy skin. *Peptides* 2002; 23: 109-16.

Harvima IT, Nilsson G. Stress, the neuroendocrine system and mast cells: current understanding of their role in psoriasis. *Expert Rev Clin Immunol.* 2012 Mar;8(3):235-41.

Harvima IT, Nilsson G, Naukkarinen A. Role of mast cells and sensory nerves in skin inflammation. *G Ital Dermatol Venereol.* 2010 Apr;145(2):195-204.

Henry J, Toulza E, Hsu CY, Pellerin L, Balica S, Mazereeuw-Hautier J, Paul C, Serre G, Jonca N, Simon M. Update on the epidermal differentiation complex. *Front Biosci.* 2012 Jan 1;17:1517-32.

Herpfer I, Lieb K. Substance P receptor antagonists in psychiatry: rationale for development and therapeutic potential. *CNS Drugs.* 2005;19:275–93.

Hickie I, Hickie C, Lloyd A, Silove D, Wakefield D. Impaired in vivo immune responses in patients with melancholia. *Br J Psychiatry.* 1993 May;162:651-7.

Hinz B, Celetta G, Tomasek JJ, Gabbiani G, Chaponnier C. Alpha-smooth muscle actin expression upregulates fibroblast contractile activity. *Mol Biol Cell.* 2001 Sep;12(9):2730-41.

Hochman B, Nahas FX, Sobral CS, Arias V, Locali RF, Juliano Y, Ferreira LM. Nerve fibres: a possible role in keloid pathogenesis. *Br J Dermatol* 2008; 158: 651-52.

Hochman B, Vilas Bôas FC, Mariano M, Ferreiras LM. Keloid heterograft in the hamster (*Mesocricetus auratus*) cheek pouch. *Acta Cir Bras.* 2005 May-Jun;20(3):200-12.

Hoffmann P, Hoeck K, Deters S, Werner-Martini I, Schmidt WE. Substance P and calcitonin gene related peptide induce TGF-alpha expression in epithelial cells via mast cells and fibroblasts. *Regul Pept.* 2010 Apr 9;161(1-3):33-7.

Hökfelt T, Kuteeva E, Stanic D, Ljungdahl A. The histochemistry of tachykinin systems in the brain. In: Holzer P (ed). *Tachykinins.* Springer: Heidelberg. 2004:63–120.

Holzer P. Neurogenic vasodilatation and plasma leakage in the skin. *Gen Pharmacol* 1998; 30:5-11.

Hölzle E. Pathophysiology of sweating. *Curr Probl Dermatol.* 2002;30:10-22.

Horan MP, Quan N, Subramanian SV, Strauch AR, Gajendrareddy PK, Marucha PT. Impaired wound contraction and delayed myofibroblast differentiation in restraint-stressed mice. *Brain Behav Immun.* 2005 May;19(3):207-16.

Hosoi J, Grabbe S, Knisely TL, Granstein RD. Aqueous humor inhibits epidermal cell antigen-presenting function. *Reg Immunol.* 1993 Sep-Oct;5(5):279-84.

Hosoi J, Tsuchiya T, Denda M, Ashida Y, Takashima A, Granstein RD *et al.* Modification of LC phenotype and suppression of contact hypersensitivity response by stress. *J Cutan Med Surg.* 1998;3:79–84.

Hulmes DJ. Building collagen molecules, fibrils, and suprafibrillar structures. *J Struct Biol.* 2002 Jan-Feb;137(1-2):2-10.

Hwa C, Bauer EA, Cohen DE. Skin biology. *Dermatol Ther.* 2011 Sep-Oct;24(5):464-70.

Indo Y. Nerve growth factor, pain, itch and inflammation: lessons from congenital insensitivity to pain with anhidrosis. *Expert Rev Neurother.* 2010 Nov;10(11):1707-24.

Irwin M. Effects of sleep and sleep loss on immunity and cytokines. *Brain Behav Immun.* 2002 Oct;16(5):503-12.

Jaffe LF. Control of development by steady ionic currents. *Fed Proc.* 1981;40:125-7.

Jaffe LF, Nuccitelli R. Electrical controls of development. *Ann Rev Biophys Bioeng.* 1977;6:445-76.

Jaffe LF, Vanable JW. Electric fields and wound healing. *Clin Dermatol.* 1984;2:34.

Jafferany M. 2007. Psychodermatology: a guide to understanding common psychocutaneous disorders. *Prim Care Companion J Clin Psychiatry* 9(3): 203–13.

Jamur MC, Oliver C. Origin, maturation and recruitment of mast cell precursors. *Front Biosci (Schol Ed).* 2011 Jun 1;3:1390-406.

Johansson A, Holmgren S, Conlon JM. The primary structures and myotropic activities of two tachykinins isolated from the African clawed frog, Xenopus laevis. *Regul Pept* 2002; 108:113-21.

Kalil-Gaspar P. Neuropeptídeos na pele [Neuropeptides in the skin]. *Anais Brasileiros de Dermatologia* 2003; 78:483-98.

Kashiwakura J, Otani IM, Kawakami T. Monomeric IgE and mast cell development, survival and function. *Adv Exp Med Biol.* 2011;716:29-46.

Kawaguchi Y, Okada T, Konishi H, Fujino M, Asai J, Ito M. Reduction of DTH response is related to morphological changes of Langerhans cells in mice exposed to acute immobilization stress. *Clin Exp Immunol.* 1997;109:397–401

Kawakami A, Fisher DE. Key discoveries in melanocyte development. *J Invest Dermatol.* 2011 Nov 17;131(E1):E2-4.

Kawana S, Liang Z, Nagano M, Suzuki H. Role of substance P in stress-derived degranulation of dermal mast cells in mice. *J Dermatol Sci.* 2006 Apr;42(1):47-54.

Kiernan JA. *The Human Nervous System: An Anatomical Viewpoint. 18th. ed.* Philadelphia: Lippincott Williams & Wilkins; 2004.

Kleyn CE, Schneider L, Saraceno R, Mantovani C, Richards HL, Fortune DG, Cumberbatch M, Dearman RJ, Terenghi G, Kimber I, Griffiths CE. The effects of acute social stress on epidermal Langerhans' cell frequency and expression of cutaneous neuropeptides. *J Invest Dermatol.* 2008 May;128(5):1273-9.

Kodali S, Ding W, Huang J, Seiffert K, Wagner JA, Granstein RD. Vasoactive intestinal peptide modulates Langerhans cell immune function. *J Immunol.* 2004 Nov 15;173(10):6082-8.

Kodali S, Friedman I, Ding W, Seiffert K, Wagner JA, Granstein RD. Pituitary adenylate cyclase-activating polypeptide inhibits cutaneous immune function. *Eur J Immunol.* 2003 Nov;33(11):3070-9.

Kono M, Nagata H, Umemura S, Kawana S, Osamura RY. In situ expression of corticotropin-releasing hormone (CRH) and proopiomelanocortin (POMC) genes in human skin. *FASEB J.* 2001 Oct;15(12):2297-9.

Krause K, Schnitger A, Fimmel S, Glass E, Zouboulis CC. Corticotropin-releasing hormone skin signaling is receptor-mediated and is predominant in the sebaceous glands. *Horm Metab Res.* 2007 Feb;39(2):166-70.

Kypriotou M, Huber M, Hohl D. The human epidermal differentiation complex: cornified envelope precursors, S100 proteins and the 'fused genes' family. *Exp Dermatol.* 2012 Feb 17; in press.

Lawson SN. Phenotype and function of somatic primary afferent nociceptive neurones with C-, Adelta- or Aalpha/beta-fibres. *Exp Physiol.* 2002 Mar;87(2):239-44.

Lee SS, Yosipovitch G, Chan YH, Goh CL. Pruritus, pain, and small nerve fiber function in keloids: a controlled study. *J Am Acad Dermatol.* 2004 Dec;51(6):1002-6.

Lee WJ, Jung HD, Lee HJ, Kim BS, Lee SJ, Kim do W. Influence of substance-P on cultured sebocytes. *Arch Dermatol Res.* 2008 Jul;300(6):311-6.

Leonard BE. The HPA and immune axes in stress: the involvement of the serotonergic system. *Eur Psychiatry.* 2005;S302-6.

Leproult R, Copinschi G, Buxton O, Van Cauter E. Sleep loss results in an elevation of cortisol levels the next evening. *Sleep.* 1997 Oct;20(10):865-70.

Liang Z, Engrav LH, Muangman P, Muffley LA, Zhu KQ, Carrougher GJ, et al. Nerve quantification in female red Duroc pig (FRDP) scar compared to human hypertrophic scar. *Burns.* 2004;30(1):57-64.

Liao S, Shang J, Tian X, Fan X, Shi X, Pei S, Wang Q, Yu B. Up-regulation of melanin synthesis by the antidepressant fluoxetine. *Exp Dermatol.* 2012;21(8):635-7.

Liezmann C, Klapp B, Peters EM. Stress, atopy and allergy: A re-evaluation from a psychoneuroimmunologic persepective. *Dermatoendocrinol.* 2011 Jan;3(1):37-40.

Ljungdahl A, Hökfelt T, Nilsson G. Distribution of substance P-like immunoreactivity in the central nervous system of the rat—I. Cell bodies and nerve terminals. *Neuroscience.* 1978;3:861–943.

Lotti T, Hautmann G, Panconesi E. Neuropeptides in skin. *J Am Acad Dermatol.* 1995 Sep;33(3):482-96.

Luger TA. Neuromediators, a crucial component of the skin immune system. *J Dermatol Sci.* 2002;30(2):87-93.

Lundy-Ekman L. *Neurociências: Fundamentos para a Reabilitação. 3. ed.* Rio de Janeiro: Elsevier Brasil; 2008.

Lynn B. Neurogenic inflammation. *Skin Pharmacol.* 1988;1(4):217-24.

Machado A. *Neuroanatomia funcional. 2. ed.* São Paulo: Atheneu; 2006.

Madden KS. Catecholamines, sympathetic innervation, and immunity. *Brain Behav. Immun.* 2003;17(Suppl 1):5–10.

Mahdavian Delavary B, van der Veer WM, van Egmond M, Niessen FB, Beelen RH. Macrophages in skin injury and repair. *Immunobiology.* 2011 Jul;216(7):753-62.

Maier SF, Watkins LR, Fleshner M. Psychoneuroimmunology. The interface between behavior, brain, and immunity. *Am Psychol.* 1994 Dec;49(12):1004-17.

Mantyh PW. Neurobiology of substance P and the NK1 receptor. *J Clin Psychiatry.* 2002;63 Suppl 11:6-10.

Manuck SB, Cohen S, Rabin BS. et al. Individual differences in cellular immune response to stress. *Psychol Sci.* 1991;2111-5.

Marshall JS, Gomi K, Blennerhassett MG, Bienenstock J. Nerve growth factor modifies the expression of inflammatory cytokines by mast cells via a prostanoid-dependent mechanism. *J Immunol.* 1999 Apr 1;162(7):4271-6.

McBain VA, Forrester JV, McCaig CD. HGF, MAPK, and a small physiological electric field interact during corneal epithelial cell migration. *Invest Ophthalmol Vis Sci.* 2003 Feb;44(2):540-7.

McLean S. Do substance P and the NK1 receptor have a role in depression and anxiety? *Curr Pharm Des.* 2005;11:1529–47.

Melzack R. Prolonged relief of pain by brief, intense transcutaneous somatic stimulation. *Pain.* 1975 Dec;1(4):357-73.

Melzack R. Possible phantom pain from childhood extremity aplasia. *Fortschr Neurol Psychiatr.* 1998 Jan;66(1):VI.

Misery L. Skin, immunity and the nervous system. *Br J Dermatol.* 1997 Dec;137(6):843-50.

Misery L. Langerhans cells in the neuro-immuno-cutaneous system. *J Neuroimmunol.* 1998 Aug 14;89(1-2):83-7.

Misery L. The neuro-immuno-cutaneous system and ultraviolet radiation. *Photodermatol Photoimmunol Photomed.* 2000 Apr;16(2):78-81.

Mycielska ME, Djamgoz MB. Cellular mechanisms of direct-current electric field effects: galvanotaxis and metastatic disease. *J Cell Sci.* 2004 Apr 1;117(Pt 9):1631-9.

Montesano R, Orci L. Transforming growth factor beta stimulates collagen-matrix contraction by fibroblasts: implications for wound healing. *Proc Natl Acad Sci U S A.* 1988 Jul;85(13):4894-7.

Munger BL and Ide C. The structure and function of cutaneous sensory receptors. *Arch Histol Cytol.*1988;51:1–34.

Myllyharju J, Kivirikko KI. Collagens and collagen-related diseases. *Ann Med.* 2001 Feb;33(1):7-21.

Nagy I, Pivarcsi A, Kis K, Koreck A, Bodai L, McDowell A, Seltmann H, Patrick S, Zouboulis CC, Kemény L. Propionibacterium acnes and lipopolysaccharide induce the expression of antimicrobial peptides and proinflammatory cytokines/chemokines in human sebocytes. *Microbes Infect.* 2006 Jul;8(8):2195-205.

Nakazato Y, Tamura N, Ohkuma A, Yoshimaru K, Shimazu K. Idiopathic pure sudomotor failure: anhidrosis due to deficits in cholinergic transmission. *Neurology.* 2004 Oct 26;63(8):1476-80.

Nauck M, Karakiulakis G, Perruchoud AP, Papakonstantinou E, Roth M. Corticosteroids inhibit the expression of the vascular endothelial growth factor gene in human vascular smooth muscle cells. *Eur J Pharmacol.* 1998 Jan 12;341(2-3):309-15.

Navarro F. *Somatopsicodinâmica das biopatias.* Brazil: Dumará; 1991.

Newbold P, Brain SD. The modulation of inflammatory oedema by calcitonin gene-related peptide. *Br J Pharmacol.* 1993 Mar;108(3):705-10.

Niessen FB, Schalkwijk J, Vos H, Timens W. Hypertrophic scar formation is associated with an increased number of epidermal Langerhans cells. *J Pathol.* 2004 Jan;202(1):121-9.

Noël F, Piérard-Franchimont C, Piérard GE, Quatresooz P. Sweaty skin, background and assessments. *Int J Dermatol.* 2012 Jun;51(6):647-55.

Nuccitelli R. Ionic currents in morphogenesis. Experientia. 1988 Aug 15;44(8):657-66.

Nuccitelli R. Endogenous ionic currents and DC electric fields in multicellular animal tissues *Bioelectromagnetics.* 1992;1:147-57.

Nuccitelli R, Smart T, Ferguson J. Protein kinases are required for embryonic neural crest cell galvanotaxis. *Cell Motil Cytoskeleton.* 1993;24(1):54-66.

Nuccitelli R. A role for endogenous electric fields in wound healing. *Curr Top Dev Biol.* 2003;58:1-26.

Oaklander AL, Siegel SM. Cutaneous innervation: form and function. *J Am Acad Dermatol.* 2005 Dec;53(6):1027-37.

Ogawa T, Sugenoya J. Pulsatile sweating and sympathetic sudomotor activity. *Jpn J Physiol.* 1993;43(3):275-89.

Olerud JE, Usui ML, Seckin D, Chiu DS, Haycox CL, Song IS, Ansel JC, Bunnett NW. Neutral endopeptidase expression and distribution in human skin and wounds. *J Invest Dermatol* 1999; 112:873-81.

Ono S, Imai T, Shimizu N, Nakayama M, Yamano T, Tsumura M. Serum markers of type I collagen synthesis and degradation in amyotrophic lateral sclerosis. *Eur Neurol.* 2000;44(1):49-56.

Onuma EK, Hui SW. Electric field-directed cell shape changes, displacement, and cytoskeletal reorganization are calcium dependent. *J Cell Biol.* 1988 Jun;106(6):2067-75.

O'Sullivan RL, Lipper G, Lerner EA. The neuro-immuno-cutaneous-endocrine network: relationship of mind and skin. *Arch Dermatol.* 1998 Nov;134(11):1431-5.

Padgett DA, Glaser R. How stress influences the immune response. *Trends Immunol.* 2003 Aug;24(8):444-8.

Parkhouse N, Crowe R, McGrouther DA, Burnstock G. Painful hypertrophic scarring and neuropeptides. *Lancet.* 1992 Dec 5;340(8832):1410.

Pavlovic S, Daniltchenko M, Tobin DJ, Hagen E, Hunt SP, Klapp BF, Arck PC, Peters EM. Further exploring the brain-skin connection: stress worsens dermatitis via substance P-dependent neurogenic inflammation in mice. *J Invest Dermatol.* 2008 Feb;128(2):434-46.

Paus R. Does prolactin play a role in skin biology and pathology? *Med Hypotheses.* 1991;36:33–42.

Paus R, Schmelz M, Biro T, Steinhoff M. Frontiers in pruritus research: scratching the brain for more effective itch therapy. *J Clin Invest.* 2006a;116:1174–86.

Paus R, Theoharides TC, Arck PC. Neuroimmunoendocrine circuitry of the "brain–skin connection". *Trends Immunol.* 2006b;27:32–9.

Peters EM. The Neuroendocrine-Immune Connection Regulates Chronic Inflammatory Disease in Allergy. *Chem Immunol Allergy.* 2012;98:240-52.

Peters EM, Arck PC, Paus R. Hair growth inhibition by psychoemotional stress: a mouse model for neural mechanisms in hair growth control. *Exp Dermatol.* 2006 Jan;15(1):1-13.

Peters EM, Handjiski B, Kuhlmei A, Hagen E, Bielas H, Braun A, Klapp BF, Paus R, Arck PC. Neurogenic inflammation in stress-induced termination of murine hair growth is promoted by nerve growth factor. *Am J Pathol.* 2004 Jul;165(1):259-71.

Peters EM, Kuhlmei A, Tobin DJ, Müller-Röver S, Klapp BF, Arck PC. Stress exposure modulates peptidergic innervation and degranulates mast cells in murine skin. *Brain Behav Immun.* 2005 May;19(3):252-62.

Peters EM, Liezmann C, Spatz K, Daniltchenko M, Joachim R, Gimenez-Rivera A, Hendrix S, Botchkarev VA, Brandner JM, Klapp BF. Nerve growth factor partially recovers inflamed skin from stress-induced worsening in allergic inflammation. *J Invest Dermatol.* 2011 Mar;131(3):735-43.

Petersen LJ, Church MK, Skov PS. Histamine is released in the wheal but not the flare following challenge of human skin in vivo: a microdialysis study. *Clin Exp Allergy* 1997;27:284-95.

Pietraszek MH, Takada Y, Takada A. Effect of mental stress on platelet aggregation: possible link to catecholamine levels. *Haemostasis.* 1991;21(6):346-52.

Pillay J, den Braber I, Vrisekoop N, Kwast LM, de Boer RJ, Borghans JA, Tesselaar K, Koenderman L. In vivo labeling with 2H2O reveals a human neutrophil lifespan of 5.4 days. *Blood.* 2010 Jul 29;116(4):625-7.

Pincelli C, Sevignani C, Manfredini R, Grande A, Fantini F, Bracci Laudiero L et al. Expression and function of nerve growth factor and nerve growth factor receptor on cultured keratinocytes. *J Invest Dermatol.* 1994;103:13-8.

Price, J. A., Pethig, R., Lai, C. N., Becker F. F., Gascoyne, P. R. and Szent-Gyorgyi, A. (1987). Changes in cell surface charge and transmembrane potential accompanying neoplastic transformation of rat kidney cells. Biochim. *Biophys. Acta* 1987;9:129-36.

Pruessner JC, Hellhammer DH, Kirschbaum C. "Burnout, perceived stress, and cortisol responses to awakening". *Psychosom Med* 61. 1999;(2):197–204.

Reed MJ, Vernon RB, Abrass IB, Sage EH. TGF-beta 1 induces the expression of type I collagen and SPARC, and enhances contraction of collagen gels, by fibroblasts from young and aged donors. *J Cell Physiol.* 1994 Jan;158(1):169-79.

Reich A, Wójcik-Maciejewicz A, Slominski AT. Stress and the skin. *G Ital Dermatol Venereol.* 2010 Apr;145(2):213-9.

Reichlin S. Neuroendocrine-immune interactions. *N Engl J Med.* 1993 Oct 21;329(17):1246-53.

Remröd C, Lonne-Rahm S, Nordlind K. Study of substance P and its receptor neurokinin-1 in psoriasis and their relation to chronic stress and pruritus. *Arch Dermatol Res.* 2007 May;299(2):85-91.

Ricard-Blum S. *The collagen family. Cold Spring Harb Perspect Biol.* 2011 Jan 1;3(1):a004978.

Rinn JL, Wang JK, Liu H, Montgomery K, van de Rijn M, Chang HY. A systems biology approach to anatomic diversity of skin. *J Invest Dermatol.* 2008 Apr;128(4):776-82.

Rojas WE, Di Martino E, Harandi B, Westhofen M. Long-term results of suture-free cutanous wound closure in head and neck incisions with octylcyanoacrylate topival skin adhesive. *Laryngorhinootologie.* 2002 Sep;81(9):644-8.

Roosterman D, Goerge T, Schneider SW, Bunnett NW, Steinhoff M. Neuronal control of skin function: the skin as a neuroimmunoendocrine organ. *Physiol Rev.* 2006 Oct;86(4):1309-79.

Rosenfeld MG, Mermod JJ, Amara SG, Swanson LW, Sawchenko PE, Rivier J, Vale WW, Evans RM . Production of a novel neuropeptide encoded by the calcitonin gene via tissue-specific RNA processing. *Nature* 1983; 304:129-35.

Rossi R, Johansson O. Cutaneous innervation and the role of neuronal peptides in cutaneous inflammation: a minireview. *Eur J Dermatol* 1998;8:299-306.

Roy SK. Regulation of transforming growth factor-beta-receptor type I and type II messenger ribonucleic acid expression in the hamster ovary by gonadotropins and steroid hormones. *Biol Reprod.* 2000 Jun;62(6):1858-65.

Ruiz MR, Quinones AG, Diaz NL, Tapia FJ. Acute immobilization stress induces clinical and neuroimmunological alterations in experimental murine cutaneous leishmaniasis. *Br J Dermatol.* 2003;149:731–8.

Rupniak NM. New insights into the antidepressant actions of substance P (NK1 receptor) antagonists. *Can J Physiol Pharmacol.* 2002;80:489–94.

Saito T, Tazawa K, Yokoyama Y, Saito M. Surgical stress inhibits the growth of fibroblasts through the elevation of plasma catecholamine and cortisol concentrations. *Surg. Today.* 1997;27:627–31.

Sakanaka M, Shiosaka S, Takatsuki K, Inagaki S, Hara Y, Kawai Y, Senba E, Tohyama M. Origins of substance P-containing fibers in the lateral septal area of young rats: immunohistochemical analysis of experimental manipulations. *J Comp Neurol.* 1982;212:268–77.

Sampogna F, Tabolli S, Abeni D; IDI Multipurpose Psoriasis Research on Vital Experiences (IMPROVE) investigators. The impact of changes in clinical severity on psychiatric morbidity in patients with psoriasis: a follow-up study. *Br J Dermatol.* 2007 Sep;157(3):508-13.

Sanders VM, Kohm AP. Sympathetic nervous system interaction with the immune system. *Int. Rev. Neurobiol.* 2002;52:17–41.

Saraceno R, Kleyn CE, Terenghi G, Griffiths CE. The role of neuropeptides in psoriasis. *Br J Dermatol.* 2006 Nov;155(5):876-82.

Saraiya H. Postburn galactorrhea with refractory hypertrophic scars: role of obesity under scrutiny. *J Burn Care Rehabil.* 2003 Nov-Dec;24(6):392-4.

Sato K, Leidal R, Sato F. Morphology and development of an apoeccrine sweat gland in human axillae. *Am J Physiol.* 1987 Jan;252(1 Pt 2):R166-80.

Sauerstein K, Klede M, Hilliges M, Schmelz M. Electrically evoked neuropeptide release and neurogenic inflammation differ between rat and human skin. *J Physiol.* 2000 Dec 15;529 Pt 3:803-10.

Schauer E, Trautinger F, Köck A, Schwarz A, Bhardwaj R, Simon M, Ansel JC, Schwarz T, Luger TA. Proopiomelanocortin-derived peptides are synthesized and released by human keratinocytes. *J Clin Invest.* 1994 May;93(5):2258-62.

Schneider MR, Paus R. Sebocytes, multifaceted epithelial cells: lipid production and holocrine secretion. *Int J Biochem Cell Biol.* 2010 Feb;42(2):181-5.

Schneider MR, Schmidt-Ullrich R, Paus R. The hair follicle as a dynamic miniorgan. *Curr Biol.* 2009 Feb 10;19(3):R132-42.

Scholzen T, Armstrong CA, Bunnett NW, Luger TA, Olerud JE, Ansel JC. Neuropeptides in the skin: interactions between the neuroendocrine and the skin immune systems. *Exp Dermatol* 1998;7:81–96.

Seiffert K, Hosoi J, Torii H, Ozawa H, Ding W, Campton K, Wagner JA, Granstein RD. Catecholamines inhibit the antigen-presenting capability of epidermal Langerhans cells. *J Immunol.* 2002 Jun 15;168(12):6128-35.

Seike M, Ikeda M, Morimoto A, Matsumoto M, Kodama H. Increased synthesis of calcitonin gene-related peptide stimulates keratinocyte proliferation in murine UVB-irradiated skin. *J Dermatol Sci.* 2002 Feb;28(2):135-43.

Sheehan TP, Chambers RA, Russell DS. Regulation of affect by the lateral septum: implications for neuropsychiatry. *Brain Res Brain Res Rev.* 2004;46:71–117.

Shertzer CL, Lookingbill DP. Effects of relaxation therapy and hypnotizability in chronic urticaria. *Arch Dermatol.* 1987 Jul;123(7):913-6.

Sivamani RK, Pullar CE, Manabat-Hidalgo CG, Rocke DM, Carlsen RC, Greenhalgh DG, Isseroff RR. Stress-mediated increases in systemic and local epinephrine impair skin wound healing: potential new indication for beta blockers. *PLoS Med.* 2009 Jan 13;6(1):e12.

Skobowiat C, Dowdy JC, Sayre RM, Tuckey RC, Slominski A. Cutaneous hypothalamic-pituitary-adrenal axis homolog: regulation by ultraviolet radiation. *Am J Physiol Endocrinol Metab.* 2011 Sep;301(3):E484-93.

Slominski A. Neuroendocrine system of the skin. *Dermatology.* 2005;211(3):199-208.

Smith KR, Thiboutot DM. Thematic review series: skin lipids. Sebaceous gland lipids: friend or foe? *J Lipid Res.* 2008 Feb;49(2):271-81.

Slominski A, Baker J, Ermak G, Chakraborty A, Pawelek J. Ultraviolet B stimulates production of corticotropin releasing factor (CRF) by human melanocytes. *FEBS Lett.* 1996;399:175–6.

Slominski AT, Botchkarev V, Choudhry M, Fazal N, Fechner K, Furkert J, Krause E, Roloff B, Sayeed M, Wei E, Zbytek B, Zipper J, Wortsman J, Paus R. Cutaneous expression of CRH and CRH-R. Is there a "skin stress response system?". *Ann N Y Acad Sci.* 1999 Oct 20;885:287-311.

Slominski A, Ermak G, Mazurkiewicz JE, Baker J, Wortsman J. Characterization of corticotropin-releasing hormone (CRH) in human skin. *J Clin Endocrinol Metab.* 1998 Mar;83(3):1020-4.

Slominski A, Mihm MC. Potential mechanism of skin response to stress. *Int J Dermatol.* 1996 Dec;35(12):849-51.

Slominski A, Paus R, Schadendorf D. Melanocytes as "sensory" and regulatory cells in the epidermis. *J Theor Biol.* 1993 Sep 7;164(1):103-20.

Slominski A, Pisarchik A, Zbytek B, Tobin DJ, Kauser S, Wortsman J. Functional activity of serotoninergic and melatoninergic systems expressed in the skin. *J Cell Physiol.* 2003 Jul;196(1):144-53.

Slominski A, Tobin DJ, Shibahara S, Wortsman J. Melanin pigmentation in mammalian skin and its hormonal regulation. *Physiol Rev.* 2004 Oct;84(4):1155-228.

Slominski A, Wortsman J. Neuroendocrinology of the skin. *Endocr Rev.* 2000 Oct;21(5):457-87.

Slominski A, Wortsman J, Paus R, Elias PM, Tobin DJ, Feingold KR. Skin as an endocrine organ: implications for its function. *Drug Discov Today Dis Mech.* 2008 Jun 1;5(2):137-44.

Slominski A, Wortsman J, Tobin DJ. The cutaneous serotoninergic/melatoninergic system: securing a place under the sun. *FASEB J.* 2005 Feb;19(2):176-94.

Slominski A, Zbytek B, Pisarchik A, Slominski RM, Zmijewski MA, Wortsman J. CRH functions as a growth factor/cytokine in the skin. *J Cell Physiol.* 2006a Mar;206(3):780-91.

Spencer RL, Hutchinson KE, Alcohol, Aging, and the Stress Response. Alcohol *Res Health.* 1999;23(4):272-83.

Stefanato CM, Yaar M, Bhawan J, Phillips TJ, Kosmadaki MG, Botchkarev V et al. Modulations of nerve growth factor and Bcl-2 in ultraviolet-irradiated human epidermis. *J Cutan Pathol.* 2003;30:351–7.

Steinhoff M, Stander S, Seeliger S, Ansel JC, Schmelz M, and Luger T. Modern aspects of cutaneous neurogenic inflammation. *Arch Dermatol.* 2003;139:1479-88.

Steinhoff M, Vergnolle N, Young SH, Tognetto M, Amadesi S, Ennes HS, Trevisani M, Hollenberg MD, Wallace JL, Caughey GH, Mitchell SE, Williams LM, Geppetti P, Mayer EA, Bunnett NW. Agonists of proteinase-activated receptor 2 induce inflammation by a neurogenic mechanism. *Nat Med.* 2000 Feb;6(2):151-8.

Sternberg EM. Neuroendocrine regulation of autoimmune/inflammatory disease. *J Endocrinol.* 2001 Jun;169(3):429-35.

Sussman C, Byl N. Electrical stimulation for wound healing. In: Sussman C, Bates-Jensen B M. *Wound Care: A colaborative practice manual for physical therapistis and nurses.* Baltimore: Lippincott Wilians & Wilkins. 2001:497-545.

Szatkowski M, Mycielska M, Knowles R, Kho AL, Djamgoz MB. Electrophysiological recordings from the rat prostate gland in vitro: identified single-cell and transepithelial (lumen) potentials. *BJU Int.* 2000 Dec;86(9):1068-75.

Szeidemann Z, Jakab RL, Shanabrough M, Leranth C. Extrinsic and intrinsic substance P innervation of the rat lateral septal area calbindin cells. *Neuroscience.* 1995;69:1205–21.

Tai G, Reid B, Cao L, Zhao M. Electrotaxis and wound healing: experimental methods to study electric fields as a directional signal for cell migration. *Methods Mol Biol.* 2009;571:77-97.

Takehara K. Growth regulation of skin fibroblasts. *J Dermatol Sci.* 2000 Dec;24 Suppl 1:S70-7.

Teunissen MB, Haniffa M, Collin MP. Insight into the immunobiology of human skin and functional specialization of skin dendritic cell subsets to innovate intradermal vaccination design. *Curr Top Microbiol Immunol.* 2012;351:25-76.

Torii H, Hosoi J, Asahina A, Granstein RD. Calcitonin gene–related peptide and Langerhans cell function. *J Investig Dermatol Symp Proc.* 1997;282-6.

Toyoda M, Luo Y, Makino T, Matsui C, Morohashi M. Calcitonin Gene-Relates Peptide upregulates melanogenesis and enhances melanocyte dendricity via induction of keratinocyte-derived melanotrophic factors. *J Invest Dermatol Symp Proc.* 1999;4(2):116-25.

Toyoda M, Morohashi M. New aspects in acne inflammation. *Dermatology* 2003; 206: 17-23.

Tranel D, Damasio H. Neuroanatomical correlates of electrodermal skin conductance responses. *Psychophysiology.* 1994 Sep;31(5):427-38.

Tsuchiya T, Kishomoto J, Granstein RD, Nakayama Y. Quantitative analysis of cutaneous calcitonin gene–related peptide content in response to acute cutaneous mechanical or thermal stimuli and immobilization-induced stress in rats. *Neuropeptides.* 1996 Apr;30(2):149-57.

Valladeau J, Saeland S. Cutaneous dendritic cells. *Semin Immunol.* 2005 Aug;17(4):273-83.

Vileikyte L. Stress and wound healing. *Clin Dermatol.* 2007 Jan-Feb;25(1):49-55.

Veldhuis JD, Iranmanesh A. Physiological regulation of the human growth hormone (GH)-insulin-like growth factor type I (IGF-I) axis: predominant impact of age, obesity, gonadal function, and sleep. *Sleep.* 1996 Dec;19(10 Suppl):S221-4.

Vgontzas AN, Papanicolaou DA, Bixler EO, Lotsikas A, Zachman K, Kales A, Prolo P, Wong ML, Licinio J, Gold PW, Hermida RC, Mastorakos G, Chrousos GP. Circadian interleukin-6 secretion and quantity and depth of sleep. *J Clin Endocrinol Metab.* 1999 Aug;84(8):2603-7.

Vileikyte L. Stress and wound healing. *Clin Dermatol.* 2007 Jan-Feb;25(1):49-55

Vitalo A, Fricchione J, Casali M, Berdichevsky Y, Hoge EA, Rauch SL, Berthiaume F, Yarmush ML, Benson H, Fricchione GL, Levine JB. Nest making and oxytocin comparably promote wound healing in isolation reared rats. *PLoS One.* 2009;4(5):e5523.

Wakamatsu K, Graham A, Cook D, Thody JH. Characterization of ACTH peptides in human skin and their activation of melanocortin-1 receptor. *Pigment Cell Res.* 1997;10:288-97.

Wallengren J. Vasoactive peptides in the skin. *J Investig Dermatol Symp Proc* 1997; 2: 49-55.

Wallengren J, Chen D, Sundler F. Neuropeptide-containing C-fibres and wound healing in rat skin. Neither capsaicin nor peripheral neurotomy affect the rate of healing. *Br J Dermatol.* 1999 Mar;140(3):400-8.

Wallengren J, Håkanson R. Effects of substance P, neurokinin A and calcitonin gene-related peptide in human skin and their involvement in sensory nerve-mediated responses. *Eur J Pharmacol.* 1987 Nov 10;143(2):267-73.

Warndorff JA. The response of the sweat glands to -adrenergic stimulation. *Br J Dermatol.* 1972 Mar;86(3):282-5.

Watson RE, Supowit SC, Zhao H, Katki KA, Dipette DJ. Role of sensory nervous system vasoactive peptides in hypertension. *Braz J Med Biol Res* 2002;35:1033-45.

Weidner C, Klede M, Rukwied R, Lischetzki G, Neisius U, Skov PS, Petersen LJ, Schmelz M. Acute effects of substance P and calcitonin gene-related peptide in human skin--a microdialysis study. *J Invest Dermatol* 2000;115:1015-20.

Weidermann CJ. Shared recognition molecules in the brain and lymphoid tissues: the polypeptide mediator network of psychoneuroimmunology. *Immunol Lett.* 1987 Dec;16(3-4):371-8.

Wilke K, Martin A, Terstegen L, Biel SS. A short history of sweat gland biology. *Int J Cosmet Sci.* 2007 Jun;29(3):169-79.

Wille JJ, Kydonieus A. Palmitoleic acid isomer (C16:1delta6) in human skin sebum is effective against gram-positive bacteria. *Skin Pharmacol Appl Skin Physiol.* 2003 May-Jun;16(3):176-87.

Willis WD, Westlund KN. Neuroanatomy of the pain system and of the pathways that modulate pain. *J Clin Neurophysiol.* 1997 Jan;14(1):2-31.

Windsor RE, Lester JP, Herring SA. Electrical stimulation in clinical practice. *Physician and Sportsmedicine.* 1993 Jun;21:85-93.

Wu H, Guan C, Qin X, Xiang Y, Qi M, Luo Z, Zhang C. Upregulation of substance P receptor expression by calcitonin gene-related peptide, a possible cooperative action of two neuropeptides involved in airway inflammation. *Pulm Pharmacol Ther* 2007; 20:513-24.

Yaar M, Grossman K, Eller M, Gilchrest BA. Evidence for nerve growth factor-mediated paracrine effects in human epidermis. *J Cell Biol.* 1991;115:821–8.

Yaar M, Park HY. Melanocytes: a window into the nervous system. *J Invest Dermatol.* 2012 Mar;132(3 Pt 2):835-45.

Yang EV, Glaser R. Stress-induced immunomodulation and the implications for health. *Int Immunopharmacol.* 2002 Feb;2(2-3):315-24.

Zbytek B, Wortsman J, Slominski A. Characterization of a ultraviolet B-induced corticotropin-releasing hormone-proopiomelanocortin system in human melanocytes. *Mol Endocrinol.* 2006 Oct;20(10):2539-47.

Zegarska B, Lelińska A, Tyrakowski T. Clinical and experimental aspects of cutaneous neurogenic inflammation. *Pharmacol Rep.* 2006 Jan-Feb;58(1):13-21.

Zhao M. Electrical fields in wound healing-An overriding signal that directs cell migration. *Semin Cell Dev Biol.* 2009 Aug;20(6):674-82.

Zhao M, Bai H, Wang E, Forrester JV, McCaig CD. Electrical stimulation directly induces pre-angiogenic responses in vascular endothelial cells by signaling through VEGF receptors. *J Cell Sci.* 2004;117:397-405.

Zhao M, Pu J, Forrester JV, McCaig CD. Membrane lipids, EGF receptors, and intracellular signals colocalize and are polarized in epithelial cells moving directionally in a physiological electric field. *FASEB J.* 2002 Jun;16(8):857-9.

Zhao Q. Mutagenesis of bovine basic fibroblast growth factor through hybrid clonemid construction: a new approach to DNA manipulation. *Br J Biomed Sci.* 1996 Dec;53(4):270-7.

Ziegler CG, Krug AW, Zouboulis CC, Bornstein SR. Corticotropin releasing hormone and its function in the skin. *Horm Metab Res.* 2007 Feb;39(2):106–9.

Zmijewski MA, Slominski AT. Neuroendocrinology of the skin: An overview and selective analysis. *Dermatoendocrinol.* 2011 Jan;3(1):3-10.

Zoccola PM, Dickerson SS. Assessing the relationship between rumination and cortisol: A review. *J Psychosom Res.* 2012 Jul;73(1):1-9.

Zouboulis CC. Acne and sebaceous gland function. *Clin Dermatol.* 2004 Sep-Oct;22(5):360-6.

Zouboulis CC. Sebaceous gland receptors. *Dermatoendocrinol.* 2009a Mar;1(2):77-80.

Zouboulis CC. The skin as an endocrine organ. *Dermatoendocrinol.* 2009b Sep;1(5):250-2.

Zoumakis E, Kalantaridou SN, Chrousos GP. The "brain-skin connection": nerve growth factor-dependent pathways for stress-induced skin disorders. *J Mol Med (Berl).* 2007 Dec;85(12):1347-9.

Zwilling BS, Hilburger ME. *Macrophage resistance genes: Bcg/Ity/Lsh. Immunol Ser.* 1994;60:233-45.

In: Psychology of Stress
Editors: Leandro Cavalcanti and Sofia Azevedo

ISBN: 978-1-62417-109-3
© 2013 Nova Science Publishers, Inc.

Chapter 2

PROFILING TASK STRESS WITH THE DUNDEE STRESS STATE QUESTIONNAIRE

Gerald Matthews[*1], *James Szalma*[2], *April Rose Panganiban*[1], *Catherine Neubauer*[1] and *Joel S. Warm*[3]

[1]Department of Psychology, University of Cincinnati, Ohio, US
[2]Department of Psychology, University of Central Florida, Orlando, Florida, US
[3]Air Force Research Laboratory, Wright-Patterson AFB, Ohio, US

ABSTRACT

Task performance is frequently stressful, especially when the task imposes high cognitive demands. Research has shown that the subjective stress response to performance is multidimensional. Different types of task demand elicit different patterns of response. This chapter reviews the use of the Dundee Stress State Questionnaire (DSSQ: Matthews et al., 2002) in the investigation of task-induced stress. The DSSQ is based on a factor model that differentiates 11 primary state factors, which cohere around three higher-order dimensions of task engagement, distress and worry. Following a review of the psychometric evidence for this factorial structure, the chapter surveys evidence on the differing profiles of state change produced by a range of basic and applied performance tasks. It also reviews evidence that links stress states to cognitive appraisal and coping processes, consistent with the transactional model of stress. Data also show that the DSSQ factors predict objective performance. These findings may be understood in relation to the emerging cognitive neuroscience of attention. The final section of the chapter covers practical issues in using the DSSQ for assessment of stress in basic and applied contexts.

---

[*] Correspondence to: Gerald Matthews, Department of Psychology, University of Cincinnati, Cincinnati, OH 45221-0376, U.S.A., Phone: (513) 556-0954, E-mail: gerald.matthews@uc.edu.

INTRODUCTION

Task performance is frequently stressful, as evidenced by laboratory studies and by research on real tasks such as vehicle driving, industrial work and military operations (Matthews, Davies, Westerman & Stammers, 2000). Tasks may be intrinsically demanding, because they impose high workload, time pressure or the likelihood of failure. The environmental context in which the task is performed may also be a source of stress. Operational settings may be noisy, hot or dangerous, or they may require prolonged, fatiguing work shifts. Social factors such as interactions between team members may also elevate task demands. Task-related stress may have a variety of consequences including acute emotional response, performance impairments and long-term impacts on the operator's health and well-being.

One way to investigate task stress is to focus on changes in the operator's mental state. For example, stress may be accompanied by negative emotions such as anxiety, anger and unhappiness. Emotions may be defined as a structured set of multiple psychological processes, including somatic responses, subjective feelings, processing biases and action tendencies that serve a functional purpose (e.g., Scherer, 2009). For example, the various components of fear promote awareness of danger and readiness for escape. An emotional *state* is thus a temporary configuration of multiple processes that may produce a variety of behavioral changes. Operationally, states may be assessed through self-reports of immediate feelings (Spielberger, 1972), or through psychophysiological response.

States also have motivational and cognitive elements. In this chapter, we will define states as a relatively transient quality permeating conscious awareness whose representation is distributed across a variety of mental processes or structures, and which has the potential to generalize across activities and contexts (Matthews et al., 2002). That is, a state such as anxiety or worry or apathy cannot be identified with any single underlying process. Also, states may persist across time periods of minutes or hours; anxiety may linger for a time following the threatening stimulus that initially elicited the state. (Note that moods are often seen as more persistent than emotions but we will not pursue this distinction here).

Various existing state measures have contributed to understanding task stress (Humrichouse, Chmielewski, McDade-Montez, & Watson, 2007). Perhaps the best known are the scales for negative emotions, such as anxiety and depression, which make up Spielberger and Reheiser's (2004) State-Trait Personality Inventory (STPI). Researchers have also developed comprehensive measures of mood or basic affects, including the Positive and Negative Affect Schedule (PANAS: Watson, Clark, & Tellegen, 1988), which reduces mood to two orthogonal dimensions. Other scales such as the Profile of Mood Scales (POMS: McNair, Lorr, & Droppleman, 1992) and UWIST Mood Adjective Checklist (UMACL: Matthews, Jones & Chamberlain, 1990a) provide more differentiated factor models. Cognitive state measures are best known from research on worry (Zeidner, 1998), such as Sarason et al.'s (1986) Cognitive Interference Questionnaire (CIQ) which discriminates intrusive thoughts related to the task from personal concerns. Motivational state measures have been rather neglected in favor of measures of goals (e.g., Eliott & Thrash, 2001), although there has been interest in the assessment of intrinsic motivation as a general state (e.g., Lustenberger & Jagacinski, 2010).

The aim of this chapter is to review performance stress research based on a comprehensive model of the various stress states that may be experienced during task performance. We describe a multifactorial stress measure, the Dundee Stress State Questionnaire (DSSQ: Matthews et al., 1999a, 2002), which builds on existing work on assessment of states. We also consider various lines of evidence intended to establish its criterion and construct validity. Evidence comes from both experiments on the factors controlling stress response, and correlational studies that link stress states to personality, cognitive stress processes and objective performance. We will also briefly consider the usage of the DSSQ in developing theories of stress and performance, and in a range of applied settings.

Key Research Issues

Emotions are popularly imagined as mysterious, sometimes fleeting experiences, and state research faces corresponding challenges. Next, we briefly set out the issues confronting those who seek to develop valid state measures, and how they are addressed in this review.

Sampling of states and multidimensional assessment. States are multidimensional. Stress may be experienced in many different ways, including a range of negative emotions, fatigue, worry and pressures to perform effectively. Unidimensional scales, such as those for state anxiety, have proved their value in performance research (e.g., Eysenck & Derakshan, 2011), but fail to provide a comprehensive assessment of the various facets of stress state. Scale development requires a strategy for systematic sampling of the domain of stress states. Matthews et al. (1999a, 2002) used the classical trilogy of mind (Hilgard, 1980) as a means for classifying the principal state constructs prevalent in the performance literature. That is, affective, motivational (conative) and cognitive constructs should be sampled in scale development. We will outline the psychometric basis for the DSSQ as a multivariate state measure.

Characterizing task situations. Contemporary performance research is interactionist in nature (Szalma, 2009a). That is, the individual's response to tasks reflects both situational demands such as workload, and personal characteristics such as traits that moderate the impact of situational factors. A state measure should be sensitive to both situational and personal factors, e.g., situational threats vs. dispositional (trait) anxiety in the case of anxiety (Spielberger, 1972). Thus, state measures should be sensitive to the key situational influences that control task stress, e.g., workload and time pressure. Validation studies must then explore the patterns of state change produced by task and environmental stressors. We will review the evidence that the DSSQ is effective in characterizing the impact of stressors on state.

Characterizing people. Individuals differ considerably in their responses to task stressors. Broadly, some are more resilient than others. People also differ qualitatively in response. For example, being evaluated might produce mostly negative affect in some individuals, but elevated worry in others (Zeidner, 1998). Various individual difference factors control state response, including broad personality traits such as neuroticism, and cognitive stress processes such as appraisal that are more proximal to the stress state. A state measure for performance research should be sensitive to individual differences as well as to situational factors. We will review studies of trait and process correlates of state.

Performance consequences. Stress has a variety of acute and chronic outcomes. Task stress may directly influence task performance, often, but not always, detrimentally. Thus, it is vital for validation that stress state measures correlate with objective performance measures. The impacts of stress state on performance signal the need for theory that ties subjective states to cognitive and neurocognitive processes. In this chapter, we will look especially at how states relate to broad neurocognitive constructs including attentional resources and working memory.

Construct validity and theory development. The early stages of scale validation are often focused on criterion validity, e.g., demonstrating associations between states and performance indices. Construct validity refers to the often more difficult process of developing a testable theoretical account of the construct. It may begin by establishing a 'nomological network' (Cronbach & Meehl, 1955) that specifies relationships between the constructs of interest and other related variables, such as appraisal and coping in the case of stress states. From this, the researcher may move to a theory that explains the relationships specified in the nomological network. The research reviewed is broadly informed by the transactional theory of stress and emotion (Lazarus, 1999; Lazarus & Folkman, 1984). In the performance context, stress is a process that accompanies the operator's attempts to manage task demands and pursue personal goals. We will examine how a transactional perspective illuminates the nature of stress states.

Applications. If states influence objective performance, various practical applications may follow. For example, studies of driver behavior may support understanding of how stress and fatigue states impact safety, leading to more effective countermeasures (Matthews et al., 2002). Similarly, studies in the work context may be informative about the effects of stress on productivity. Stress state assessment may also be useful to designers in evaluating novel human-machine interfaces. We will conclude the chapter with a brief review of some practical applications of stress state research.

A PSYCHOMETRIC MODEL OF STRESS STATES

Initial development work on the DSSQ (Matthews et al., 1999a) focused on 'primary' scales defined by sets of items. Constructs of interest were sampled on the basis of the trilogy of mind (Hilgard, 1980) and relevant studies of stress and fatigue (Matthews et al., 2000). Some of the items were taken from existing scales such as UMACL (Matthews et al., 1990a) and CIQ (Sarason et al., 1986). An item-based factor analysis ($N = 767$) extracted 10 correlated factors similar to those initially hypothesized. Each factor related to one of the three Hilgard (1980) domains: affect, motivation or cognition. Only a single motivation dimension was extracted in this study. Subsequent work (Matthews, Campbell & Falconer, 2001a) divided motivational state into two factors related to intrinsic interest and striving for success, consistent with the distinction made between mastery and performance goals in current motivation theory (e.g., Elliot & Thrash, 2001). Subsequently, we report some studies using the single motivation scale, and others using both. The DSSQ has been translated into languages including German (Langner et al., 2010a), Hebrew (Matthews & Zeidner, 2012), Hindi (Tiwari, Singh & Singh, 2009), Kazakh (Zholdassova, Matthews, Kustubayeva, &

Jakupov, 2012), Russian (Kamzanova, Matthews & Kustubayeva, 2012), and Japanese (Okamura, Tsuda, & Yajima, 2004).

The final set of primary scales included in the DSSQ is illustrated in Table 1, organized in relation to the higher order factor structure we discuss next. The table shows alpha coefficients in the normative sample, together with longer-term test-retest correlations where available (Matthews et al., 1999a). With a state measure, the expectation is that internal consistencies should be high, but test-retest reliability over several weeks should be low (Zuckerman, 1976).

Table 1. Scales of the Dundee Stress State Questionnaire

Factor	Scale	Example item	Scale α	3-week retest r[1]
Task Engagement	Energetic arousal	I feel... Vigorous	.80	.14
	Task Interest	The content of the task is interesting	.75	-
	Success Motivation	I want to perform better than most people do	.87	-
	Concentration	My mind is wandering a great deal (negative item)	.85	.52
Distress	Tension	I feel... Nervous	.82	.48
	Hedonic Tone (low)	I feel... Contented	.86	.42
(low)	Confidence-Control	I feel confident about my abilities	.80	.54
Worry	Self-Focus	I am reflecting about myself	.85	.41
	Self-Esteem	I am worrying about looking foolish (negative item)	.87	.66
	CI (task-relevant)	I have thoughts of... How much time I have left	.78	.37
	CI (task-irrelevant)	I have thoughts of... Personal worries	.86	.49

Note. CI = Cognitive Interference. [1]Data from Matthews et al. (1999a; $N = 112$).

Primary scales were inter-correlated, and so Matthews et al. (2002) conducted second-order factor analyses in several data samples. A consistent three-factor solution was found, as shown in Table 2. The three factors represent broad state syndromes corresponding to (1) task engagement vs. fatigue, (2) distress vs. calmness and confidence, and 3) worry vs. peace of mind. Factors were allowed to correlate, but, in fact, inter-factor correlations were small. Together, these factors comprise an economical description of the performer's state of mind. The first two factors cross Hilgard's (1980) domain boundaries. For example, engagement binds together affect (energetic arousal), cognition (concentration) and task motivation.

The emergence of multiple higher-order factors confirms that characterizing subjective state in terms of global 'stress' is simplistic; stress states are fundamentally multi-dimensional. Indeed, the factor structure corresponds to two major divisions prevalent in the existing literature. The distinction between task engagement and distress corresponds to that between positive and negative affect (Watson et al., 1988), and the separation of distress from worry corresponds to the emotionality-worry distinction prevalent in the anxiety literature (Zeidner, 1998).

Table 2. Secondary factor structure of the DSSQ, in post-task data (pattern matrix)

	Factor		
	Task Engagement	**Distress**	**Worry**
Energetic arousal	**.71**	-.22	-.02
Motivation	**.84**	.02	.17
Concentration	**.68**	-.02	**-.46**
Tense arousal	.29	**.82**	.03
Hedonic Tone	.34	**-.75**	-.01
Confidence-Control	.29	**-.67**	.05
Self-Focus	-.03	-.23	**.85**
Self-Esteem	-.26	-.24	**-.71**
CI (task-relevant)	.01	.31	**.64**
CI (task-irrelevant)	**-.47**	-.07	**.58**

Note. CI = Cognitive Interference, Loadings exceeding ±0.4 are in bold.

Recent research (Guznov, Matthews, Funke & Dukes, 2011; Guznov, Matthews & Warm, 2010; Matthews & Zeidner, 2012) has employed a short version of the DSSQ, which measures only the three secondary factors with 7-item scales (see Helton, 2004, for an alternate short DSSQ). The initial report on the short scale (Matthews, Emo & Funke, 2005) reported scale alphas ranging from $0.78 - 0.83$ ($N = 564$). The short version may be useful when the time available for administration is short, as may be the case in applied settings. Table 3 provides example items.

Table 3. Example items from the short DSSQ

Factor Scale	Example items
Task Engagement	I was determined to succeed on the task.
	My attention was directed towards the task.
	I felt tired. (negative item)
	I felt bored. (negative item)
Distress	I felt tense.
	I felt that I could not deal with the situation effectively.
	I felt relaxed. (negative item)
	I felt confident about my performance. (negative item)
Worry	I felt concerned about the impression I was making.
	I reflected about myself.
	I thought about something that happened earlier today.
	I thought about personal concerns and interests.

ASSESSMENT OF STRESS RESPONSE IN PERFORMANCE SETTINGS

One of the aims of the DSSQ is to afford measurement of the state changes induced by task and environmental stressors. State may be measured before and after exposure to the stressor, in order to determine the state change.

A lower-stress control condition may be run for comparison. There are a variety of study designs in which such measurement may be useful:

- *Task-induced stress.* The cognitive demands of tasks may themselves be stressful. Laboratory studies have investigated workload factors such as stimulus modality and time on task (Szalma et al., 2004), time pressure (Matthews & Campbell, 2009), display uncertainty (Szalma & Teo, 2012), and display configurality (Szalma, 2011), whereas work with an applied focus has investigated real and simulated vehicle driving (Desmond & Matthews, 2009; Funke et al., 2007), human-automation interaction (Szalma & Taylor, 2011), and samples of real or simulated work activities (Horner et al., 2011; Matthews & Falconer, 2000, 2002).
- *Evaluative stressors.* Stress may also be generated by stimuli that signal the operator's level of performance, relative to some personal target or socially-defined norm. Test anxiety, computer anxiety and sports anxiety appear to be fundamentally evaluative in nature, for example (Zeidner & Matthews, 2005). Studies have investigated the impact on state of failure experiences (Matthews et al., 2006), and feedback manipulations (Fairclough & Venables, 2006; Kustubayeva, Matthews & Panganiban, 2011), as well as assessing how anxiety following a real test is expressed as a multidimensional state (Matthews, Hillyard & Campbell, 1999b).
- *Environmental stressors.* Manipulations of psychophysically defined stressors, such as loud noise (Szalma & Hancock, 2011), temperature extremes (Hancock, Ross, & Szalma, 2007), and glare are common in the research literature (Matthews et al., 2000). A broader conception of stressors would take in other agents that potentially impact mood such as drugs, illnesses and nutrients. DSSQ studies of this kind have focused on loud noise (Helton, Matthews & Warm, 2009a), hypoglycemia in a sample of diabetics (McAuley et al., 2006), and cold infection (Matthews et al., 2001b).
- *Prolonged work.* Stress overlaps with task-induced fatigue, which is typically induced by extended work durations. Like stress, fatigue appears to be a multi-faceted construct provoking a variety of different responses (Desmond & Hancock, 2001; Matthews, Desmond & Hitchcock, 2012). In addition to studies of monotonous tasks such as vigilance (Matthews et al., 2010a), research has also been directed towards the states associated with driver fatigue (Matthews & Desmond, 2002; Neubauer, Langheim, Matthews, & Saxby, in press).

Existing studies within the various subfields of stress research have used a variety of scales and indices to assess state change. The lack of any common metric makes it difficult to compare findings across studies in any systematic way. Use of the DSSQ may provide a metric that allows for comparisons to be made across studies and various task domains. Matthews et al. (1999a, 2002) proposed that change scores be standardized using the standard deviations of the scales in the original normative sample. State changes can then be compared across scales and across studies, providing direct effect size indices.

Figure 1 shows the standardized change profiles for 10 of the DSSQ primary scales in two studies, one using a demanding working memory task, and the other a vigilance task (Matthews et al., 1999a). The primary scales are arranged in relation to the secondary factors with which they are most strongly associated (though note some scales have additional factor loadings). Different tasks elicit qualitatively different state changes. The working memory task (Turner & Engle, 1989) required the person to check the accuracy of arithmetic problems while maintaining an ordered list of words in short term storage. A speeded version of the task was used to overload participants with information. The predominant state changes were increased tense arousal, decreased hedonic tone (unpleasant mood) and loss of confidence; a pattern of change signaling increased distress. Scales associated with worry such as self-focus of attention also tend to decline, because the high rate of information input forces attention outward, towards the task rather than inward, towards self-related concerns. The small increase in task-related cognitive interference likely reflects the secondary loading of this scale on distress.

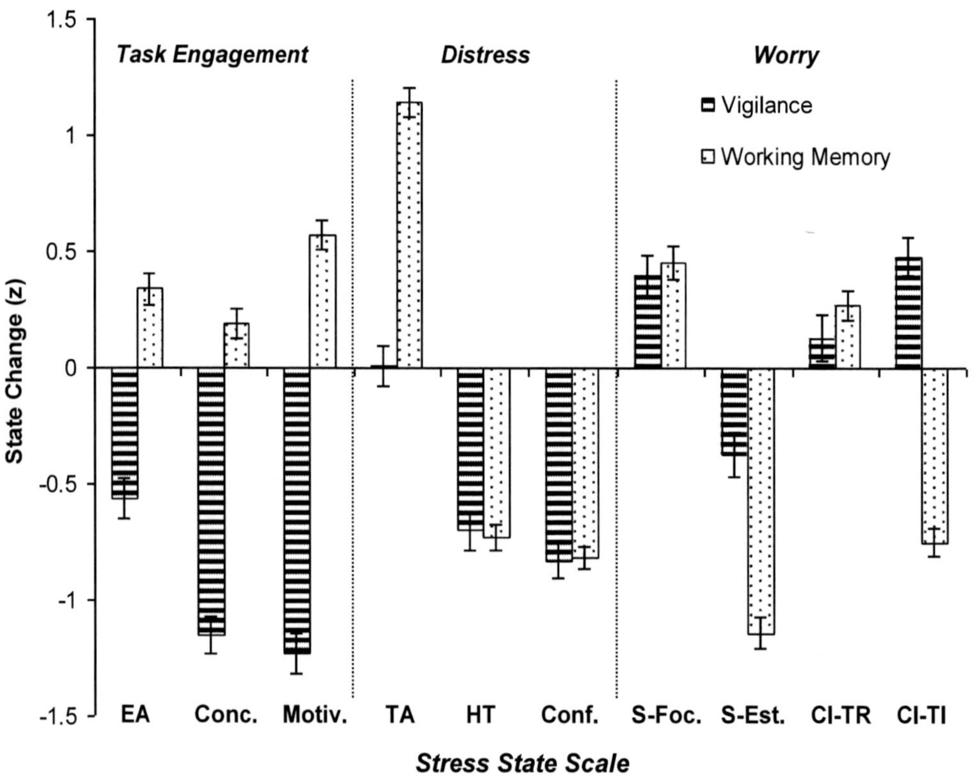

Figure 1. Change scores for DSSQ scales for vigilance ($N = 229$) and working memory ($N = 137$). Error bars indicate standard errors. EA = Energetic Arousal, Conc. = Concentration, Motiv. = Motivation, TA = Tense Arousal, HT = Hedonic Tone, Conf. = Confidence-Control, S-Foc. = Self-Focus, S-Est. = Self-Esteem, CI = Cognitive Interference, TR = Task-Related, TI = Task-Irrelevant.

Performing the vigilance task induced a different pattern of state change. The task required detection of small changes in the lengths of flickering lines, which is apt to be monotonous. The major state changes were those associated with loss of task engagement (fatigue); loss of energy, motivation and concentration. Worry scales showed a mixed pattern of response, with self-esteem increasing but task-irrelevant interference also increasing. Relative to working memory, vigilance may afford more opportunity to reflect on personal concerns.

The profiles shown in Figure 1 represent a fine-grained approach to characterizing task stress. A simpler, but coarser-grained approach is to work with scores for the three secondary factors only, estimated using a regression method (Matthews et al., 2002). Figure 2 illustrates data of this kind, in a study comparing three different task stressors (Matthews et al., 2006). A control condition (reading magazines) was also included. A working memory task provoked high levels of distress, whereas vigilance induced loss of task engagement. The distress response elicited by vigilance may reflect use of a higher-workload task version than in the Matthews et al. (1999a) study. A third task – attempting to solve impossible anagrams – was associated with the highest levels of post-task worry. The task provides both a failure experience, and ample time to reflect on failure.

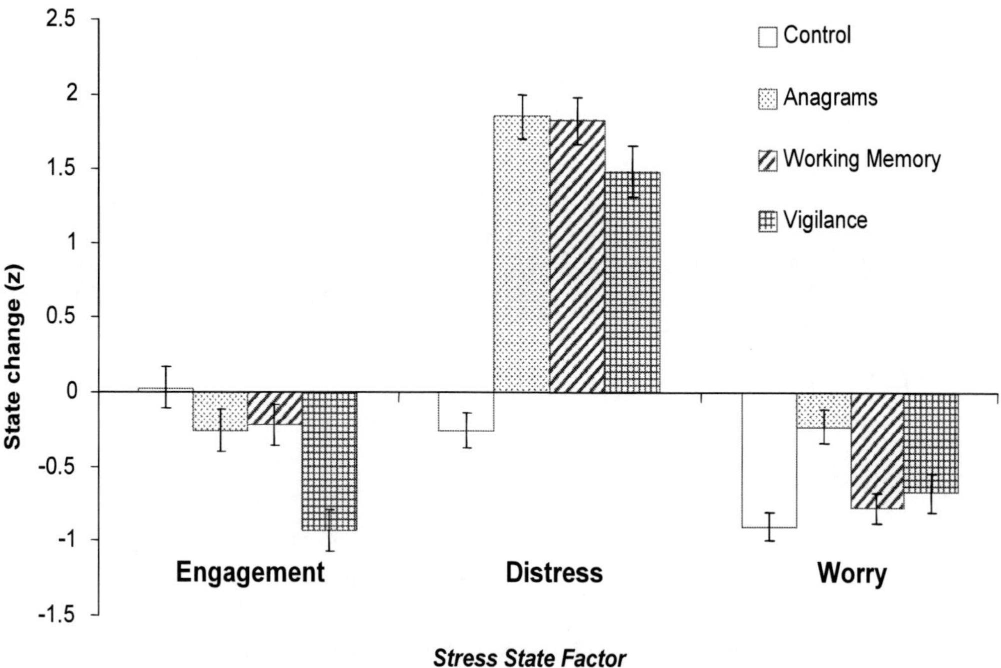

Figure 2. Change scores for DSSQ state factors in four task conditions ($N = 50$, in each). Error bars indicate standard errors.

Figure 3 shows profiles for several complex tasks, representing simulations of real-world operational performance. A fatiguing drive (Neubauer et al., in press) elicited both distress and engagement; we discuss below evidence that different kinds of fatigue manipulations produce different stress profiles. A simulation of customer service work (Matthews & Falconer, 2000) elicited both distress and decreased worry. The Roboflag command-and-control (C2) simulation, requiring control of multiple robots to play a 'capture-the-flag' game, produced a similar pattern of response (Guznov et al., 2010). The final task was designed to provide a positive experience (Kustubayeva et al., 2011). Participants searched a map display to determine the best route for a search-and-rescue mission, and were given positive feedback, leading to elevated task engagement and no change in distress (negative feedback lowered engagement and increased distress).

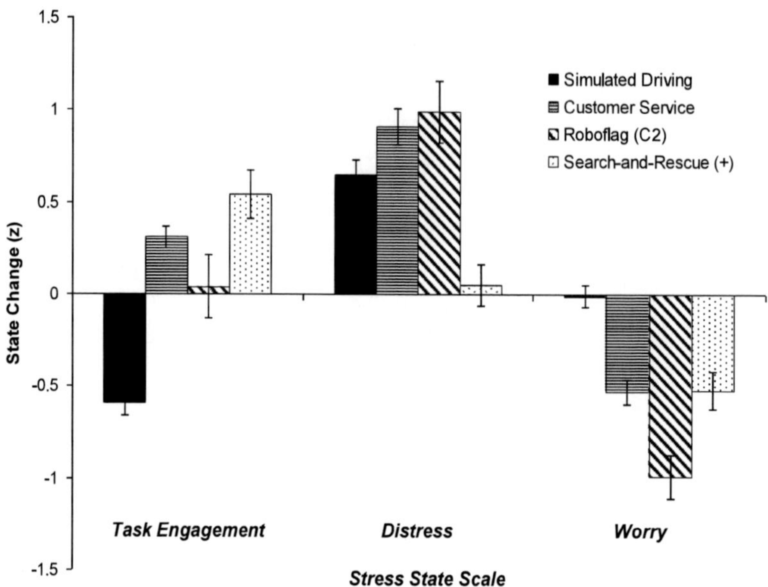

Figure 3. Change scores for DSSQ state factors in four complex tasks. Error bars indicate standard errors. Data are taken from the following sources. Simulated driving: Neubauer et al. (in press; normal driving condition; $N = 91$). Customer service: Matthews and Falconer (2000; $N = 86$). Roboflag: Guznov et al. (2010; solo condition; $N = 50$). Search-and-rescue: Kustubayeva et al. (2011; positive feedback condition; $N = 80$).

Task Engagement

Large-magnitude decreases in task engagement are reliably found with a range of monotonous tasks requiring sustained attention (Warm, Matthews, & Finomore, 2008). In a typical study, Matthews et al. (2010a) investigated two tasks: a sensory vigilance task and a cognitive vigilance task. The sensory vigilance task required participants to detect within a simulated air traffic control display an alignment of two lines representing two aircraft on a collision path. The cognitive vigilance task required the participant to mentally transform letter strings in order to detect a target letter sequence. Across 36 minutes, both tasks showed substantial declines in task engagement relative to baseline, approximately 1.5 SD during sensory vigilance, and 1.3 SD during cognitive vigilance. Similarly, Teo and Szalma (2011) reported that task engagement declined for both a cognitive and sensory version of a 32-minute vigilance task. Typically, in vigilance studies, the primary scales associated with engagement show declines of similar magnitude to one another (e.g., Szalma et al., 2004). Short-duration vigilance tasks also elicit loss of task engagement, although effect sizes tend to be smaller; for example, Shaw et al. (2010) found a 0.4 SD decline for a 12-min task. Langner et al. (2010a) reported decreased engagement on a presumably monotonous, 51 minute simple reaction time task.

Declines in task engagement are also seen on complex tasks that may be monotonous. Prolonged vehicle driving produces loss of task engagement in both field (Desmond & Matthews, 2009) and simulator studies, especially at longer task durations (Saxby et al., 2007). Automation of a battlefield engagement task reduced energy and motivation in a simulation study conducted by McGarry, Rovira, and Parasuraman (2003). Szalma and Taylor (2011) reported that change in task engagement varied as a function of task load in a simulated uninhabited vehicle threat detection task using decision automation. Specifically, task engagement declined when task load was decreased from four video displays to be monitored to a 2 video display condition, and increased in a subsequent block in which the task load was increased to four displays.

Several factors moderate loss of task engagement on monotonous tasks, including display uncertainty (the number of displays to be monitored, ranging from 1-8) and stimulus event rate (Szalma & Teo, 2012). The short-duration, cognitive vigilance task required discriminations of pairs of digits, in which critical signals were cases in which a pair of digits were the same or differed by +/- 1. Post-task engagement exhibited a curvilinear increase as a function of event rate, but only for the lowest level of display uncertainty (i.e., monitoring a single display; see Figure 4). Loss of engagement during vigilance is alleviated by providing a cue to target arrival (Hitchcock et al., 2002), knowledge of results (Szalma, Hancock, Dember, & Warm, 2006), and the opportunity to acquire and destroy targets following detection (Parsons et al., 2007). Generally providing operators with more task-relevant information and personal control helps to maintain engagement, at least to some degree. External stressors also play a role; simulated jet-engine noise elevates engagement (Helton et al., 2009a), whereas cold infection has the opposite effect (Matthews et al., 2001b).

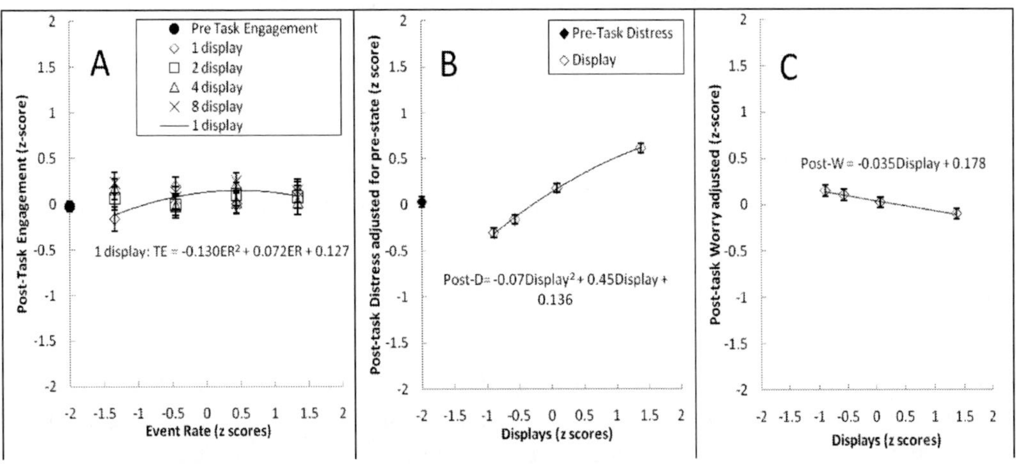

Figure 4. Post-task stress (z-scores of means adjusted for pre-task state) as a function of event rate for post-task engagement (A), and display uncertainty for post-task distress (B), and post-task worry (C). In each case the functions were fitted to the data points. Error bars indicate standard errors.

In the vehicle driving context, Saxby et al. (2007, 2008) investigated Desmond and Hancock's (2001) distinction between passive fatigue, elicited by monotony and underload, and active fatigue, associated with overload. As hypothesized, a passive fatigue manipulation (automated driving) produced larger-magnitude declines in task engagement than an active fatigue manipulation (frequent wind gusts). Effect sizes exceeded 1 SD in the most fatiguing conditions. Disturbingly, from a road safety perspective, Neubauer, Matthews and Saxby (2012) found that texting produced a larger loss of task engagement than either driving without phone use, or driving while talking on the phone. By contrast, Matthews, Quinn and

Mitchell (1998) found that loud rock music tended to elevate engagement during a simulated drive.

Other commonly used information-processing tasks such as working memory (Matthews & Campbell, 2010), selective attention (Matthews & Zeidner, 2012), and discrimination learning (Fellner et al., 2012) often show little or no change in task engagement. Simple tasks used for control purposes such as card-sorting and reading magazines also do not change engagement (Matthews et al., 2002, 2006). Complex tasks that have a game-like element to them may elevate task engagement (even if they also impose high workload). For example, Guznov et al. (2011) reported elevated engagement and increased distress during performance of the 'Roboflag' command-and-control simulation. Positive feedback effects are illustrated in Figure 3; Venables and Fairclough (2009) obtained similar enhancements in engagement following positive feedback, with a restricted set of DSSQ primary scales.

The interest of the task to the participant appears to be the strongest influence on engagement; indeed, Saxby et al. (2007) found that changes in engagement were closely paralleled by changes in challenge appraisals. Using a rapid information-processing task, Matthews and Campbell (2009) found that imposing a near-impossible level of time pressure (150 stimuli/minute) depressed task engagement, as well as challenged appraisal and task-focused coping. Similarly, Ewing and Fairclough (2010) reported that excessive demand reduced scores on the DSSQ motivation scale; an external incentive had the opposite effect. Finally, social factors may also influence engagement; performing in a two-person team produces higher levels of engagement than performing alone (Guznov et al., 2010).

Distress

Increases in distress are fairly easy to produce in the laboratory. The key factor appears to be workload, and even short-duration high workload tasks will elevate distress and its components (high tension, low hedonic tone, low confidence). For example, Matthews et al. (2010a) administered a task battery comprised of three demanding 2-minute tasks (signal detection, working memory, psychomotor tracking), raising distress by 1.46 SD. Increases in distress of varying but often substantial magnitude have also been observed in a range of tasks including vigilance (Warm et al., 2008), simple reaction time (Langner et al., 2010a), working memory (Matthews et al., 2002, 2006; Matthews & Campbell, 2010), and selective attention (Matthews & Zeidner, 2012). Teo and Szalma (2011) found that relative to a sensory discrimination task, a cognitive discrimination task induced higher post-task distress (1.39 SD), compared to 0.79 SD for the sensory discrimination). Helton et al. (2009a) demonstrated the role of task workload directly; decreasing signal salience on a vigilance task elevated distress (without affecting task engagement). External stress factors including loss of control (Funke et al., 2007), cold infection (Matthews et al., 2001b) and negative feedback on performance (Kustubayeva et al., 2011, unpublished analysis; Venables & Fairclough, 2009) also raise distress.

Workload may also be the primary driver of distress response on complex tasks. Even challenging, enjoyable game-like tasks may elevate distress if workload is high; high distress and high task engagement may coexist (Guznov et al., 2011). Simulated vehicle driving often elevates distress, depending on workload (e.g., Stanton & Young, 2005). Saxby et al.'s (2007, 2008) active fatigue manipulation (wind gusts), which increased workload through increasing the difficulty of vehicle control, increased distress over a normal-driving control condition. Texting, and to a lesser degree, speaking on the phone, also seem to elevate distress during driving (Neubauer et al., 2012). Funke et al. (2007) showed that partial vehicle automation both reduced workload and decreased distress, relative to free control of driving. However, full automation, even under the driver's voluntary control, does not seem to be effective in reducing distress (Neubauer et al., in press). Although the primary effect of such manipulations is to increase fatigue (decreased task engagement), prolonged driving under fatiguing conditions appears also to be associated with distress, in both simulated and real driving (Desmond & Matthews, 2009; Matthews & Desmond, 2002).

Display size appears to be an important influence on distress in visual attention. Increasing the field of view of robots under the operator's control, which tended to highlight additional enemy robots, increased distress in Guznov et al.'s (2011) Roboflag study. In the context of decision automation for a threat detection task, Szalma and Taylor (2011) found that post-task distress increased as demand was increased from two to four displays to be monitored, but declined in later blocks of trials in which demand decreased from four to two displays and increased again to four displays. Szalma and Teo (2012), in a study of sustained attention, also found that larger display size was associated with a larger distress response (see Figure 4).

Studies focusing on job-related tasks also show the potential for elevated distress in work settings. Matthews and Falconer (2000, 2002) conducted two studies of customer service agents employed by major British corporations, who performed simulations of their work activities. In both studies, the primary influence of customer service work was to increase distress, by about 0.8 SD. The 7-month longitudinal study conducted by Matthews and Falconer (2000) showed that the distress response did not attenuate over time. (By contrast, Matthews and Campbell's, 2010, laboratory study of working memory did show response attenuation with repeated testing). Medical practitioners may experience high levels of work intensity that are associated with distress: Horner et al. (2011) reported pilot data on the use of the DSSQ to assess stress states during patient encounters in the clinic. Klein et al. (2008) focused on one of the higher-workload components of surgical work, use of a TV image to perform laparoscopic surgery. Performing with the use of a simulated 'surgical field' elevated distress relative to a control condition. A follow-up study (Klein et al., 2012) suggested that stress could be alleviated by a robotic interface, the da Vinci system, which was designed to be more user-friendly for surgeons.

Increases in distress, sometimes exceeding 1 SD, are commonly found across a range of high-workload tasks. However, distress may not be directly driven by workload, as defined in relation to objective task characteristics. For example, Guznov et al. (2011) found that decreasing the maneuverability of robots in their simulation impaired performance but did not impact distress. The effects of display size on a threat detection task obtained by Szalma and Taylor (2011) were independent of the provision of automation, and whether or not the automation was reliable. Szalma (2011) observed that pre-post distress increased for a demanding vigilance task, but this increase did not depend on the discrimination required or the perceptual demands (i.e., configurality) of the display. Szalma et al. (2006) reported that although a demanding vigil increased pre-post-task distress, provision of knowledge of results did not affect this stress dimension.

Helton et al. (2008) conducted a vigilance study in which a workload parameter (signal salience) was switched to either a higher or lower level during the vigil. Compared to control participants for whom workload was constant, switched participants reported higher distress, even when switching from higher to lower workload. In other words, distress appeared to reflect the need to adapt to changing workload, rather than the absolute level of workload per se. Using an air defense simulation, Panganiban, Matthews, Knott, and Funke (2011, unpublished analysis) showed that while the high cognitive demands of the task appeared to increase distress, so too did an external anxious mood induction involving music and guided imagery, although the induction did not affect the actual demands of the task. As discussed below, although high task loads are frequently associated with distress, it may be how the operator interprets and copes with task load that is the critical factor driving distress.

Worry

By contrast with distress, worry typically decreases during task. With both undemanding 'control tasks' (card-sorting and reading magazines), and time-pressured working memory tasks, worry declines by about 1 SD (Matthews et al., 2002, 2006). The majority of tasks show congruent changes in three of the four DSSQ primary scales associated with worry; self-focus decreases, self-esteem increases, and task-irrelevant cognitive interference decrease. Task-related interference sometimes increases (Matthews et al., 1999a), which may reflect its secondary loading on the distress factor. Increases in worry – or in components of worry – may be seen in task paradigms that encourage mind-wandering (Finnigan, Schulze & Smallwood, 2007; Langner et al., 2010b). As shown in Figure 1, task-irrelevant interference may be the scale most likely to show task-induced elevation, for example, during vigilance. Alcohol ingestion may increase task-irrelevant cognitive interference (Finnigan et al., 2007).

Such trends are partly a function of the design of studies of task-induced stress. The shift from anticipating performance to actually processing the task stimuli necessarily shifts attention from internal concerns to external stimuli, reducing self-focus and reflection on personal concerns. In addition, exposure to the task reduces uncertainty, which may reduce evaluative concerns (Stöber, 2004; Zeidner, 1998), increasing self-esteem. Real-life tasks may produce more worry than artificial laboratory tasks, where the person has little at stake. However, in a study in which the DSSQ assessed state during a real examination (Matthews et al., 1999b), scores on the worry-related scales were broadly similar to those seen in laboratory studies. Indeed, self-focused attention was about 0.5 SD below the normative value, although task-related interference was elevated.

The issue is, then, the factors that govern the extent of decline in worry during performance. Tasks that overload attention with frequent stimuli, such as time-pressured working memory tasks (Matthews et al., 2002; Matthews & Campbell, 2010) and complex command-and-control tasks (Guznov et al., 2010, 2011) tend to reduce worry because they force attention outwards, away from personal concerns. Selective and sustained attention tasks (e.g., Matthews et al., 2010a; Matthews & Zeidner, 2012) commonly show drops in worry of around 0.5 SD or so, although short, high event rate vigilance tasks may show greater declines (e.g., Shaw et al., 2010). Tiwari et al. (2009) found that increasing event rate tended to lower some elements of worry, in a vigilance study. By contrast, worry tends to drop only modestly on tasks that allow the respondent to reflect on personal failure, such as attempting to solve impossible anagrams while an experimenter looks on (Matthews et al., 2006). Worry may also be maintained on tasks with a high rate of stimulus input if the task is unusually difficult (Matthews & Campbell, 2009). Szalma and Teo (2012) reported that worry declined as a function of display uncertainty (see Figure 4), possibly because higher numbers of displays to be monitored may divert attention from the self to the task. However, there have also been cases in which variations in task discrimination or display configurality (Szalma, 2011), in task load and decision automation (Szalma & Taylor, 2011), or in variations in KR format (Szalma et al., 2006) did not moderate the decline in pre-post task worry. As with distress, the impact of task parameters may depend on how they are understood by the performer.

Variation in worry response is also seen on tasks relevant to the real world. Funke et al. (2007) recorded declines in worry of about 0.5 SD during several versions of a simulated driving task, a result typical of this paradigm. Worry tends to be more strongly maintained during fatiguing drives; for example, Neubauer et al. (in press) found no change in worry from pre- to post-task. A study of long-haul truckers found that task-irrelevant interference actually increased significantly during work shifts of around 12 hours or so (Desmond & Matthews, 2009). Stanton and Young (2005) reported increases in task-irrelevant cognitive interference associated with use of adaptive cruise control. In the occupational context, Matthews and Falconer (2000, 2002) found decreases of worry of around 0.5 SD in their studies of customer service agents. External stressors including loud noise (Helton et al., 2009a) and cold infection (Matthews et al., 2001b) have little effect on worry, although Smallwood, Fitzgerald, Miles and Phillips (2009) found that a negative mood induction (video of a seriously ill dog) elicited higher scores on both cognitive interference scales.

In sum, worry typically declines during performance, and is less sensitive to manipulations of task demand than are distress and task engagement. Often, distress and worry responses are dissociated, most dramatically during working memory in which they change in opposite directions (Matthews & Campbell, 2010). Such findings confirm the value of separating distress and worry, rather than using the broader state anxiety construct. The extent of task-related decline in worry may reflect the balance between internal and external focus of attention. High task demands drive attention towards external stimuli; failure and lack of stimulation drive attention inward.

CORRELATES OF STRESS STATES

In support of construct validation, relationships between the DSSQ scales and various other constructs have been obtained. In this section, we review correlational data on (1) other state measures, (2) stable personality traits and (3) stress process measures (appraisal and coping). Theories of personality traits predict that certain traits should predict states, but divergent evidence supporting the distinctiveness of trait and state measures is required (Zuckerman, 1976). By contrast, states should converge more strongly with stress process measures, given that within the cognitive model of states, state response should be closely tied to appraisal and coping (Lazarus, 1999).

Convergence with Other State Measures

Table 4 shows correlates of the DSSQ secondary factors with two other leading state measures, the state scales of the STPI (Spielberger & Reheiser, 2004) and the PANAS-X (Watson & Clark, 1991). The latter scale provides measures of both overall positive and negative affect, as well as scores on 11 specific affects. It was administered in an unpublished study of decision-making conducted with undergraduate participants (Grove, 2012; $N = 96$), using a task similar to that of Kustubayeva et al. (2011). The data shown are for post-task assessments, representing states experienced during task performance.

**Table 4. Correlations between DSSQ factors and affect scales
from the STPI and PANAS**

	Task Engagement	Distress	Worry
STPI			
Anxiety	-.10	.62**	.45**
Anger	-.19*	.36**	.40**
Depression	-.27**	.53**	.35**
Curiosity	.40**	.35**	.08
PANAS			
Positive Affect	.47**	-.35**	.03
Negative Affect	-.21*	.51**	.42**
Fear	.19	.09	.28**
Hostility	-.30**	.57**	.33**
Guilt	-.21*	.53**	.40**
Sadness	-.33**	.39**	.30**
Joviality	.45**	-.41**	-.03
Self-Assurance	.25*	-.43**	-.04
Attentiveness	.51**	-.23*	-.06
Shyness	-.08	.14	.22*
Fatigue	-.43**	.17	.09
Serenity	.10	-.58**	-.17
Surprise	.17	.15	.27**

Note. * $p < .05$, ** $p < .01$. STPI correlations from Matthews & Campbell (2010, $N = 144$); PANAS correlations from Grove (2012).

Task engagement correlated most strongly with positive affect, and specific affects including attentiveness, joviality and low fatigue. However, task engagement was not very highly correlated with any affective scale, a divergence that may reflect the wider scope of the DSSQ, the inclusion of DSSQ items that are tied to the performance assessment context, and the use of monopolar scales in the PANAS-X (despite evidence for bipolarity of mood: Matthews et al., 1990a; Thayer, 1989). Notably, the interest and success motivation scales that contribute to task engagement correlated at only .31 ($p<.01$) and .24 ($p<.05$) with positive affect, respectively.

Distress correlated most strongly with state anxiety, as well as state depression, negative affect, hostility and guilt. Distress was also associated with low serenity, a scale resembling low tense arousal in content. These findings were expected, although, as with task engagement, they were not so high as to suggest identity between distress and any specific affect. Neither the STPI nor the PANAS provided a scale that was strongly associated with *worry*; state anxiety, state anger, negative affect and guilt showed the largest-magnitude correlations. The divergence of worry from STPI and PANAS may reflect the limited sampling of cognitive state constructs in these instruments. By contrast, Smallwood et al. (2004a, 2004b) found that an element of worry (task-irrelevant cognitive interference) correlated substantially with task-unrelated thoughts measured using a thought probe technique.

Studies have also investigated psychophysiological correlates of the state factors. Early studies of mood showed that both energetic arousal (similar to engagement) and tense arousal (similar to distress) correlated with various measures of autonomic arousal, including heart rate and skin conductance (Thayer, 1978). A study of state response to multi-tasking (Fairclough & Venables, 2006) revealed a more differentiated picture of state response. Approximately 40% of the variance in task engagement was predicted by psycho-physiological variables. Engagement was positively related to respiration rate, and negatively associated with EEG α power, the 0.1 Hz component of sinus arrhythmia and eye-blink frequency. Distress, however, was positively associated with EEG α and the 0.1 Hz component of sinus arrhythmia, a pattern of response that Fairclough and Venables (2006) interpret as an attempt to conserve mental effort. Worry was unrelated to the psycho-physiological predictors.

Matthews et al. (2010a) investigated individual differences in the cerebral bloodflow velocity (CBFV) response to a short battery of demanding tasks. CBFV was measured using transcranial Doppler sonography (TCD: Warm, Tripp, Matthews & Helton, 2012). The response correlated modestly but significantly with task engagement. Furthermore, pre-task engagement predicted CBFV response magnitude, suggesting the subjective state indexes a neurological state of readiness to attend. As further discussed below, both CBFV and task engagement may index the mobilization and utilization of information-processing resources during attentional task performance.

Neurological bases for worry are not well understood, though recent brain-imaging studies implicate medial prefrontal and anterior cingulate regions (Paulesu et al., 2010). Barron, Riby, Greer and Smallwood (2011) showed that high task-irrelevant cognitive interference (a component of worry) was associated with reduced P300 response during a visual oddball task. They interpreted the data in terms of the decoupling hypothesis, which suggests preserving an internal train of thought requires suppression of the processing of external stimuli. Thus, worry may correlate with brain activity in circuits specialized for internalized thinking that is disconnected from immediate stimulus input (Christoff et al., 2009).

Personality Trait Correlates

Three categories of stable personality traits are linked to stress response. First, there are broad personality traits influenced by basic temperaments, notably those of the Five Factor Model (FFM: McCrae & Costa, 2008). Table 5 shows the FFM correlates of the DSSQ secondary factors during four representative studies, using a range of tasks and alternate scales for the FFM. We focus on linear associations here, but the relationship of the FFM traits to distress and worry also depends on interactions among the traits (Szalma, 2008).

Second, there are more narrowly defined traits, which may be linked structurally to the FFM within hierarchical trait models (Matthews, Deary & Whiteman, 2009). Here, we will discuss traits for fatigue (Finomore, Matthews, Shaw & Warm, 2009) and for mood-regulation (Salovey et al., 1995) as examples. Third, there are traits linked to specific contexts; we will refer to data from studies of test anxiety and vehicle driving here. The data reviewed here establish some meaningful associations between the states experienced during performance, but they also show that trait – state associations are modest in magnitude (usually <.4), providing divergent evidence.

Task engagement is not strongly correlated with the FFM. Conscientiousness appears to be the most reliable correlate of task engagement (e.g., Matthews & Zeidner, 2012; Shaw et al., 2010; Szalma & Taylor, 2011), although correlation magnitudes are typically low and not always significant in our studies. Agreeableness and low neuroticism also show a weak tendency towards correlating with engagement. Although extraversion is commonly linked to reward sensitivity and positive affect (e.g., Corr, 2009), this trait is not a reliable predictor of task engagement, even on tasks that actually elevate task engagement. However, Guznov et al. (2010) found a significant extraversion – engagement correlation of 0.28 in a team condition, and Szalma, Oron-Gilad, and Hancock (2005) reported a positive relationship between task engagement and extraversion among police officers engaged in a firearms training task. At most, extraversion is weakly predictive of engagement prior to performance, but typically fails to predict post-task engagement (e.g., Matthews et al., 2006).

Table 5. FFM correlates of the three DSSQ state factors assessed pre-and post- task

	Study	Neuroticism		Extraversion		Agreeableness		Conscientious-ness		Openness	
		Pre	Post	Pre	Post	Pre	Post	Pre	Post	Pre	Post
Task Engage-ment	1	.03	-.09	.09	.03	.22**	.25**	.28**	.32**	.19**	-.04
	2	-.22**	-.18**	.12*	.05	.17*	.21**	.30**	.23**	.05	.08
	3	-.34**	-.17*	.32**	.13	.26**	.11	.38**	.11	.04	.12
	4	-.21**	-.10	.04	-.01	.13	.03	.28**	.06	.04	.10
Distress	1	.20**	.31**	-.38**	-.17**	-.22**	-.04	-.22**	-.15*	-.20**	.01
	2	.44**	.23**	-.32**	-.19**	-.27**	-.04	-.16**	.00	-.24**	-.03
	3	.61**	.25**	-.38**	-.03	-.26**	-.05	-.34**	.01	-.13	-.10
	4	.54**	.31**	-.11	-.09	-.20**	-.09	-.24**	-.17*	-.18*	-.12
Worry	1	.22**	.20**	-.05	.06	.01	-.22**	-.08	-.22**	-.03	-.02
	2	.26**	.23**	-.10	-.05	-.08	-.06	.02	.11	.02	.00
	3	.40**	.26**	-.06	.04	-.02	.00	-.03	.03	.09	.07
	4	.47**	.33**	.03	.05	-.07	-.10	-.20**	-.15*	-.12	.06

Note. *p<.05, **p<.01. Some data are unpublished in the cited articles.

Study 1: Matthews et al. (1999a, Study 2, $N = 229$). Task: Visual vigilance. FFM scale: Goldberg's (1992) adjectival markers.

Study 2: Matthews et al. (2010a, $N = 294$). Task: Short task battery. FFM scale: Saucier's (2002) adjectival markers.

Study 3: Matthews et al. (2006, $N = 200$). Task: Four tasks used. FFM scale: NEO-FFI (Costa & McCrae, 1992).

Study 4: Shaw et al. (2010, $N =210$). Task: Visual vigilance. FFM scale: NEO-FFI (Costa & McCrae, 1992).

Looking at personality using more fine-grained dimensional models, Shaw et al. (2010) addressed personality predictors of fatigue states during a monotonous vigilance task. A factor analysis of 17 scales linked to fatigue-proneness identified four factors labeled cognitive disorganization, impulsivity, heightened awareness and sleep quality. These factors showed a number of significant correlations in the .15 - .30 range with the DSSQ secondary factors. With the FFM traits controlled, the cognitive disorganization factor (e.g., cognitive failures, mind-wandering) remained significantly correlated with lower post-task engagement. Mood-regulation may play a role in maintaining energy. Salovey et al.'s (1995) Trait Meta-Mood Scale (TMMS) assesses attention to emotion, clarity of thinking about emotion, and mood repair. These traits may contribute to 'emotional intelligence'. Matthews and Fellner (2012) pooled data from three studies that measured the TMMS, as well as stress state during performance (N = 608). Clarity and repair tended to be associated with higher post-task engagement, although effect sizes were small.

The impact of traits on states may be explored in specific performance contexts. Matthews, Desmond, Joyner and Carcary (1997) developed the Driver Stress Inventory (DSI) to assess driving-related traits associated with stress and emotion, and confirmed that this measure predicts moods during real and simulated drives. Studies using DSSQ scales to assess states in real (Desmond & Matthews, 2009) and simulated driving (Funke et al., 2007; Matthews et al., 2002; Neubauer et al., in press) have typically found that the DSI fatigue-proneness trait is a reliable predictor of loss of task engagement during driving.

Distress is most reliably predicted by neuroticism (Table 5), although effect sizes tend to be larger in pre-task than in post-task data, and for studies using the NEO-FFI questionnaire (Costa & McCrae, 1992) to assess the trait. Additional studies have also shown neuroticism – distress correlations in the 0.2 – 0.4 range (e.g., Matthews & Campbell, 2009, 2010; Szalma & Taylor, 2011; Szalma & Teo, 2010), suggesting adequate divergence of the trait from the state. Guznov et al. (2010) found that neuroticism was most strongly related to distress in a 'team player' condition, consistent with a link between the trait and vulnerability to social stress (Matthews et al., 2009). Agreeableness and Conscientiousness tend to be modestly associated with lower distress in pre- but not post-task data (Table 5).

More narrowly defined traits may predict distress over and above the FFM, including cognitive disorganization (Shaw et al., 2010) and (low) TMMS clarity (Matthews & Fellner, 2012). Pessimism has also been observed to correlate with both distress and worry, although the relationships vary as a function of knowledge of results provided (Szalma, 2009b; Szalma et al., 2006). In the vehicle driving context, the DSI (Matthews et al., 1997) assesses a dislike of driving trait which correlated with distress during driving (Desmond & Matthews, 2009). A recent study of fatigue in the automated vehicle (Neubauer, et al., in press) found that DSI fatigue-proneness predicted distress as well as reduced task engagement, especially when the driver initiated automation. There may be dynamic interaction between stress and fatigue, such that fatigue-prone drivers have heightened awareness of the discomforts associated with fatigue states, elevating distress.

Worry consistently relates to neuroticism, as shown in Table 5, but not to any other FFM trait (Szalma & Taylor, 2011; Szalma & Teo, 2010). Shaw et al. (2010) found that a 'heightened experience' trait linked to schizotypal personality predicted worry, with the FFM controlled. Clarity of thought on the TMMS is associated with lower worry (Matthews & Fellner, 2012). In a study of test anxiety, Matthews et al. (1999b) defined a factor associated with dysfunctional metacognitions (Wells, 2000), including worry about worry and beliefs about the importance of attending to negative thoughts. The factor predicted levels of task-related and task-irrelevant cognitive interference during an exam. Sarason's (1984) measure of trait test anxiety also predicted several DSSQ scales in this study. In driver behavior studies, DSI dislike of driving predicts higher worry (Desmond & Matthews, 2009).

Stress Process Correlates

States of stress have both physiological and psychological aspects, and we have already discussed evidence linking states to physiological responses (Matthews et al., 2010a; Fairclough & Venables, 2006). From the psychological standpoint, the leading theory is the transactional theory of stress and emotion (Lazarus, 1999). In brief, Lazarus saw emotions as reflecting 'core relational themes' that express the current meaning of an encounter for the person. The core relational theme is associated with patterns of appraisal and coping that are characteristic of each emotion. The present research has used appraisal and coping scales appropriate to the performance setting that may elucidate the cognitive process underpinnings of stress states.

Lazarus and Folkman (1984) distinguished primary appraisal of the immediate personal significance of an event from secondary appraisal of one's own capabilities for coping with the event. Our research has used the Assessment of Life Events scale (ALE: Ferguson, Matthews & Cox, 1999) to measure primary appraisal dimensions of threat and challenge, as well as an additional secondary appraisal scale for the perceived controllability of the task situation (Matthews et al., 2001a). Our approach to coping follows that of Endler and Parker (1990) who discriminated broad factors of task-focus, emotion-focus and avoidance. Matthews and Campbell (1998) developed the Coping Inventory for Task Stress-Situational (CITS-S) which assesses the three Endler and Parker strategies in relation to the specific context of task performance. We focus here on these measures of the appraisal and coping elicited by a specific task, although, in the occupational context, there is evidence too that stress states are associated with the person's typical styles of appraising and coping with work demands (Matthews et al., 2002). We will present an overview of our relevant research first, and then outline the principal stress process correlates of the three secondary DSSQ factors.

Table 6 shows typical results from three representative studies, chosen to sample different tasks and populations. Data are taken from (1) a study of a high workload vigilance task (Shaw et al., 2010), (2) a pooled sample of customer service agents performing work simulations (Matthews & Falconer, 2000, 2002), and (3) a pooled sample of participants performing simulated drives of various task configurations, most of which were fatiguing (Saxby et al., 2007, 2008). All data were taken post-task (see Matthews et al., 2006, and Matthews and Campbell, 2009, for similar results).

In these and other studies, workload data were secured. Although workload is typically seen as a property of tasks rather than people, use of standard instruments such as the NASA Task Load Index (TLX: Hart & Staveland, 1988) reveals substantial individual differences for any given task. There may be individual differences in appraisal of task demands and of one's own reactions to those demands, such as committing effort or becoming frustrated. Table 7 shows correlations in a pooled data set between the DSSQ and the six rating scales for the various workload components that make up the TLX (Matthews et al., 1999a).

Table 6. Appraisal (ALE) and coping (CITS-S) correlates of the three DSSQ state factors assessed post- task

	Study	Appraisal			Coping		
		Challenge	Threat	Controll ability	Task-focus	Emotion -focus	Avoidance
Task Engagement	1	.53**	-.07	.28**	.65**	-.21**	-.53**
	2	.45**	-.02	.26**	.49**	-.15*	-.33**
	3	.60**	.07	.12*	.41**	.22**	-.47**
Distress	1	-.32**	.27**	-.41**	-.40**	.41**	.31**
	2	-.24**	.52**	-.42**	-.06	.63**	.14
	3	-.08	.38**	-.36**	-.14*	.42**	.27**
Worry	1	.30**	.38**	-.32**	.29**	.67**	.26**
	2	.17*	.51**	-.44**	.23**	.66**	.21**
	3	.20**	.33**	-.47*	.25**	.57**	.50**

Note. *p<.05, **p<.01. Some data are unpublished in the cited articles.
Study 1: Shaw et al. (2010, $N = 210$).
Study 2: Data (total $N = 177)$ pooled from Falconer et al. (2000, 2002) samples.
Study 3: Data (total $N = 288)$ pooled from Saxby et al. (2007, 2008) samples.

Table 7. Correlations between workload components assessed by the NASA-TLX and DSSQ state factors assessed post-task ($N = 567$)

	Engagement	Distress	Worry
Mental demands	.46**	23**	.08
Physical demands	.20**	28**	.18**
Temporal demands	.29**	.37**	.13**
Poor performance	-.44*	43**	.14**
Effort	.57**	.13**	-.01
Frustration	-.29**	.58**	.25**
Total Workload	.21**	.58**	.23**

Note. *p<.05, **p<.01.

Each of the DSSQ factors relates to multiple appraisal and coping processes. *Task engagement* is most reliably associated with challenge appraisal, task focused coping and low use of avoidance (Table 6). Engagement is moderately associated with higher overall workload on the NASA-TLX, consistent with the idea that task demands lead to mobilization of processing resources (Young & Stanton, 2002), but it also relates to a characteristic pattern of ratings: higher perceived demands and higher effort, but also lower performance concerns and frustration. Thus, engagement may relate to the qualitative nature of perceptions of task demands; those that encourage effort and performance attainment appear to be engaging.

Distress correlates most reliably with threat appraisal, low perceived controllability and use of emotion-focus. Its correlations with the other appraisal and coping dimensions are less consistent. Distress is also generally associated with higher workload ratings on the NASA-TLX, evident for all six rating scales to varying degrees. Like distress, *worry* correlates with threat, low controllability and emotion-focus, but it is also consistently related to avoidance. Intriguingly, two processes that are normally adaptive in performance environments, challenge appraisal and task-focused coping are also associated with higher worry. Correlations between the NASA-TLX and worry are small, verging on the trivial.

Correlation magnitudes are in some cases quite substantial, consistent with the Lazarus (1999) hypothesis that appraisal and coping are drivers of emotion. Several studies (e.g., Matthews et al., 2006; Matthews & Falconer, 2000, 2002; Matthews & Campbell, 2009; Shaw et al., 2010) used multiple regression methods to predict post-task state from appraisal and coping, with pre-task state controlled. Appraisal and coping consistently explained about 30-40% of the variance in post-task state. In addition, each study identifies multiple independent predictors of states, which are thus non-isomorphic with any given appraisal or cognitive process. Outcomes of regressions vary somewhat across studies. However, the most consistent predictors of task engagement in the regressions are challenge appraisal, task-focus and low avoidance; of distress, emotion-focus and low controllability; of worry, emotion-focus and avoidance. Each state corresponds to a distinct patterning of processing.

Pre-task states also predict subsequent appraisal and coping, to a modest degree (Matthews et al., 2010b). Thus, the relationship between states and stress processes may be seen as bidirectional. For example, in line with Thayer's (1989) view that subjective energy has an internal signaling function, high pre-task engagement encourages challenge appraisals and task-focused coping, which tend to elevate engagement further.

PERFORMANCE STUDIES

Contemporary studies of stress states and performance are guided by cognitive science, and, increasingly, cognitive neuroscience. Figure 5 shows an outline conceptual framework for research into the relationships between multidimensional stress states and performance (Matthews, Hancock & Desmond, 2012). States include both subjective states, measured by the DSSQ, and physiological states associated with the activation of functional brain systems. There is some overlap between subjective and physiological states, but the latter cannot be fully indexed using subjective measures. Stress states are sensitive both to physical agents (e.g., noise), and to operators' appraisal of task demands and their competency in managing those demands. States, in turn, influence information-processing characteristics which are expressed in observed performance. Stressor effects can thus be mitigated either by reducing the operator's sensitivity to the stressor (state-directed mitigators), or by reducing the impact of the state on performance (performance-directed mitigators).

Performance may be understood dynamically (Hancock & Warm, 1989) or transactionally (Matthews, 2001), in that the operator attempts to exert control over the task environment, which itself influences operator state. Two types of state influence on information-processing may be distinguished (Matthews, 2001). First, states may influence basic parameters of the cognitive and neural architectures, such as the capacity of a memory store, or the speed with which a process is executed. Second, states may influence the person's understanding of the task, their performance goals, and the strategies employed to attain those goals (cf., Hockey, 1997). Relationships between states and strategy use may be understood in terms of Lazarus's (1999) appraisal and coping processes (Matthews & Desmond, 2002).

We will briefly survey studies that have demonstrated correlations between the three state factors and objective performance indices. Caution is needed in inferring causal impacts of states from such data, given that appraisal of performance may feed back to influence states, but in some cases a causal argument can be advanced. The research reviewed has focused primarily on task engagement and its relationships with attention, but we will also refer to findings on distress and worry.

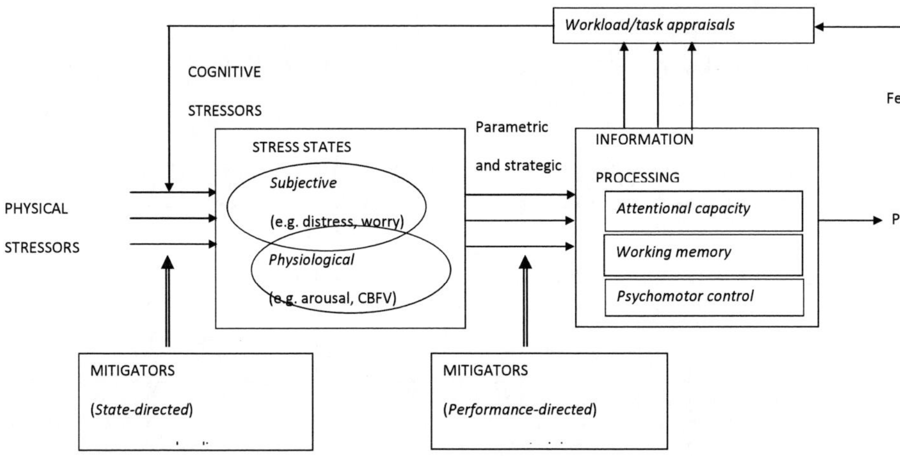

Figure 5. An outline multivariate stress state model.

Task Engagement

Much stressor research has contrasted the typically beneficial effects on performance of energizing agents such as stimulants and incentives with the fatiguing effects of sleep deprivation, sedatives and prolonged work periods. Space limitations prevent any review of this research (see Ackerman, 2011; Matthews, Desmond, Neubauer & Hancock, 2012). Relevant to the current studies is the resource theory of Humphreys and Revelle (1984), which proposes that high arousal increases the availability of processing resources for attention or 'sustained information transfer'. Matthews, Davies and Lees (1990b) identified 'arousal' with energetic arousal. They showed that pre-task energetic arousal predicted performance on a range of attentionally demanding tasks, consistent with the Humphreys and Revelle theory. Importantly, high energy was beneficial only when tasks were highly demanding and presumably most strongly resource-dependent. These and other studies (Matthews & Davies, 1998) suggested the value of using resource models to understand subjective state effects. Schell, Melton, Woodruff, and Corbin (2004) reported a similar result.

Subsequent research has shown that task engagement is similarly predictive of demanding attentional task performance (see Matthews et al., 2010b, for a review). Table 8 summarizes some relevant studies, using a variety of tasks, in which the engagement – performance correlation was typically around 0.3. The table also indicates how fatiguing the task was in relation to the change in engagement resulting from performance. In fact, associations between engagement and performance are found in both fatiguing and non-fatiguing settings. Several of the studies used fatiguing vigilance tasks that lowered task engagement by 1 SD or more. In studies of this kind, task engagement measured pre-task reliably predicts perceptual sensitivity (Matthews et al., 2010a, 2010c; Shaw et al., 2010). Funke et al. (2007) found that engagement was associated with superior vehicle control during a moderately fatiguing simulated drive. However, engagement – performance associations are also seen for tasks that do not lower engagement substantially, including visual search (Fellner et al., 2007), working memory (Matthews & Campbell, 2010), reading comprehension (Helton & Garland, 2006) and discrimination learning (Fellner et al., 2012). Schell, Woodruff, Corbin, and Melton (2005), using a subset of DSSQ primary scales, found that motivation, but not energy was associated with accuracy of detecting errors on a simulation of prescription checking in a pharmacy.

Table 8. Examples of studies showing positive correlations between DSSQ task engagement and performance indices

Study	N	Task (and performance index)	Duration (min)	Task-induced engagement change	Performance correlation with engagement
Matthews et al. (2010a)	187	Sensory vigilance: air traffic control display (A')	36	-1.59	.32**
Matthews et al. (2012c)	462	Sensory vigilance: battlefield monitoring task (d')	60	-1.50	.29**
Matthews et al. (2010a)	108	Cognitive vigilance: letter decoding task (A')	36	-1.26	.29**
Funke et al. (2007)	168	Simulated driving (SD of lateral position)	20	-.76	-.24**
Matthews & Campbell (2009)	144	Rapid Information Processing task (A')	15	-.53	.31**
Fellner et al. (2007)	129	Visual search of faces for emotion target (RT)	c. 10	-.13	-.21*
Fellner et al. (2012)	180	Discrimination learning using facial cues (% correct, final trial block)	c. 20	-.21	.20**
Helton et al. (2009a)	192	Sensory vigilance: short task with degraded stimuli (correct detections)	12	.03	.39**
Matthews & Campbell (2010)	111	Working memory (ordered word recall)	12	.43	.28**

Note. *p<.05, ** p<.01

Multivariate modeling has shown that task engagement mediates the impacts of external stressors on vigilance including loud noise (Helton et al., 2009a) and cold infection (Matthews et al., 2001b), consistent with the model shown in Figure 5. The structural equation model (SEM) fitted by Helton et al. (2009a) is shown in Figure 6. Matthews et al. (2012a) fitted an SEM to data obtained from sensory and cognitive vigilance tasks. A measure of CBFV response was also secured, to provide a physiological index of resource mobilization. The SEM suggested that, although correlated, CBFV and task engagement influenced subsequent vigilance independently. State effects were associated with the higher-order engagement factor, rather than of its specific primary state components (energy, motivation, concentration).

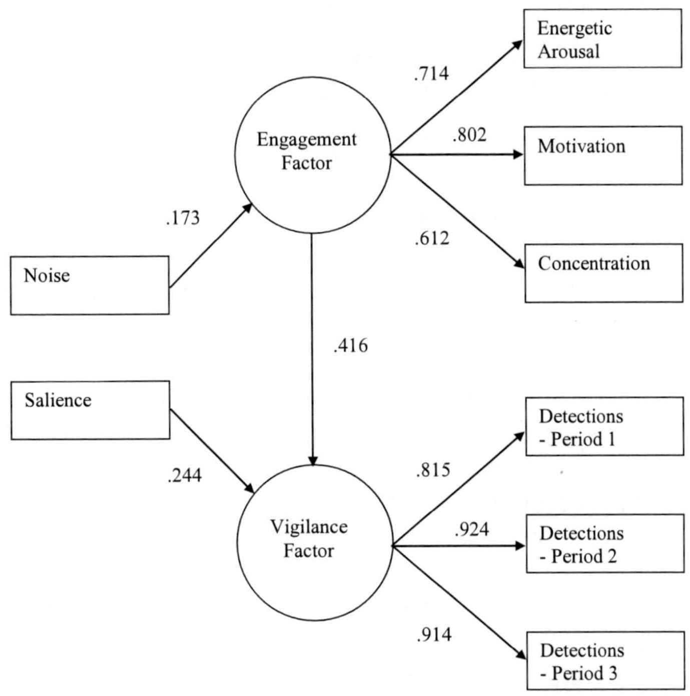

Figure 6. Path coefficients for a structural equation model defining engagement and vigilance as latent factors (Model 1).

'Resources' is a diffuse concept that may be expressed through multiple indices, including but not limited to subjective state. Elaborating resource models may require more precise specification of processing mechanisms. One approach is to explore executive control processes that may govern performance on attentional and working memory tasks (Matthews et al., 2010b). Matthews and Zeidner (2012) confirmed that task engagement was associated with superior executive control using Fan et al.'s (2002) Attention Network Test (ANT). Task engagement also mediated facilitative effects of the conscientiousness trait on the ANT index (whereas extraversion showed an independent effect).

Another issue for resource models is the extent to which performance effects reflect changes in the total size of the resource pool (availability) versus changes in the person's deployment of resources (allocation). Whereas vigilance findings tend to support a resource availability interpretation (Matthews et al., 2010b), other lines of research implicate resource allocation. Matthews and Campbell (2009) found that performance on a rapid information processing task was associated with higher use of task-focused coping and lower avoidance, suggesting strategic influences on performance. Matthews et al. (2012a) replicated these associations for vigilance. Neubauer et al. (in press) showed that drivers low in task engagement were more prone to voluntarily use vehicle automation, presumably as a strategy for reducing task load. Fatigue may lead to lowered goals for performance (Hockey, 1997).

Thus, the low-engagement operator may reduce effort accordingly, even if resources are available. One possibility is that changes in resource availability and allocation operate in tandem. Level of engagement may signal resource availability to the operator who regulates effort accordingly. In underload conditions, the fatigued operator may 'overshoot' and reduce effort more than actual shrinkage of the resource pool warrants (Matthews & Desmond, 2002).

Distress

Both distress and worry might be expected to impair attention, given their overlaps with state anxiety (Matthews & Campbell, 2010). However, while significant negative associations between distress and performance are sometimes found in our vigilance studies (Matthews et al., 2012a; Shaw et al., 2010), they are less consistent across studies than for task engagement. However, in a real life context, police officers performing a handgun shooting exercise, distress was found to correlate with greater accuracy (Stafford, Oron-Gilad, Szalma, & Hancock, 2004), although the distress elicited by the firearms task may depend to some extent on personality characteristics (Szalma, 2008; Szalma et al., 2005).

Eysenck and Derakshan's (2011) Attention Control Theory (ACT) proposes that anxiety interferes with executive control, and specifically with inhibition of task-irrelevant stimuli. In their study of the ANT, Matthews and Zeidner (2012) confirmed that distress was associated with poorer inhibition. The ANT index of executive functioning is based on inhibition of competing responses during a stimulus discrimination task. Distress was also associated with stronger orienting to a spatial cue, perhaps corresponding to enhanced exogenous control of attention.

Matthews and Campbell (2010) showed consistent associations between higher distress and poorer working memory, using the Turner and Engle (1989) task. This was a longitudinal study in which subjects performed the task on four successive days. Structural equation modeling allowed day-to-day state variation in distress to be separated from a more stable, trait-like component linked to neuroticism. The SEM showed that it was state rather than trait distress that was associated with working memory impairment.

Worry

Detrimental effects of worry are best-known from test anxiety research, which suggests a variety of impacts on attention, working memory, and retrieval from long-term memory (Zeidner, 1998). In our studies, like distress, worry is sometimes but not always associated with poorer vigilance (e.g., Helton et al., 2009a; Shaw et al., 2010). If worry occupies verbal short-term memory (Eysenck, 1992), it may be especially detrimental to verbally-mediated tasks. Consistent with this idea, Matthews et al. (2012a) found that worry was related to perceptual sensitivity on a cognitive but not a sensory vigilance task. Matthews and Falconer (2002) had customer service agents perform a task requiring updating of records in a database, during a call from a customer. Agents high in worry prior to performance were less accurate on both declarative and procedural aspects of the task.

On the other hand, Matthews and Campbell (2010) found that pre-task worry predicted impairment of one of two components of their working memory task, i.e., arithmetic, but not verbal recall. Funke et al. (2007) showed that worry was associated with poorer vehicle control (i.e., nonverbal performance). Helton and Garland (2006) found that worry was unrelated to reading comprehension but was associated with poor navigation during an orienteering competition (although their version of the DSSQ differs somewhat from the standard one). The task-irrelevant interference component of worry was related to poorer performance during a traverse of a climbing wall (Green & Helton, 2011). One of the major cognitive process correlates of worry, avoidance coping, seems to be more strongly related to impaired vigilance than is worry itself (Shaw et al., 2010), presumably reflecting strategic withdrawal of effort from the task. Where worry is found to impact attention, it may be as a proxy for this mode of coping, as the more direct influence.

Effects of worry may be more subtle than a simple loss of functional resources. Johnson (2009) showed that worry was associated with slower switching from a neutral to an emotional set on a task requiring discriminations to be made on facial stimuli. Worry may thus influence executive control of task-switching. Another perspective on worry comes from work on mindwandering (see Smallwood & Schooler, 2006, for a review). In these studies (e.g., Smallwood et al., 2004a, 2004b), the cognitive interference scales of the DSSQ were used to supplement experience-sampling measures of mindwandering.

Subsequent studies (Helton, Kern & Walker, 2009b; Helton & Warm, 2008) confirmed a negative association between DSSQ task-irrelevant interference and performance on the sustained attention task used in the Smallwood et al. (2004a, 2004b) studies. Helton et al. (2009b) attributed these effects to impulsive responding associated with disruption of executive control of motor response rather than to the resource mechanism underpinning task engagement effects on vigilance. Taken together, these studies suggest that mindwandering is associated with deficits in sustained attention when the task requires executive control. Mind wandering is also associated with more superficial encoding of external stimuli. As noted previously, linking worry to decoupling of internal processing from immediate task demands is compatible with neuroscience models of networks for attention (Christoff et al., 2009).

USE OF THE DSSQ: THEORY DEVELOPMENT AND PRACTICAL APPLICATION

The DSSQ may be of use both in developing theoretical accounts of stress, fatigue and performance, and for assessment of stress in applied settings. We will conclude by summarizing some key issues for researchers and practitioners

Theoretical Issues

It is not our purpose here to provide anything resembling a comprehensive theory of stress and performance. Instead, our aim is to highlight some of the main theoretical frameworks relevant to interpreting stress state data. We will follow the tri-level framework suggested by Matthews (2001; Matthews et al., 2000). In recognition of the diversity and complexity of stress effects on performance, multiple levels of explanation are needed. For example, a stressor such as noise (Szalma & Hancock, 2011) may influence psychophysiological functioning (via activation of the hypothalamic-pituitary-adrenal axis: HPA), parameters of information-processing, and strategic adaptation to the perceived demands imposed by the stressor. Different levels of theory are needed to explain these different impacts, and different theories may be appropriate for different problems in stress research. States index multiple mechanisms, and it is an open question whether the state is best treated as an integrated whole, or as a collection of distinct processes that can be decomposed.

Biological perspective. States are often characterized as expressions of activity in underlying brain systems, consistent with the neuroscience of emotion (Thayer, 1989). In addition to broad arousal and motivation systems, theory may also refer to more specialized circuits, such as those controlling sleep and circadian rhythms (Banks, Jackson, & Van Dongen, 2012), and to executive systems in frontal cortex with a higher-level regulative function (Killgore, 2012). Studies of the DSSQ have investigated stressors with direct impacts on brain functioning including cold infection (Matthews et al., 2001b), hypoglycemia (McAulay et al., 2006) and alcohol (Finnigan et al., 2007). Work of this kind may identify the neural bases for state factors. Matthews et al. (2010b) linked task engagement to subcortical dopaminergic afferents to prefrontal areas for executive control. Although not a focus of our work, the HPA is a plausible basis for distress. A promising approach to understanding worry may be in relation to the 'default network' of medial prefrontal structures that are associated with internally focused thought, including mind-wandering (Christoff et al., 2009). There are also parallels between task engagement, distress and worry and three brain systems featuring in current neurological models of personality: behavioral approach, fight/flight/freeze and behavioral inhibition, respectively (Corr, 2009; Matthews, 2008).

The capability of purely neurological theories to account for data on stress and performance is controversial. It is certainly important to determine the role in performance of brain systems associated with subjective states, but predictive models require a cognitive psychological element to account for the role of task factors in stressor effects (Matthews, 2001). For example, predicting associations between task engagement and executive function requires an account of the information-processing mechanisms supported by prefrontal cortex (Matthews & Zeidner, 2012). Cognitive neuroscience theories of anxiety (Eysenck & Derakshan, 2011) may suggest mechanisms for distress and worry effects on performance.

Biological theories may be most useful for integrating psychophysiological and subjective data. Extensive research on CBFV and other hemodynamic indices (Warm et al., 2012) suggests that CBFV indexes resource utilization during sustained attention. In other words, a metabolic index (CBFV) may be interpreted in relation to a cognitive construct (resources). As previously described, 'resources' can then be characterized as a multifaceted construct expressed both in CBFV response and in subjective task engagement (Matthews et al., 2010a).

An intriguing recent development in theory is the use of molecular genetic assays to investigate individual differences in task-induced stress response (Parasuraman & Jiang, 2011). These authors report that different alleles of the Dopamine Beta Hydroxylase (DBH) gene predicted DSSQ responses on a stressful military command-and-control simulation. Those with genotypes conferring lower enzyme activity reported relatively higher task-induced engagement and lower distress and worry, relative to those with higher enzyme activity genotypes. The former group also performed better on the task, in some respects.

Information-processing perspective. Both the origins of stress states and their impact on performance may be understood in relation to 'virtual' cognitive architectures that specify how information is processed. The importance of appraisal, coping and perceptions of workload in generating subjective states points towards information-processing mechanisms. However, these self-report measures are only indirectly related to processing in the computational sense. Contemporary appraisal theories (Scherer, 2009) provide explicit accounts of how processing generates emotions, and they may be extended to explain stress states more generally. Scherer's theory includes multiple appraisal processes, which may be simulated computationally; some processes may be inaccessible to consciousness.

Cognitive psychological accounts of performance correlates of states are quite well-developed. As discussed previously, task engagement and distress effects can be understood in relation to existing cognitive theories of the impacts on processing of arousal and emotion (Eysenck & Derakshan, 2011; Humphreys & Revelle, 1984). While predictively useful, such theories utilize fairly broad constructs such as working memory and resources. Computational models that specify quantitative parameters of processing may provide more precise accounts of stress state effects (Gunzelmann & Gluck, 2009; Matthews & Harley, 1993). Ideally, cognitive neuroscience models will succeed in quantifying both the neural and information-processing impacts of stress states.

Self-regulative perspective. A third theoretical perspective is to understand states as signaling modes of adaptation to stress (Hancock & Warm, 1989). In terms of Hockey's (1997) control theory, distress may be associated with a 'strain' mode as the person adapts to cognitive overload, and loss of engagement with adaptation through lowering performance goals (Matthews et al., 2002). Such perspectives are also compatible with the transactional theory of stress (Lazarus, 1999), as the state signals the relation between person and task demands. Building on Lazarus' (1999) theory, Matthews et al. (2002) suggested that task engagement corresponds to a core relational theme of commitment to effort, distress to a theme of management of cognitive overload, and worry to self-evaluation in the task context.

The data reviewed above show that task engagement, distress and worry are each associated with characteristic patterns of appraisal and coping which reflect the core transactional themes. There are likely to also be unconscious or implicit elements of appraisal that also contribute to stress state response. Thus, while computational appraisal models (Scherer, 2009) attribute states to specific processes or process sets, an alternate perspective is to identify the states with broader states of adaption supported by a variety of self-regulative processes.

Self-regulative models also contribute to understanding the performance correlates of states. Associations between appraisal and coping and objective performance (Matthews & Campbell, 2009; Matthews et al., 2010a) suggest that the task strategies associated with states influence performance. The allocation of effort may be under strategic control, as suggested by studies of fatigue and simulated driving (Matthews & Desmond, 2002; Neubauer et al., in press). In the case of distress and worry, emotion-focused and avoidance strategies may divert attention from the task (Wells & Matthews, 1994). Indeed, worry may be seen as the hijacking of task-related processing by a more pressing, personally relevant goal (Smallwood & Schooler, 2006).

Practical Applications

The DSSQ has been used to assess stress response in applied contexts including transportation (Desmond & Matthews, 2009; Neubauer et al., in press), work simulations (Matthews & Falconer, 2000, 2002; Schell et al., 2005), military operations (Shingledecker et al., 2009; Szalma & Taylor, 2011), and medicine (Horner et al., 2011; Klein et al., 2012). The advantage of the DSSQ is that assessment of multivariate state responses to performance environments may be more informative about operator well-being and performance competency than more global measures of 'stress'.

Some limitations of the method must be acknowledged. Subjective measures are necessarily unsuitable for measuring unconscious or implicit qualities of the person. They are also unsuitable for measuring state change over short time durations (less than a few minutes), for which psychophysiological recording may be more appropriate. Mood measures are not generally vulnerable to social desirability bias (Matthews et al., 1990a), but more could be done to investigate response biases across the spectrum of states. There are also issues surrounding the appropriate level of granularity. Often, working with the three higher-order factors seems to capture the essential features of the stress response, but sometimes the more fine-grained assessment provided by the primary DSSQ scales may be more appropriate. For example, in studies of the relationship between mindwandering and performance, researchers have used the task-irrelevant cognitive interference scale in preference to the broader worry factor (e.g., Helton et al., 2009b; Smallwood et al., 2004b). The DSSQ is also not intended to measure specific emotions, although it does include a separate anger scale useful in studies of driver aggression (Emo, Funke, Matthews, & Warm, 2004). With these cautions in mind, we will set out various applications for the DSSQ.

Evaluation of tasks. The simplest application is evaluating the patterns of stress state elicited by specific operational tasks. We have described how the DSSQ has been used to investigate the stress produced by the cognitive demands of vehicle operation (Funke et al., 2007), customer service work (Matthews & Falconer, 2002), air defense (Panganiban et al., 2011) and surgical procedures (Klein et al., 2012). Typically, measurement of the three higher-order factors provides a reasonable if simplified picture of task induced stress, although use of the full DSSQ provides additional detail (Klein et al., 2008; Stanton & Young, 2005; Szalma et al., 2004).

Such assessments have various applications. Knowing which specific dimensions of state are impacted by the task allows for task redesign (Szalma, 2008; 2009a). High distress suggests a need to reduce workload, loss of task engagement a need to reduce monotony and increase challenge, and high worry a need to support attentional focus through design features or providing reassurance to the operator.

Use of the DSSQ also allows specific sources of task load to be evaluated. Guznov et al. (2011) found that changing operator field of view had stronger impacts on stress response than changing maneuverability, in a simulation of remotely piloting robots. Spiridon and Fairclough (2009) investigated effects of a malfunctioning keyboard on stress state response. Stanton and Young (2005) explored the impact of adaptive cruise control on stress during driving. The impact of vehicle automation was also studied by Funke et al. (2007), Neubauer et al. (2012, in press) and Saxby et al. (2007, 2008), whereas McGarry et al. (2003) showed effects of automation on stress response during a battlefield engagement task.

Thus, the DSSQ is useful for designers to assess the impact of system features.

Evaluation of performance environments. In operational settings, operator stress reflects not only the immediate demands of the task, but also the macroenvironmental context, including environmental stressors. The DSSQ may also be used to evaluate stress factors extrinsic to the task, as demonstrated in studies of cold infection (Matthews et al., 2001b), jet engine noise (Helton et al., 2009a) and hazardous driving conditions (Funke et al., 2007). Social factors may also be assessed, as in studies of the impact of teamwork on stress (Guznov et al., 2010). Such findings might be used to drive stress management interventions targeted towards the most salient elements of the stress response (Matthews & Falconer, 2002). Indeed, the DSSQ may be used to assess training protocols (Ross, Ganey & Broadway, 2004) and virtual training environments (Taylor & Barnett, 2010) intended to reduce stress.

The DSSQ may also be used to test functional fidelity of simulations of operational tasks. Simulations may faithfully reproduce cognitive demands of tasks but fail to elicit stress responses characteristic of the real environment (Matthews et al., 2011). In our vehicle driving research, we have shown that stress manipulations on the simulator appear to reproduce state responses seen in real driving (e.g., Desmond & Matthews, 2009; Emo et al., 2004), supporting functional fidelity.

Diagnostic monitoring. The DSSQ also supports diagnostic monitoring for tasks requiring sustained performance. Monitoring of operator cognitive fitness is 'diagnostic' if it indicates the nature or origins of vulnerability to loss of performance. In the military context, Grier (2011) describes the need for assessment of tactical combat readiness, defined as the individual's potential for performance in environments that may be impose high levels of stress and workload. Reinerman-Jones, Matthews, Warm and Langheim (2011) advocated a two-stage evaluation, such that stress response to a short but cognitively challenging task is used to diagnose operator fitness for a subsequent, longer-duration period of work. The evaluation of response to cognitive challenge might also include psychophysiological assessments. Consistent with this approach, studies of vigilance have confirmed that stress response to cognitive challenge predicts subsequent performance (Matthews et al., 2010a, 2010c). On this basis, the DSSQ might be part of a field kit used to assess groups such as soldiers or truckers for levels of fatigue sufficient to impair sustained attention.

In tasks requiring extended work shifts, such as operation of remotely pilot vehicles (Guznov et al., 2011), periodic administration of the DSSQ allows tracking of the development of fatigue. (The short form of the scale may be more suitable for this purpose). For example, Saxby et al. (2007) were able to plot the time course of driver stress and fatigue across different drive durations. The DSSQ might also contribute to augmented cognition, on tasks where needs for machine support, such as automation of some operator functions, is evaluated over relatively long timespans (Kustubayeva et al., 2011). The DSSQ also seems promising for performance prediction in other work settings (Matthews & Falconer, 2002; Schell et al., 2005).

Multivariate assessment is especially important for diagnosis of potential performance vulnerabilities, given that different stress state dimensions attach to different components of performance. Loss of task engagement especially threatens vigilance (Matthews et al., 2010b), whereas distress may signal overload of working memory (Matthews & Campbell, 2011). Similarly, in fatiguing settings, it may be important for maintaining safety to differentiate passive from active fatigue (Desmond & Hancock, 2001). Saxby et al. (2008) confirmed that only the former leads to loss of alertness, as evidenced by slowed braking to an emergency event. Global measures of stress or fatigue may be less effective in identifying impending loss of performance.

Table 9. A summary of some of the principal attributes of the three state factors

	Task Engagement	Distress	Worry
Key task factors that influence the state	Challenge, task interest, personal control, positive feedback, teamwork Vs. Monotony, long task duration, system automation, passive fatigue	High workload, multiple display elements, low-salience signals, active fatigue, workload transition, negative feedback	Failure, opportunity for personal reflection, lack of stimulation Vs. High stimulus frequency, task complexity
Personality correlates	Conscientiousness, clarity, mood repair Vs. Cognitive disorganization, dispositional fatigue-proneness	Neuroticism, pessimism, cognitive disorganization Vs. Clarity	Neuroticism, pessimism, evaluative anxiety, dysfunctional metacognition
Stress process correlates	Challenge appraisal, task focused coping Vs. Avoidance coping	Threat appraisal, emotion-focused coping, perceived workload Vs. Perceived controllability	Threat appraisal, emotion-focused coping Vs. Avoidance coping, perceived controllability
Mechanisms for performance effects	Attentional resource mobilization, executive processing, task-directed effort	Working memory, impaired executive functioning, exogenous attention	Mindwandering, withdrawal of effort
Core relational theme	Commitment to effort	Management of cognitive overload	Self-evaluation in the performance context

Evaluation of stress vulnerability and resilience. The research reviewed demonstrated a variety of personality predictors of stress, but also showed the limitations of standard trait measures for predicting task stress. For example, in Shaw et al.'s (2010) study, standard dispositional measures (e.g., Big Five) predicted up to 10% of the variance in post-task state, with the more specialized cognitive-energetic trait factors adding another 7-8%. Thus, even the more predictive traits are not very effective in picking out those individuals who may be especially resilient or vulnerable to task stress. In relation to occupational health (Matthews, Panganiban & Gilliland, in press), it may be useful to detect stress-prone individuals even if they do not show overt performance deficits, given that organizational stress is implicated in health problems, burnout and absenteeism (e.g., Halbesleben, 2006).

The DSSQ provides direct assessment of both individual differences in anticipatory stress (measured pre-task) and stress experienced during task performance (post-task). Pre-task state is typically at least moderately predictive of post-task state (Matthews et al., 1999a), so that the DSSQ can be used to screen for stress vulnerability prior to a demanding task assignment. Predictive validity may be improved by assessing state response to a practice task or other short task (Reinerman-Jones et al., 2011). It remains to be determined how effective the

DSSQ is for long-range prediction of stress vulnerability; how best to identify an employee who will be persistently stressed by a given task. Stress responses to a customer service task showed moderate stability (rs ranging from 0.35 – 0.51) over a seven-month period (Matthews & Falconer, 2000). Repeated testing at the initial phase might provide more reliable assessment of stable stress vulnerability within the specific work context.

CONCLUSION

Understanding the stress of task performance requires a multivariate perspective. The DSSQ provides a means for assessing the main subjective elements of stress and fatigue responses in a range of laboratory and applied performance settings. We have emphasized especially the use of the three higher-order factors as a framework for understanding stress state response. Table 9 summarizes some of the main findings on these factors. The Table is not intended to be definitive or comprehensive. Rather, it highlights some of the main causes, concomitants and consequences of stress states that we believe are best supported by existing studies, and worth pursuing in future research.

Use of the scale may be of value in theory development, in testing neuroscience, information-processing and self-regulative models of performance stress. In theory testing, the DSSQ is best used in conjunction with objective measures such as those provided by psychophysiology and performance assessment. Nevertheless, state assessment may provide information on operator functioning that cannot easily be derived from other sources. The DSSQ also provides a general metric for evaluating the impact of environmental and person factors on operator stress in a range of applied settings. Subject to the normal limitations of self-report scales, the DSSQ may be of value in identifying and mitigating task stressors, in monitoring for performance vulnerabilities, and in discriminating stress-vulnerable from resilient operators.

ACKNOWLEDGMENTS

Thanks are due to our graduate students past and present who have contributed to this research: Amanda Emo, Vic Finomore, Greg Funke, Rebecca Grier, Slava Guznov, Deak Helton, Ted Hitchcock, Tina Klein, Lisa Langheim, Kelly Parsons, Lauren Reinerman-Jones, Dyani Saxby, Tyler Shaw and Grace Teo. Contact Gerald Matthews for information on the availability of the DSSQ.

REFERENCES

Ackerman, P. L. (Ed.) (2011). *Cognitive fatigue: Multidisciplinary perspectives on current research and future applications.* Washington, DC: American Psychological Association.

Banks, B., Jackson, M. L., & Van Dongen, H. P. A. (2012). Neuroscience of sleep and circadian rhythms. In G. Matthews, P.A. Desmond, C. Neubauer & P.A. Hancock (Eds.), *Handbook of operator fatigue* (pp. 173-184). Aldershot, UK: Ashgate Press.

Barron, E., Riby, L. M., Greer, J., & Smallwood, J. (2011). Absorbed in thought: The effect of mind wandering on the processing of relevant and irrelevant events. *Psychological Science*, 22, 596-601.

Christoff, K., Gordon, A. M., & Smallwood, J. (2009). Experience sampling during fMRI reveals default network and executive system contributions to mind wandering. *Proceedings of the National Academy of Sciences of the United States of America*, 106, 8719-8724.

Corr, P.J. (2009). The Reinforcement Sensitivity Theory of personality. In P.L. Corr & G. Matthews (Eds.), *Cambridge handbook of personality* (pp. 347-376). Cambridge: Cambridge University Press.

Costa, P. T., Jr., & McCrae, R. R. (1992) *NEO PI-R Professional Manual.* Odessa, FL: Psychological Assessment Resources.

Cronbach, L. J., & Meehl, P. E. (1955). Construct validity in psychological tests. *Psychological Bulletin*, 52, 281-302.

Desmond, P.A., & Hancock, P.A. (2001). Active and passive fatigue states. In P.A. Hancock & P.A. Desmond (Eds.), *Stress, workload, and fatigue* (pp. 455-465). Mahwah, NJ: Lawrence Erlbaum.

Desmond, P.A., & Matthews, G. (2009). Individual differences in stress and fatigue in two field studies of driving. *Transportation Research Part F*, 12, 265-276.

Elliot, A. J., & Thrash, T. M. (2001). Achievement goals and the hierarchical model of achievement motivation. *Educational Psychology Review*, 13, 139-156.

Emo, A.K., Funke, G., Matthews, G., & Warm, J.S. (2004). Stress vulnerability, coping, and risk-taking behaviors during simulated driving. *Proceedings of the Human Factors and Ergonomics Society*, 48, 1228-1232.

Endler, N., & Parker, J. (1990) Multidimensional assessment of coping: A critical review. *Journal of Personality and Social Psychology*, 58, 844–54.

Ewing, K.C., & Fairclough, S.H. (2010). The effect of an extrinsic incentive on psychophysiological measures of mental effort and motivational disposition when task demand is varied. *Proceedings of the Human Factors and Ergonomics Society,* 54, 259-263.

Eysenck, M. W. (1992). *Anxiety:The cognitive perspective.* Hillsdale, NJ: Lawrence Erlbaum.

Eysenck, M. W., & Derakshan, N. (2011). New perspectives in attentional control theory. *Personality and Individual Differences*, 50, 955-960.

Fairclough, S. H., & Venables, L. (2006). Prediction of subjective states from psychophysiology: A multivariate approach. *Biological Psychology*, 71, 100-110.

Fan, J., McCandliss, B.D., Sommer, T., Raz, A., & Posner, M.I. (2002). Testing the efficiency and independence of attentional networks. *Journal of Cognitive Neuroscience*, 14, 340-347.

Fellner, A., Matthews, G., Funke, G.J., Emo, A.K., Zeidner, M., Pérez-González, J.C., & Roberts, R.D. (2007). The effects of emotional intelligence on visual search of emotional stimuli and emotion identification. *Proceedings of the Human Factors and Ergonomics Society*, 51, 845-849.

Fellner, A.N., Matthews, G., Shockley, K.D., Warm, J.S., Zeidner, M., Karlov, L., & Roberts, R.D. (2012). Using emotional cues in a discrimination learning task: Effects of trait emotional intelligence and affective state. *Journal of Research in Personality*, 46, 239–247.

Ferguson, E., Matthews, G., & Cox, T. (1999) The Appraisal of Life Events (ALE) Scale: Reliability and validity. *British Journal of Health Psychology*, 4, 97-116.

Finnigan, F., Schulze, D., & Smallwood, J. (2007). Alcohol and the wandering mind: A new direction in the study of alcohol on attentional lapses. *International Journal on Disability and Human Development*, 6, 189-199.

Finomore, V.S., Matthews, G., Shaw, T., & Warm, J.S. (2009). Predicting vigilance: A fresh look at an old problem. *Ergonomics*, 52, 791-808.

Funke, G. J., Matthews, G., Warm, J.S., & Emo, A. (2007). Vehicle automation: A remedy for driver stress? *Ergonomics*, 50, 1302-1323.

Goldberg, L. R. (1992). The development of markers for the Big-Five factor structure. *Psychological Assessment*, 4, 26–42.

Green, A. L., & Helton, W. S. (2011). Dual-task performance during a climbing traverse. *Experimental Brain Research*, 215, 307.

Grier, R. A. (2011). Military cognitive readiness at the tactical level: A review of measures. *Proceedings of the Human Factors and Ergonomics Society*, 55, 404–408.

Grove, J. (2012). *Trait self-esteem and stress response to feedback.* Unpublished undergraduate honors thesis, University of Cincinnati.

Gunzelmann, G., & Gluck, K. A. (2009). An integrative approach to understanding and predicting the consequences of fatigue on cognitive performance. *International Journal of Cognitive Technology*, 14, 14-25.

Guznov, S., Matthews, G., Funke, G., & Dukes, A. (2011). Use of the RoboFlag synthetic task environment to investigate workload and stress responses in UAV operation. *Behavior Research Methods*, 43, 771-780.

Guznov, S., Matthews, G., & Warm, J.S. (2010). Team member personality, performance, and stress in a Roboflag synthetic task environment. *Proceedings of the Human Factors and Ergonomics Society*, 54, 1679-1683.

Halbesleben, J. R. B. (2006). Sources of social support and burnout: A meta-analytic test of the conservation of resources model. *Journal of Applied Psychology*, 91, 1134-1145.

Hancock, P.A., Ross, J.M., & Szalma, J.L. (2007). A meta-analysis of performance response under thermal stressors. *Human Factors*, 49, 851-877.

Hancock, P.A., & Warm, J.S. (1989). A dynamic model of stress and sustained attention. *Human Factors*, 31, 519-537.

Hart, S.G., & Staveland, L.E. (1988) Development of a multidimensional workload rating scale: Results of empirical and theoretical research. In P. A. Hancock & N. Meshkati (Eds.), *Human mental workload* (pp. 139-183). Amsterdam: Elsevier.

Helton, W.S. (2004). Validation of a short stress state questionnaire. *Proceedings of the Human Factors and Ergonomics*, 48, 1238-1242.

Helton, W.S., & Garland, G. (2006). Short stress state questionnaire: Relationships with reading comprehension and land navigation. *Proceedings of the Human Factors and Ergonomics Society*, 50, 1731–1735.

Helton, W. S., Kern, R. P., & Walker, D. R. (2009b). Conscious thought and the sustained attention to response task. *Consciousness and Cognition: An International Journal*, 18, 600-607.

Helton, W.S., Matthews, G., & Warm, J.S. (2009a). Stress state mediation between environmental variables and performance: The case of noise and vigilance. *Acta Psychologica*, 130, 204-213.

Helton, W.S., Shaw, T.H., Warm, J.S., Matthews, G., Dember, W.N., & Hancock, P.A. (2008). Effects of warned and unwarned demand transitions on vigilance performance and stress. *Anxiety, Stress and Coping*, 2, 173-184.

Helton, W. S., & Warm, J.S. (2008). Signal salience and the mindlessness theory of vigilance. *Acta Psychologica*, 129, 18-25.

Hilgard, E.R. (1980). The trilogy of mind: Cognition, affection, and conation. *Journal of the History of the Behavioral Sciences*, 16, 107-117.

Hitchcock, E.M., Warm, J.S., Matthews, G., Dember, W.N., Shear, P.K., Mayeben, D.W., & Parasuraman, R. (2002). Automation cueing modulates cerebral blood flow and vigilance in a simulated air traffic control task. *Theoretical Issues in Ergonomics Science*, 4, 89-112.

Hockey, G.R.J. (1997). Compensatory control in the regulation of human performance under stress and high workload: A cognitive-energetical framework. *Biological Psychology*, 45, 73-93.

Horner, R.D., Szaflarski, J.P., Jacobson, C.J., Elder, N., Bolon, S., Matthews, G., Ying, J., Meganathan, K., & Raphaelson, M. (2011). *Clinical work intensity among physician specialties: How might we assess it? What do we find? Medical Care*, 49, 108-113.

Humphreys, M. S., & Revelle, W. (1984). Personality, motivation, and performance: A theory of the relationship between individual differences and information processing. *Psychological Review*, 91, 153-184.

Humrichouse, J., Chmielewski, M., McDade-Montez, E.A., & Watson, D. (2007). Affect assessment through self-report methods. In J. Rottenberg & S.L. Johnson (Eds.), *Emotion and psychopathology: Bridging affective and clinical science* (pp. 13-34). Washington, DC: APA.

Johnson, D. R. (2009). Emotional attention set-shifting and its relationship to anxiety and emotion regulation. *Emotion*, 9, 681-690.

Kamzanova, A.T., Matthews, G., & Kustubayeva, A. M. (2012). Diagnostic monitoring of vigilance decrement using EEG workload indices. *Proceedings of the Human Factors and Ergonomics Society*, 56.

Killgore, W.D.S. (2012). Socio-emotional and neurocognitive effects of sleep loss. In G. Matthews, P.A. Desmond, C. Neubauer & P.A. Hancock (Eds.), *Handbook of operator fatigue* (pp. 227-243). Aldershot, UK: Ashgate Press.

Klein, M.I., Warm, J.S., Riley, M.A., Matthews, G., Gaitonde, K., Doarn, C.R., & Donovan. J. F. (2012). Perceived mental workload and stress experienced by medical students working with the laparoscopic and robotic minimally invasive surgical systems. *Endourology*, 26, 1089-1094.

Klein, M. I., Warm, J. S., Riley, M. A., Matthews, G., Gaitonde, K., & Donovan. J. F. (2008). Perceptual distortions produce multidimensional stress profiles in novice users of an endoscopic surgery simulator. *Human Factors*, 50, 291-300.

Kustubayeva, A., Matthews, G., and Panganiban, A.R. Emotion and information search in tactical decision-making: moderator effects on feedback. *Motivation and Emotion*. Published Online First: 18 December 2011. doi:10.1007/s11031-011-9270-5.

Langner, R., Steinborn, M. B., Chatterjee, A., Sturm, W., & Willmes, K. (2010a). Mental fatigue and temporal preparation in simple reaction-time performance. *Acta Psychologica*, 133, 64-72.

Langner, R., Willmes, K., Chatterjee, A., Eickhoff, S. B., & Sturm, W. (2010b). Energetic effects of stimulus intensity on prolonged simple reaction-time performance. *Psychological Research/Psychologische Forschung*, 74, 499-512

Lazarus, R. S., & Folkman, S. (1984) *Stress, appraisal and coping*. New York: Springer.

Lazarus, R.S. (1999) *Stress and emotion: A new synthesis*. New York: Springer.

Lustenberger, D. E., & Jagacinski, C. M. (2010). Exploring the effects of ostracism on performance and intrinsic motivation. *Human Performance*, 23, 283-304.

Matthews, G. (2001). Levels of transaction: A cognitive sciences framework for operator stress. In P.A. Hancock & P.A. Desmond (Eds.*), Stress, workload, and fatigue* (pp. 5-33). Mahwah, NJ: Erlbaum.

Matthews, G. (2008). Reinforcement Sensitivity Theory: A critique from cognitive science. In P.L. Corr (Ed.), *The Reinforcement Sensitivity Theory of personality* (pp. 482-527). Cambridge: Cambridge University Press.

Matthews, G., & Campbell, S.E. (1998). Task-induced stress and individual differences in coping. *Proceedings of the Human Factors and Ergonomics Society*, 42, 821-825.

Matthews, G., & Campbell, S.E. (2009). Sustained performance under overload: Personality and individual differences in stress and coping. *Theoretical Issues in Ergonomics Science*, 10, 417-442.

Matthews, G., & Campbell, S.E. (2010). Dynamic relationships between stress states and working memory. *Cognition and Emotion*, 24, 357-373.

Matthews, G., Campbell, S., Falconer, S. (2001a) Assessment of motivational states in performance environments. *Proceedings of the Human Factors and Ergonomics Society*, 45, 906-910.

Matthews, G., Campbell, S.E., Falconer, S. Joyner, L., Huggins, J., Gilliland, K., Grier, R., & Warm, J.S. (2002). Fundamental dimensions of subjective state in performance settings: Task engagement, distress and worry. *Emotion*, 2, 315-340.

Matthews, G., & Davies, D.R. (1998). Arousal and vigilance: The role of task demands. In R.R. Hoffman, M.F. Sherrick, & J.S. Warm (Eds.), *Viewing psychology as a whole: The integrative science of William N. Dember* (pp. 113-144). Washington, DC: American Psychological Association.

Matthews, G., Davies, D. R., & Lees, J. L. (1990b). Arousal, extraversion, and individual differences in resource availability. *Journal of Personality and Social Psychology*, 59, 150-168.

Matthews, G., Davies, D. R., Westerman, S. J., & Stammers, R. B. (2000). *Human performance: Cognition, stress, and individual differences*. Hove, UK: Psychology Press.

Matthews, G., Deary, I.J., & Whiteman, M.C. (2009). *Personality traits (3rd ed.)*. Cambridge: Cambridge University Press.

Matthews, G., & Desmond, P.A. (2002). Task-induced fatigue states and simulated driving performance. *Quarterly Journal of Experimental Psychology*, 55A, 659-686.

Matthews, G., Desmond, P.A., & Hitchcock, T. (2012). In G. Matthews, P.A. Desmond, C. Neubauer & P.A. Hancock (Eds.), *Handbook of operator fatigue* (pp. 139-154). Aldershot, UK: Ashgate Press.

Matthews, G., Desmond, P.A., Joyner, L.A., & Carcary, B. (1997). A comprehensive questionnaire measure of driver stress and affect. In E Carbonell Vaya & J.A Rothengatter (Eds.*), Traffic and transport psychology: Theory and application* (pp. 317-324). Amsterdam: Pergamon.

Matthews, G., Desmond, P.A., Neubauer, C.E., & Hancock, P.A. (Eds.) (2012). *Handbook of operator fatigue*. Aldershot, UK: Ashgate Publishing.

Matthews, G., Emo, A.K., & Funke, G. J. (2005). A short version of the Dundee Stress State Questionnaire. *Presented at the Twelfth Meeting of the International Society for the Study of Individual Differences*, Adelaide, Australia, July 2005.

Matthews, G., Emo, A.K., Funke, G., Zeidner, M., Roberts, R.D., Costa, P.T., Jr., & Schulze, R. (2006). Emotional intelligence, personality, and task-induced stress. *Journal of Experimental Psychology: Applied*, 12, 96-107.

Matthews, G., & Falconer, S. (2000). Individual differences in task-induced stress in customer service personnel. *Proceedings of the Human Factors and Ergonomics Society*, 44, 145-148.

Matthews, G., & Falconer, S. (2002) Personality, coping and task-induced stress in customer service personnel. *Proceedings of the Human Factors and Ergonomics Society*, 46, 963-967.

Matthews, G., & Fellner, A.N. (2012). The energetics of emotional intelligence. In M.W. Eysenck, M. Fajkowska, & T. Maruszewski (Eds.), *Warsaw Lectures on personality, emotion, and cognition* (Vol. 2, pp. 25-45). Clinton Corners, NY: Eliot Werner Publications.

Matthews, G., Hancock, P.A., & Desmond, P.A. (2012). Models of individual differences in fatigue for performance research. In G. Matthews, P.A. Desmond, C. Neubauer & P.A. Hancock (Eds.), *Handbook of operator fatigue* (pp. 155-170). Aldershot, UK: Ashgate Press.

Matthews, G., & Harley, T.A. (1993) Effects of extraversion and self-report arousal on semantic priming: A connectionist approach. *Journal of Personality and Social Psychology*, 65, 735-756.

Matthews, G., Hillyard, E.J., & Campbell, S.E. (1999b). Metacognition and maladaptive coping as components of test anxiety. *Clinical Psychology and Psychotherapy* 6, 111-125.

Matthews, G., Jones, D. M., & Chamberlain, A. G. (1990a). Refining the measurement of mood: The UWIST Mood Adjective Checklist. *British Journal of Psychology*, 81, 17-42

Matthews, G., Joyner, L., Gilliland, K., Campbell, S.E., Falconer, S., & Huggins, J. (1999a). Validation of a comprehensive stress state questionnaire: Towards a state "Big Three." In I. Mervielde, I.J. Deary, F. DeFruyt, & F. Ostendorf (Eds.), *Personality psychology in Europe* (Vol. 7, pp. 335-350). Tilburg: Netherlands Tilburg University Press.

Matthews, G., Panganiban, A.R., & Gilliland, K. (in press). Cognitive assessment: Implications for occupational health psychology. In L. Tetrick, R. Sinclair & M. Wang (Eds.), *Research methods in occupational health psychology: State of the art in measurement, design, and data analysis*. London: Routledge.

Matthews, G., Quinn, C.E.J., & Mitchell, K.J. (1998). Rock music, task-induced stress and simulated driving performance. In G. B. Grayson (Ed.), *Behavioural research in road safety VIII* (pp. 20-32). Crowthorne, Berkshire, UK: Transport Research Laboratory.

Matthews, G., Warm, J.S., Dember, W.N., Mizoguchi, H., & Smith, A.P. (2001b). The common cold impairs visual attention, psychomotor performance, and task engagement. *Proceedings of the Human Factors and Ergonomics Society*, 45, 1377-1381.

Matthews, G., Warm, J.S., Reinerman, L.E., Langheim, L.K., & Saxby, D.J. (2010b). Task engagement, attention and executive control. In A. Gruszka, G. Matthews & B. Szymura (Eds.), *Handbook of individual differences in cognition: Attention, memory and executive control* (pp. 205-230). New York: Springer.

Matthews, G., Warm, J.S., Reinerman, L.E., Langheim, L, Washburn, D.A., & Tripp, L. (2010a). Task engagement, cerebral blood flow velocity, and diagnostic monitoring for sustained attention. *Journal of Experimental Psychology: Applied*, 16, 187–203.

Matthews, G., Warm, J.S., Reinerman-Jones, L.E., Langheim, L.K., Guznov, S., Shaw, T.H., & Finomore, V.S. (2011). The functional fidelity of individual differences research: The case for context-matching. *Theoretical Issues in Ergonomics Science,* 12, 435-450.

Matthews, G., Warm, J.S., Shaw, T.H., & Finomore, V.S. (2010c). A multivariate test battery for predicting vigilance. *Proceedings of the Human Factors and Ergonomics Society*, 54, 1072-1076.

Matthews, G., & Zeidner, M. (2012). Individual differences in attentional networks: Trait and state correlates of the ANT. *Personality and Individual Differences.* 53, 574-579.

McAulay, V., Deary, I.J., Sommerfield, A.J., Matthews, G., & Frier, B.M. (2006). Effects of acute hypoglycaemia on motivation and cognitive interference in people with type 1 diabetes. *Journal of Clinical Pharmacology*, 26, 143-150.

McCrae, R.R., & Costa, P.T. (2008). Empirical and theoretical status of the five-factor model of personality traits. In G.J. Boyle, G. Matthews & D.H. Saklofske (Eds.), *Sage handbook of personality theory and testing: Volume 1: Personality theories and models* (pp. 273-294). Thousand Oaks, CA: Sage.

McGarry, K., Rovira, E., & Parasuraman, R. (2003). Effects of task duration and type of automation support on human performance and stress in a simulated battlefield engagement task. *Proceedings of the Human Factors and Ergonomics Society,* 47, 548-552.

McNair, D. M., Lorr, M., & Droppleman, L. F. (1992*). Revised Manual for the Profile of Mood States.* San Diego, CA: Educational and Industrial Testing Service.

Neubauer, C., Langheim, L., Matthews, G., & Saxby, D. (in press). Fatigue and voluntary utilization of automation in simulated driving. *Human Factors.* doi: 10.1177/ 0018720811423261.

Neubauer, C., Matthews, G., & Saxby, D. (2012). The effects of cell phone use and automation on driver performance and subjective state in simulated driving. *Proceedings of the Human Factors and Ergonomics Society*, 56.

Okamura, N., Tsuda, A., & Yajima, J. (2004). Stress State Questionnaire. In M. Oshima, K. Takada, M. Ueda, & T. Kono (Eds.), *Stress scale guidebook* (pp. 214–220). Tokyo: Jitsumu Kyoiku-Shuppan.

Panganiban, A.R., Matthews, G., Knott, B., & Funke, G. (2011). Effects of anxiety in an air defense task. *Proceedings of the Human Factors and Ergonomics Society,* 55, 909-913.

Parasuraman, R., & Jiang, Y. (2011). Individual differences in cognition, affect, and performance: Behavioral, neuroimaging, and molecular genetic approaches. *NeuroImage*, [No Volume/Issue], No Pagination Specified. doi:10.1016/j.neuroimage.2011.04.040

Parsons, K.S., Warm, J.S., Nelson, W.T., Riley, M., & Matthews, G. (2007). Detection-action linkage in vigilance: Effects on workload and stress. *Proceedings of the Human Factors and Ergonomics Society*, 51, 1291-1295.

Paulesu, E., Sambugaro, E., Torti, T., Danelli, L., Ferri, F., Scialfa, G., Sberna, M., Ruggiero, G.M., Bottini, G., & Sassaroli, S. (2010). Neural correlates of worry in generalized anxiety disorder and in normal controls: A functional MRI study. *Psychological Medicine: A Journal of Research in Psychiatry and the Allied Sciences*, 40, 117-124.

Reinerman-Jones, L.E., Matthews, G., Warm, J.S., & Langheim, L.K. (2011). Selection for vigilance assignments: A review and proposed new direction. *Theoretical Issues in Ergonomics Science*, 12, 273-296.

Ross, J.M, Ganey, H.C. &. Broadway, R.S. (2004). Efficacy of stress exposure training on target acquisition in combat simulations. *Proceedings of the Human Factors and Ergonomics Society*, 48, 2187-2190.

Salovey, P., Mayer, J. D, Goldman, S., Turvey, C., & Palfai, T. (1995). Emotional attention, clarity, and repair: Exploring emotional intelligence using the Trait Meta-Mood Scale. In J. W. Pennebaker (Ed.*), Emotion, disclosure, and health* (pp. 125-154). Washington, DC: American Psychological Association.

Sarason, I. G. (1984). Stress, anxiety, and cognitive interference: Reactions to tests. *Journal of Personality and Social Psychology*, 46, 929-938.

Sarason, I. G., Sarason, B. R., Keefe, D. E., Hayes, B. E., & Shearin, E. N. (1986) Cognitive interference: situational determinants and traitlike characteristics. *Journal of Personality and Social Psychology*, 31, 215-226.

Saucier, G. (2002). Orthogonal markers for orthogonal factors: The case of the Big Five. *Journal of Research in Personality*, 36, 1-31.

Saxby, D.J., Matthews, G., Hitchcock, E.M., & Warm, J.S. (2007). Development of active and passive fatigue manipulations using a driving simulator. *Proceedings of the Human Factors and Ergonomics Society*, 51, 1237-1241.

Saxby, D.J., Matthews, G., Hitchcock, E.M., Warm, J.S., Funke, G.J., & Gantzer, T. (2008). Effects of active and passive fatigue on performance using a driving simulator. *Proceedings of the Human Factors and Ergonomics Society*, 52, 1252-1256.

Schell, K. L., Melton, E. C., Woodruff, A., & Corbin, G. B. (2004). Self-regulation, engagement, motivation, and performance in a simulated quality control task. *Psychological Reports*, 94, 944-954.

Schell, K. L., Woodruff, A., Corbin, G. B., & Melton, E. C. (2005). Trait and state predictors of error detection accuracy in a simulated quality control task. *Personality and Individual Differences*, 39, 47-60.

Scherer, K. R. (2009). The dynamic architecture of emotion: Evidence for the component process model. *Cognition and Emotion*, 23, 1307-1351.

Shaw, T.H., Matthews, G., Warm, J.S., Finomore, V., Silverman, L., & Costa, P.T., Jr. (2010). Individual differences in vigilance: Personality, ability and states of stress. *Journal of Research in Personality*, 44, 297-308.

Shingledecker, S., Weldon, D.E., Behymer, K., Simpkins, B., Lerner, E., Warm, J., Matthews, G., Finomore, V., Shaw, T., & Murphy, J.S. (2009). Measuring vigilance abilities to enhance combat identification performance. In D.H Andrews, R.P. Herz & M.B. Wolf (Eds.), *Human factors in combat identification performance* (pp. 47–65). Aldershot, UK: Ashgate Publishing.

Smallwood, J., Fitzgerald, A., Miles, L. K., & Phillips, L. H. (2009). Shifting moods, wandering minds: Negative moods lead the mind to wander. *Emotion*, 9, 271-276.

Smallwood, J. M., Davies, J. B., Heim, D., Finnigan, F., Sudberry, M., O'Connor, R., & Obonsawin, M. (2004a). Subjective experience and the attentional lapse: Task engagement and disengagement during sustained attention. *Consciousness & Cognition*, 13, 657-690.

Smallwood, J. M., O'Connor, R. C., Sudberry, M. V., Haskell, C., & Ballantyne, C. (2004b). The consequences of encoding information on the maintenance of internally generated images and thoughts: The role of meaning complexes. *Consciousness & Cognition*, 13, 789-820.

Smallwood, J. M., & Schooler, J. W. (2006). *The restless mind. Psychological Bulletin*, 132, 946-958.

Spielberger, C. D. (1972). Current trends in theory and research on anxiety. In C. D. Spielberger (Ed.), *Anxiety--Current trends in theory and research* (Vol. 1, pp. 3-19). New York: Academic Press.

Spielberger, C. D., & Reheiser, E. C. (2004). Measuring anxiety, anger, depression, and curiosity as emotional states and personality traits with the STAI, STAXI and STPI. In M. J. Hilsenroth & D. L. Segal (Eds.), *Comprehensive handbook of psychological assessment, Vol. 2. Personality assessment* (pp. 70-86). Hoboken, NJ: John Wiley.

Spiridon, E., & Fairclough, F. (2009). Detection of anger with or without control for affective computing systems. *Proceedings of the 3rd International Conference on Affective Computing and Intelligent Interaction* (pp. 1-6). Amsterdam: ACII 2009.

Stafford, S. C., Oron-Gilad, T., Szalma, J. L., & Hancock, P. A. (2004). Individual differences related to shooting performance, in a police night-training shooting exercise. *Proceedings of the Human Factors and Ergonomics Society*, 48, 1131-1135.

Stanton, N. A., & Young, M. S. (2005). Driver behaviour with adaptive cruise control. *Ergonomics*, 48, 1294-1313.

Stöber, J. (2004). Dimensions of test anxiety: Relations to ways of coping with pre-exam anxiety and uncertainty. *Anxiety, Stress, & Coping*, 17, 213-226.

Szalma, J.L. (2008). Individual differences in stress reaction. In: P.A. Hancock and J.L. Szalma (Eds.), *Performance under stress* (pp. 323-357). Aldershot, Hampshire, UK: Ashgate.

Szalma, J.L. (2009a). Individual differences in human-technology interaction: Incorporating variation in human characteristics into human factors research and design. *Theoretical Issues in Ergonomics Science*, 10, 381-397.

Szalma, J.L. (2009b). Individual differences in performance, workload, and stress in sustained attention: Optimism and pessimism. *Personality and Individual Differences*, 47, 444-451.

Szalma, J.L. (2011). Workload and stress in vigilance: The impact of display format and task type. *American Journal of Psychology*, 124, 441-454.

Szalma, J.L., & Hancock, P.A. (2011). Noise effects on human performance: A meta-analytic synthesis. *Psychological Bulletin*, 137, 682-707.

Szalma, J.L., & Taylor, G.S. (2011). Individual differences in response to automation: The big five factors of personality. *Journal of Experimental Psychology: Applied,* 17, 71-96.

Szalma, J.L., & Teo, G.W.L. (2010). The joint effect of task characteristics and neuroticism on the performance, workload, and stress of signal detection. *Proceedings of the Human Factors and Ergonomics Society*, 54, 1052-1056.

Szalma, J.L., & Teo, G.W.L. (2012). Spatial and temporal task characteristics as stress: A test of the dynamic adaptability theory of stress, workload, and performance. *Acta Psychologica*, 139, 471-485.

Szalma, J.L., Hancock, P.A., Dember, W.N., & Warm, J.S. (2006). Training for vigilance: The effect of KR format and dispositional optimism and pessimism on performance and stress. *British Journal of Psychology*, 97, 115-135.

Szalma, J.L., Oron-Gilad, T., & Hancock, P.A. (2005). Individual differences in workload, stress, and coping in police officers engaged in shooting tasks. In: P. Carayon, M. Robertson, E. Kleiner, and P.L.T. Hoonakker (Eds.), *Human factors in organizational design and management VIII* (pp. 587-592). Santa Monica, CA: IEA Press.

Szalma, J. L., & Taylor, G. S. (2011). Individual differences in response to automation: The five factor model of personality. *Journal of Experimental Psychology: Applied,* 17, 71-96.

Szalma, J.L., Warm, J.S., Matthews, G., Dember, W.N., Weiler, E.M., Meier, A., & Eggemeier, F.T. (2004) Effects of sensory modality and task duration on performance, workload, and stress in sustained attention. *Human Factors*, 46, 219-233.

Taylor, G.S., & Barnett, J.S. (2010). *Proceedings of the Human Factors and Ergonomics Society,* 54, 2267-2271.

Teo, G., & Szalma, J.L. (2011). The effects of task type and source complexity on vigilance performance, workload, and stress. *Proceedings of the Human Factors and Ergonomics Society*, 55, 1180-1184.

Thayer, R. E. (1978). Toward a psychological theory of multidimensional activation (arousal). *Motivation and Emotion*, 2, 1-34.

Thayer, R.E. (1989) *The biopsychology of mood and arousal*. New York: Oxford University Press.

Tiwari, T., Singh, A.L., & Singh, I.L. (2009). Task demand and workload: Effects on vigilance performance and stress. *Journal of the Indian Academy of Applied Psychology*, 35, 265-275.

Turner, M. L., & Engle, R. W. (1989). Is working memory capacity task dependent? *Journal of Memory and Language*, 28, 127-154.

Venables, L., & Fairclough, S. H. (2009). The influence of performance feedback on goal-setting and mental effort regulation. *Motivation and Emotion*, 33, 63-74.

Warm, J.S., Matthews, G., & Finomore, V.S. (2008) Workload and stress in sustained attention. In P.A. Hancock & J.L. Szalma (Eds.), *Performance under stress* (pp. 115-141). Aldershot, UK: Ashgate Publishing.

Warm, J.S., Tripp, L.D., Matthews, G., & Helton, W.S. (2012). Cerebral hemodynamic indices of operator fatigue in vigilance. In G. Matthews, P.A. Desmond, C. Neubauer & P.A. Hancock (Eds.), *Handbook of operator fatigue* (pp. 197-207). Aldershot, UK: Ashgate Press.

Watson, D., & Clark, L. A. (1991). *The PANAS-X: Manual for the Positive and Negative Schedule: Expanded Form.* Iowa City: University of Iowa.

Watson, D., Clark, L. A., & Tellegen, A. (1988). Development and validation of brief measures of positive and negative affect: The PANAS scales. *Journal of Personality and Social Psychology,* 54, 1063-1070.

Wells, A. (2000). *Emotional disorders and metacognition: Innovative cognitive therapy.* Chichester: Wiley.

Wells, A., & Matthews, G. (1994) *Attention and emotion: A clinical perspective.* Hove: Erlbaum.

Young, M. S., & Stanton, N. A. (2002). Malleable attentional resources theory: A new explanation for the effects of mental underload on performance. *Human Factors,* 44, 365-375.

Zeidner, M. (1998). *Test anxiety: The state of the art.* New York: Plenum Press.

Zeidner, M., & Matthews, G. (2005). Evaluation anxiety. In A.J. Elliot & C.S. Dweck (Eds.), *Handbook of competence and motivation* (pp. 141-163). New York: Guilford Press.

Zholdassova, M. K., Matthews, G., Kustubayeva, A. M., & Jakupov, S. M. (2012). The cognitive neuroscience of vigilance – A test of temporal decrement in the Attention Networks Test (ANT). *International Journal of Social and Human Sciences,* 6, 467-472.

Zuckerman, M. (1976) General and situation-specific traits and states: New approaches to assessment of anxiety and other constructs. In M. Zuckerman & C. D. Spielberger (Eds.), *Emotions and anxiety: New concepts, methods and applications* (pp. 133–74.) Hillsdale, NJ: Erlbaum.

In: Psychology of Stress
Editors: Leandro Cavalcanti and Sofia Azevedo

ISBN: 978-1-62417-109-3
© 2013 Nova Science Publishers, Inc.

Chapter 3

STRESS IN ADOPTIVE PARENTHOOD

Yolanda Sánchez-Sandoval
Developmental and Educational Psychology
University of Cádiz, Spain

ABSTRACT

This chapter focuses on the stress that parents experience in raising adoptive children. Parenting stress is linked to the familiar functioning and to the children and adolescent psychological adjustment. Parenting stress is both condition and consequence of the family and psychological well being. On the one hand, for example, higher emotional or behavioral problems manifested by children affect parental stress. On the other hand, when parents face the task of rearing a child in a very stressful situation, it is more probable that child-rearing practices are affected. Through parental stress, it is possible to analyze bidirectional effects of individual and family processes involved.

Life in adoptive families is very similar to life in the non-adoptive ones. Nevertheless, they have to deal with challenges or tasks added by the fact of adoption. We are interested in learning how being an adoptive family affects parental stress. This chapter is based on the findings of the current empirical research with adoptive families, which counted on the participation of 260 adoptive families from Spain in our own longitudinal research. The most widely used measures for parenting stress (Parent Stress Index (Abidin, 1995), and Stress Index for Parents of Adolescents (Sheras, Abidin, & Konold, 1998)) were applied. These measures are designed to identify parent/child or adolescent systems at-risk for dysfunctional parenting and problematic child adjustment.

When the analyzed adoptive families are not clinical but rather a representative sample of adoptive families, the picture they present is, broadly speaking, that of a good adjustment and a high satisfaction. Differences between families with adopted children and families with adopted adolescents are discussed. We identified several predictors of parenting stress. Consistent with the research findings on adoptive families, characteristics of the children, characteristics of the parents and context in which adoption takes place are significantly predictive scores for adoptive parenthood. So, for example, the parental stress is related to the age of arrival of the adopted children, to the parent educational levels, to the child-rearing practices and to the support and resources used regarding adoption.

This analysis allows us to focus the intervention into high stress areas and predicts children's future psychosocial adjustment. Important implications for the current and future adoptions are suggested. To sum up, identifying the most stressful aspects in the adoptive parenthood is useful to work in the pre-adoptive phases, but it is also necessary for organizing post-adoption services.

INTRODUCTION

"Almost from the start of our relationship, my partner and I talked about having children"

Mother of a son adopted when he was two years old

"We knew that adopting two girls would not be easy..., but I have to admit that it has been much more difficult than we thought"

Mother of two girls adopted aged 4 and 6 years old

Becoming parents is one of the greatest desires of a large number of people in our society. In fact, certain psychological theories have outlined access to paternity or maternity as one of the key developmental tasks to perform during adulthood. The now classic Havighurst (1972) theory included that building a family and caring for children among the nine developmental tasks during early adulthood (selecting a mate, learning to live with a partner, starting a family, rearing children, managing a home, getting started in an occupation, taking on civic responsibility, finding a congenial social group). Havighurst emphasized the importance of the achievement of developmental tasks. In the case of failure, there would be an adverse repercussion in later aspects of development.

Several decades have passed since this theory was suggested; undoubtedly, things have changed in many senses, but not in others. Nowadays, to become father or mother, especially in industrialized societies, responds, in a good number of cases, to a personal option of life. Some people, however, do not include parenthood among their life priorities or objectives, with many people never having children. Moreover, it does not appear that not having them obligatorily implies an adverse repercussion in later aspects of development, as the aforementioned theory postulated. In addition, the access routes to paternity have changed, and family models have diversified.

What has probably not changed is that when a person decides to become a parent, the would-be parent invests a great deal of hope and effort in the process; without a doubt some more than others, because the route to achieve this goal can be more complicated and slower on some occasions, more satisfactory and easy on others. In part, this chapter is the story of people who one day decided to become parents through a different route other than conception, as is adoption. Although this chapter will focus on the stress that parents experience in raising adoptive children, we will begin with a brief introduction to the concept of Parenting Stress.

Parenting Stress

As parents, adults find that daily demands their attention in a number of matters. Parenting stress is a specific kind of stress, perceived by parents, and emanating from the demands of being parents (Abidin, 1990). As Deater-Deckard indicates (2004), the demands of parenting are many and varied, and they include *meeting children's needs for survival like feeding, sheltering, and protection, but also include psychological demands for attention, affection, and help in controlling or regulating emotion* (p.5). Mothers and fathers can find difficulties in adjusting to the parenting role. As Deater-Deckard (1998) indicates, parenting stress is those aversive feelings experienced by most parents that are associated with the demands of the parenting role. All parents experience some degree of parenting stress. Individual differences in parenting stress have been shown to be an important aspect of parent, child, and family function. This concept is linked to family function and child and adolescent psychological adjustment: higher parenting stress has been linked with parent reports of less optimal parenting and child outcomes (Abidin, 1992; Anthony, et al., 2005).

The first models seeking to analyze and explain the stress within family contexts was conceived from lineal and causal positions, such as the already classic ABCX model by Hill (1958). Family stress is understood as a state that arises due to an imbalance between the perception of the demands and the ability to face that demand. The impact of a stressor and its subsequent crisis or adaptation is the product of a group of interacting factors. In the ABCX model described by Hill, factor A (stressor event) interacting with factor B (the family's resources for dealing with stressors and transitions) interacting with factor C (the definition the family makes of this situation) produce X (crisis). Numerous studies have demonstrated the relationship between these elements. For example, as indicated by Leigh & Milgrom (2008), in the case of parents of children with disabilities (A) the existence of a concurrent association between social support (B) and parental stress (X) during both the early childhood and school-age periods is well documented. This support-stress relationship is particularly evident for high risk groups (Deater-Deckard, 1998).

Despite the richness of the model, it seems to be an extremely static and hardly sensitive explanation about the efforts made by families when faced with the new demands that arise throughout family life. McCubbin and Patterson (1983) up-dated the concept and proposed *the Double ABCX Model of Family Adjustment and Adaptation Response.* The aA factor (family demands: stressor event and/or accumulation of demands) in interaction with the bB factor (family adaptive resources: resources existent before the crisis and new resources) and with the cC factor (family definition and meaning: understood as what the family attributes to the stressful event and its ability to handle it) produces an adaptation result or xX factor (family adaptation balancing, stress level). This model has been tested on families with very different characteristics (eg. Pozo, Sarriá & Mendez (2006), with mothers of individuals with autistic spectrum disorders).

A second criticism that could be made regarding the initial models explaining parental stress is their lineal, causal and mechanic character. We agree with the idea that when parents face the task of rearing a child in a very stressful situation, it is more probable that child-rearing practices are affected. Family stress directly affects family function, and with this, the psychological adjustment of parents and children. Gagnon-Oosterwaal et al. (2012), for instance, have shown that maternal stress mediates links between pre-adoption adversity and behavior problems. But, it does not affect the family function in a single direction. In other words, parenting stress is both an antecedent and a consequence of family and psychological well being. For example, higher emotional or behavioral problems manifested by children affect parental stress. The greatest feeling of stress perceived by the parents of children with behavior problems can lead to less successful educational practices, and with this, behavior by their children's behavior being less adjusted. It is in this sense that we state that parenting stress could be an antecedent to or a cause of poorer family function, but also a consequence of this. The educational styles of the parents are sensitive to the characteristics of their children. In this regard, we incorporate the dialectical perspective to our understanding the role of family stress in the functioning of the group and individual adjustment. Through parental stress, it is possible to analyze bidirectional effects of individual and family processes involved. Recently, a cross-lagged panel analysis supported a bidirectional relationship between parenting stress and child behavior problems for mothers and fathers (Neece, Green & Baker, 2012).

A third aspect to incorporate in the explanatory models of parental stress is that, at present, psychological processes tend to be analyzed from much more systemic theoretical perspectives. Thus, the explanation of parental stress has been progressively built, and completed, from more multidimensional models. Parenting stress arises from many sources: child characteristics, parent characteristics and context characteristics (Abidin, 1990). In the theoretical model elaborated by Richard Abidin to explain the determinants of dysfunctional parenting, the total stress a parent experiences would be a function of certain salient child characteristics, parental characteristics, and situational variables that were directly related to the role of being a parent (Abidin, 1995, p.29). Different models have tried to identify the implied variables, and the way they interact. Östberg & Hagekull (2000), for example, tested a multidimensional model of predictors of parenting stress on mothers with children ages 6 months to 3 years. High workload, low social support, perception of child as fussy-difficult, negative life events, child caretaking hassles, more children in the family, and high maternal age related directly more stress. As can be seen, this model bears in mind both the variable of the child itself (e.g. fussy-difficult child), that of the parents (e.g. maternal age) and the context (number of children in the family).

Parenting Stress in Adoptive Families

Life in adoptive families is very similar to life in the non-adoptive ones. Adoptive parents have to take on and respond to the tasks inherent in all upbringings and the education of a child within the family context. Nevertheless, they have to deal with challenges or tasks added by the fact of adoption. Therefore, we asked about the way in which parents face typical parenting demands, together with the demands characteristic of adoption. We were interested in learning how they manage the tensions involved in the process, and what the repercussion were on the family and individual adjustment of those adopted, once they has been living together for a certain time. Nevertheless, as indicated by Tan, Camras, Deng, Zhang & Lu (2012), few studies have examined the influence of post-adoption family experiences on adopted children's behavioral adjustment.

Traditionally, research has been devoted to explaining the adjustment of adoptions being based solely on children's characteristics, solely on parents' characteristics, of the families, or on a specific area of the relationship between parents and children; in other words, research tends to understand adoptions fundamentally with a one-dimensional perspective. In the last two decades, the panorama has become richer, in such a way that explanatory models adopting a multidimensional perspective to explain the adjustment in adoptive families have proliferated. In the models based on *stress and coping theory*, families are seen as a dynamic system. Families continuously face diverse challenges, which they try to respond in an effort to maintain a healthy balance. When the resources available to families were insufficient to attend to the demands made, families would enter a crisis phase. Based on the hypothesis that stressful factors occur in all families, Patterson (1988) defines the stress situation as a vital event that takes place at a discreet point in time and produces, or can produce, changes in the family system. To respond to stressful situations, families have personal, family and community resources.

This model endeavors to be applicable to the adoptive families to understand why some families are able to adapt to stressful situations and function well as a family, while for others, the integration of adopted children is not as successful. Different authors have identified variables that could be acting as tension or stressful factors in adoptive families and others that could be useful resources for adaptation (Brodzinsky, 1990; Groze, 1994; Katz, 1986; Mainemer, Gilman & Ames, 1998; Palacios, 1997; Pinderhughes, 1996; Rosenthal & Groze, 1992). Recently, several explanatory models about stress in the paternity perceived by Spanish families involved in international adoptions have been presented (Berástegui, 2007; León, 2011).

A. Stressful Elements

As said, among the tensions affecting adoptive families, there may be, in addition to those any other family might experience, specific factors imposed by the adoption. These could be factors related to the adopted children, the adoptive parents, the family system or the community.

> "(With regards to previous experiences). A person's life is everything. The previous two years and a half years (before the adoption) undoubtedly have an influence. It is like a little tree that you plant, and since it was tiny you water it, you keep it growing straight, you take care of it... it is not the same as if you just leave it there (careless). It is not the same thing. Perhaps, also, with that one (the second case), with work, it will blossom and you have a stupendous tree... but...."

> Mother of identical twin boys, adopted at 2 years; they are currently 13 years old.

Among the *tensions contributed by the adopted children,* studies with non-adoptive families have shown that certain characteristics in the children are related to greater life stress in the parents. Higher levels of parenting stress have been found in mothers of handicapped children born prematurely (Beckman & Pokorni, 1998), in parents of autistic children (Estes et al., 2009; Silva & Schalock, 2012), those with developmental delay (Baker, Blacher, & Olson, 2005; Tervo, 2012; Webster, Majnemer, Platt, & Shevell, 2008), and with an intellectual disability (Hassall, Rose, & McDonald, 2005). In a review on this topic, stress and child psychopathology were positively correlated in over 88% of the 60 studies examined (Grant, Compass, Thurm, McMahon, & Gipson, 2004). One can assume that, if the presence of disease, disability or other difficulties in the development of the children generates higher stress levels in non-adoptive families, these circumstances will also be predictors of a higher level of stress in adoptive families. Thus, Judge (2003) for example, demonstrated the higher stress levels in the parents when the adopted children presented chronic medical problems or developmental delays. It is not only physical and health problems that are related to an increase in the level of stress in the parents. Behavior problems, difficulties in creating safe and healthy bonds of affection, the lack of social abilities or difficulties in carrying out the role of children, among others, can also increase the levels of stress in non-adoptive (eg. Tervo, 2012; Neece, Green, & Baker, 2012) and adoptive (León, 2011; Rijk, Hoksbergen, ter Laak, van Dijkum, & Robbroeckx, 2006) parents.

The pre-adoptive characteristics of the children plays a specific role as stressful events in these families; among other aspects, the age when the child was adopted and prior events (abuse, institutionalization, previous placing). Gagnon-Oosterwaal et al. (2012) have recently demonstrated that pre-adoption adversity is related to maternal stress and child behavior problems. On the other hand, Mainemer et al. (1998) studied the effect of institutionalization in early childhood on the adoptive experience. For this, they analyzed families that had adopted children from Romanian orphanages who had been institutionalized for at least eight months and compared with another two groups, one made up of families with biological children and another by families that had adopted Romanian children who had spent less than four months in orphanages. In each of the three samples, the average age of the children at the time of the study was 30 months of age. They analyzed the relative magnitude of the stress in the family system through the Parenting Stress Index (Abidin, 1995). While they did not find differences in this measure of family stress between the biological families and adoptive families with children that had been institutionalized for less than four months, the families that had adopted children who had experienced institutionalization for periods exceeding eight months presented more stress in the areas related to the children than the other two comparison groups. For example, the families with children with the longer period of institutionalization scored higher (p < .05) on the acceptability sub-scale or, what is the same thing, there were more of them who felt that their children were not completely what they had expected. The authors concluded that it was not the adoption itself that was the source of stress and problems in the families, but rather, the critical variable was the duration of the institutionalization before the adoption.

Among *stressors coming from the families,* it is necessary to bear in mind the desire to have a child and infertility; an absence of roles that guide them in their adoptive paternity, difficulties in creating affective bonds, non-realistic expectations for their children and about the adoption, the non-acceptance of the individuality of the adopted children, and inflexibility in the family norms and rules. Bejanaru & Roth (2012) demonstrated that deficient communication about adoption causes a constant level of stress in families. Other aspects that these authors found, which worked as stressors for adoptive families, were the adoption procedure, uncertainty regarding the moment of placement, the instant adoption of the parental role-status, the lack of information about the child, and the costs.

The role played by the sociodemographic characteristics of the parents is not clear. Studies with non-adoptive families have shown that, according to socioeconomic status, the low-income mothers experienced higher levels of maternal parenting stress compared to their high-income counterparts (Se & Moon, 2012). While in adoptive families, Mainemer et al. (1998) substantiate what has already been detailed by other authors, in such that in the group of parents that adopted children with an adverse previous history, stress in the parents correlated negatively with the family income; the lower the income, the families perceived the adoptive experience as more complicated and more difficult. Other studies, however, did not find a relationship between the sociodemographic characteristics of the adoptive parents (age, income, educational level) and the level of stress in the adoptive parents Viana & Welsh (2010) or their satisfaction with the adoption (Groothues, Beckett, & O'Connor, 1998).

The results of some studies regarding the role of the age of the adoptive parents are interesting. In this sense, Mainemer et al. (1998) showed that the mother's age correlated negatively with the stress in the parents in the group with adopted children over eight months of age and with a prior history of adversity, while there was no relationship between the other two comparison groups of adopted children. Thus, in those cases in which children had been adopted with a more negative history, the older mothers perceived the situation as less complicated than the younger mothers. Somewhat similar conclusions can be extracted from a study with a sample of children with special needs (Rosenthal & Groze, 1992); although the correlation between the age of the parents and the impact of the adoption is not significant, it can be seen that when the averages are compared between three age groups of mothers, there are significant differences. Older mothers (45 years or over) perceive the impact of the adoption on their families as very positive (49% of the cases); the percentage among mothers of 35 to 44 years reduces to 42%, and it is the youngest mothers, up to 34 years, who consider it very positive to a greater degree (55%). The differences between the groups are significant, and the authors consider that the good results observed in the youngest mothers could be partly due to the fact that it was also more frequent that they has adopted younger children. Both studies appear to show that in certain types of adoptions the older mothers adapt better to the process, assessing the adoption in a more positively.

Of the *tensions coming from the community*, examples include certain stereotypes, social rejections or lack of appreciation for the adoptive parents, or the obligation of demonstrating their suitability as parents openly and with the use of intermediaries.

B. Support and Resources

Among the resources that appear to facilitate the adaptation of the families to such demands we found, on the one hand, *personal resources* of children and parents, such as positive states of health, knowledge, skills, personality features and problem coping strategies. International adoption families have shown that, when faced with stressful situations, they make more use of coping strategies based on problem solving and searching for help (Levy-Shiff, Zoran, & Shulman, 1997). These strategies are seen more in adoptive families with good family function (Bird, Peterson, & Miller, 2002). Other family resources include cohesion, flexibility, having a clear and coherent family organization, as well as communicative abilities. Bejenaru & Roth (2012) have shown, for example, how affection shown by the child is an important resource for the adoptive family. In addition, parenting stress has been found to be a significant correlate of parenting styles, with parents who are stricter and less nurturing obtaining higher stress scores (Anthony et al., 2005; Karras, VanDeventer, & Braungart-Ricker, 2003).

There are, in addition to these, *community resources,* which would correspond to the formal and informal social networks that provide emotional, informative and instrumental support. These could come from the partner, family, friends, the neighborhood, the adoption teams and services or other groups of parents. Studies with non-adoptive samples have shown the relationship between parenting stress and social support. Thus, for example, Visconti

(2005), in a sample of children with congenital heart disease, found support for the hypothesis that parents who reported more social support would also report less stress, since there were significant negative correlations between parent perceptions of stress and social support. Having a social support network is an important resource when accessing biological paternity (see, for example, Hidalgo, 1994); similarly, this is very beneficial when coping with the challenges that adoptive paternity imposes. Having other people's help and support can be an important resource predicting success among adoptive families (Katz, 1986; Rosenthal & Groze, 1992). This fact is documented by Cohen et al. (1994): the adoptive mothers of clinical groups perceived less support from their in-laws family that those of the non-clinical group. In the case of families that adopt special needs children, Cohen and Westhues (1990) stress the importance of the woman having her partner's help, so that the demands of such adoptions can be shared between both; this is a team effort in which the men would have to take on roles that the women have traditionally carried out. These authors also point out the importance that these family members are able to "recharge their batteries" with activities and friends outside of the family setting.

In addition to these support networks, which may be common with non-adoptive families, there are specific resources for adoptive parents: private agencies or public bodies that intervene in the assessment study of the adoptive families and adoption procedure. In this sense, the literature tends to agree: a better performance of these teams is associated with more successful adoptions. And, it appears that it is not only the pre-adoption contacts are important throughout the course of the adoption but also those following the adoption. As Mainemer et al. (1998) detail, there is a strong relationship between stress in the parents and behavior problems and post-adoption services must be sensitive to such needs. In fact, the families from clinical groups more than agree that there should be greater support services once the children are integrated into the families (Cohen, Duvall & Coyne, 1994; Groze, 1994). Equally, Palacios, Sánchez-Sandoval, & Sánchez-Espinosa (1996) show that the more the families experience greater complications during the initial moments of integration, whether legal, health or behavior problems, the greater the dissatisfaction with the work of the adoption teams.

C. Parent Perceptions and Interpretations

Negative perceptions about the child and child behavior are implicit in parenting stress (McMahon & Meins, 2012). These authors examined the extent to which individual differences in mothers' mental representations of their children (mind-mindedness) were related to parenting stress and observed parenting behavior. Mothers who used more mental-state words when describing their child reported lower parenting stress and showed less hostility when interacting with their children. Mothers who used more positive mental state descriptors were rated as more sensitive during interaction. The relation between mind-mindedness and negative maternal behavior was indirect, and mediated through parenting stress.

As McCubbin and Patterson (1983) outlined in the Double ACBX Model of Adjustment and Adaptation, family stress is not only explained by the conjunction between stressors and resources, but rather the C factor is also important or, the meaning that the family attributes to the stressful event and its capacity to handle it. When adapting this model to that of adoptive families, we dare say that this C factor could incorporate the vision that the adoptive families themselves have of the adoption and the peculiarities the adoption offers them.

In this sense, we revert back to an old concept that arose in the 1950s. It was a much more social vision of adoption than those that have arisen to date, and this interpretation was led by H. David Kirk and then crystallized in his books *Shared Fate* (1964) and *Adoptive Kinship* (1985). The starting point for this author is that the adoptive relationship is objectively different to the biological relationship, and he identifies some dissenting situations between the two types of paternities. These include the fact that adoptive paternity does not always benefit from the same medical and legal benefits and the same social support, the future adoptive parents have to demonstrate their suitability as parents and they have to count on brokers to be able to have children and there is a less gradual preparation and the few external signs that their status is changing (from not being parents to being parents), to mention a few. These differences are the cause of added stress for the adoptive parents, corroborated by the attitudes and feelings of other people within the community who benevolently discriminate against adoption. In other words, public opinion perceives the adoptive relationship as different to the biological one, even though this is expressed in a benign, understanding and tolerant way. Adoptive parents react to the opposing tensions using a number of mechanisms, which are found between two poles: "acknowledgement of differences," when the families identify peculiarities in the adoptive situation, and "rejection of differences," when the families think that the adoptive experience does not make them any different from other families. These parental attitudes will give rise to different family relationships; thus, the families that reject the differences empathize less with the situation of their adopted children and, in these homes, there will be a much poorer communication regarding subjects related with adoption. These situations will have negative consequences on the parent-children relationships. On the contrary, attitudes recognizing the differences would benefit family dynamics.

This theory has been revised by other authors, not always finding coinciding data. A generation later, Kaye (1990) explored the coping strategies formulated a by Kirk, and obtained quite different results. He used the low or high distinction dimension as a measure, since acceptance or rejection of the differences would mean that all the families experience major differences with some recognizing these differences while others did not. His data seem to show that when people say they have found greater differences, it is probably true, since this usually correlates with a higher presence of difficulties soon after the adoption. Based on these studies with adopted adolescents, it can be concluded, contrary to Kirk, the fact that adoptive families find differences when compared to biological families would not necessarily be preventive by nature, but rather, this recognition would be the result of the problems faced following adoption, while feeling similar to the rest would be a consequence of a well functioning family. Therefore, his theoretical proposal is quite the contrary to that of Kirk, holding that the more problems the families found, the more they attributed these problems to the adoption and talked about the biological parents. This last problem coping strategy in adoptive homes does not appear to be an adaptive strategy.

We interpret that, while for Kirk, greater acceptance of the differences would lead to good family function, for Kaye it would nevertheless be a consequence of poor family function. Brodzinsky (1987) sheds some light on this dilemma, also suggesting certain critique and modifications to Kirk's theory. First of all, while the social role theory suggests a lineal relationship between recognition of differences and psychological well-being, Brodzinsky suggests that the relationship between beliefs or attitudes and family adjustment are much more complex. This author introduces a new concept known as "insistence upon differences," which represents the adoptive families that not only recognize their differences from biological families, but rather, they emphasize these to the point that they become the central nucleus of their coexistence, thus, these differences are used to explain all the problems they experience. The less adaptive attitudes will be those that adopt extreme visions in this continuum (rejection - acceptance - insistence), therefore, rather than lineal, Brodzinsky suggests a curvilinear relationship between the attitudes to the differences and family adjustment. A second critique refers to the suggestion by Kirk of a static model in which each family is located at one of the two poles on the continuum, with two exclusive patterns. Brodzinsky suggests that families can modify the way in which they face tasks, so that at the beginning, when the family objective is to create unity and confidence in its center, rejecting differences would perhaps be more convenient; as the years go by and the children begin to be interested in their adoption, it is probable that the parents start acknowledging the differences. An insistence on the differences usually appears in families that are facing many problems; and since these difficulties usually occur more frequently during school and adolescent years, it is not probable that these insistent attitudes emerge before these ages.

In this regard, the work of Viana & Welsh (2010) is noteworthy, who suggest that the parental cognitive processes, such as attitudes, beliefs and expectations, affect the parental behavior and the subjective experience of parenting stress. Specifically, they analyze the role of pre-adoption expectations of child problems on parenting stress six months post-adoption. While the hypothesis of the authors was that those families who "prepare for the worst" in terms of expectations for their children's behavior and development may have the best outcomes, they found that higher pre-adoption expectations of developmental and behavioral/emotional problems were significantly related to higher parenting stress. This study is a clear example of the danger of developing extremely negative expectations about the future adjustment of adopted children. In part, these expectations could self-fulfill, as the behavior of the parents toward their children is modified. These families could feel less influential in the development of their children; they have less trust in their own possibilities of intervening in this development.

X. Stress in Adoptive Families

Despite the various tensions and difficulties that families might encountered, families that adopt are, in general, very satisfied with their decision, the process and the repercussions of the adoption in their family life (Sánchez-Sandoval, 2011). Most studies (Bird, Peterson, & Miller, 2002; Ceballo, Lansford, Abbey, & Stewart, 2004; Judge, 2003, 2004; Levy-Shiff, Zoran, & Shulman, 1997) have reported lower levels of stress in adoptive compared to non-adoptive parents. Sánchez-Sandoval & Palacios (2012) hypothesized that, at the time of their study, these parents were still in the "honeymoon" period, with more difficult times ahead. In addition, research into parental stress and adoption has frequently focused on parents who are involved in more difficult adoptions, such as those involving special-needs children (McGlone, Santos, Kazama, Fong & Mueller, 2002), children who have been institutionalized for extended periods of time (Judge, 2003, 2004; Mainemer et al., 1998), or parents who have sought help from adoptive parents' support groups (Bird et al., 2002). Most of these studies (Judge, 2003; Mainemer et al., 1998; McGlone et al., 2002) have reported a clear association between the children's behavioral problems and parental stress. With very few exceptions (Levy-Shiff et al., 1997), there is little information available regarding the experience of stress in parents engaged in less problematic adoptions and it is difficult to determine whether the stress is linked to the adoption itself, or to the behavioral problems of the adopted children whose parents are being studied.

Even today, literature based on this model is far from abundant with regards to adoptive families; as mentioned, studies usually research the independent affect of how isolated variables on the adoptive processes. Despite this, we believe that from this perspective a much more real vision of adoptions as a complex process is offered, the success of which not only depends on the characteristics of the children, nor on the characteristics of the parents, but rather, it will be the balance between these that can predict the integration of the children, the satisfaction of all those involved and good family function. As will be shown throughout this chapter, this theoretical perspective is, in fact, the inspiration and upon which it is based. It is necessary to develop comprehensive models to integrate effects of various stressor types in parenting.

Our Research

We are interested to know how being an adoptive family affects parental stress. This chapter is based on the findings of the current empirical research with adoptive families. 260 adoptive families from Spain have participated in our own longitudinal research. The most widely used measures of parenting stress (Parent Stress Index (Abidin, 1995), and Stress Index for Parents of Adolescents (Sheras, Abidin, & Konold, 1998) were applied. These measures are designed to identify parent/child or adolescent systems at risk for dysfunctional parenting and problematic child adjustment.

METHOD

Participants

The sample for the current analysis was drawn from the Phase 2 (or Time 2) of a longitudinal study on the development of domestically adopted children in Spain (see eg. Sánchez-Sandoval, 2011). Between 1987 (the year in which the new adoption laws came into force) and 1994, 568 children were adopted in Andalusia, Southern Spain. The original sample (Phase 1) consisted of 393 families and included 88% of all of the adoptive parents contacted, since 12% decided not to participate in the study. All of the children were adopted through domestic adoption programs. The data collection for the study (Phase 2) reported here took place six years after the first one. Parenting stress was assessed in 260 of these families (104 families completed the PSI (children), and 156 families the SIPA (adolescents)). No difference in child and family characteristics was found between families who participated in Phase 2 surveys and those who did not. Data about these two groups have been published (Palacios & Sánchez-Sandoval, 2006; Sánchez-Sandoval & Palacios, 2012).

Below are the socio-demographic characteristics. Regarding the children and adolescents, 52.3% were boys and 47.7% were girls. The average age at the time of adoption was 1.92 years (sd = 3.16) and 13.01 (sd = 4.36) at the time when the data was collected. They had been living for an average of 11.10 years (sd= 2.60) with their adoptive parents. 16.2%

(n=42) were adopted above the age of 6 years; 13.5% (n= 35) were adopted with a biological sibling; 10.4% (n=27) had special physical, psychological or sensorial needs, and 7.7% (n=20) were from different ethnic groups. Some children are in more than one of these categories (e.g., older than 6 and adopted with a sibling). It is known that at least 23.8% (n=62) had suffered maltreatment prior to the adoption, and a 53.8 % (n= 140) had been institutionalized.

As for the adoptive parents, 91.2% (n=237) of the families were two-parent families and 8.8% (n=23) were single-parent ones. At the time of the child's arrival in the adoptive home, on average fathers were 38.55 years old (sd= 6.42) and mothers were 36.60 years old (sd= 6.23). At the time of the study, on average fathers were 50.13 years old (sd= 7.31) and mothers were 48.17 years old (sd= 7.06). The educational level of the families (measured taking into account the parent with the highest educational level) were as follows: 45.8% (n=119) had a low educational level (primary studies); 23.8% (n=62) had a middle educational level (more than primary and less than university); and 30.4% (n=79) had a high or university educational level.

Procedure

The study described here is a prospective longitudinal study that included interviews and questionnaire measures with the adoptive parents after placement. We re-contacted the adoptive families studied in Phase 1 six years later. The families were visited at home and interviewed. The semi-structured questionnaire and the 4er were answered by father and mother together. The mothers completed the parenting stress measures.

Measures

- The *semi-structured questionnaire* explored the parents' socio-demographic characteristics, the type of adoption (single or siblings, for example), the experience of the child before adoption (existence of abuse/neglect, institutionalization), the adoption process (including communication about the adoption, for example), the acknowledgement/rejection of differences (see below) and the availability and use of resources and support (professional services, for example). The questionnaires were carried out by trained psychologists and lasted 60-90 minutes. The parents' answers were written down as they were produced and later coded.
- The most widely used measures of parenting stress, *Parent Stress Index* (Abidin, 1995), and *Stress Index for Parents of Adolescents* (Sheras, Abidin, & Konold, 1998) were applied. These measures are designed to identify parent/child or adolescent systems at-risk for dysfunctional parenting and problematic child adjustment.

The *Parenting Stress Index* is a 120-item questionnaire that was standardized for use with parents of children aged 1 month to 12 years. These items are rated on a 5-point Likert-type scale that ranges from 1 (strongly agree) to 5 (strongly disagree). Higher scores indicate higher parenting stress.

The PSI yields three scores: one for the stress related to the child (CD), one for the stress associated with the characteristics of the parents (PS) and a third that indicates a total score for parenthood stress (TS). There are 6 *Child Domain* subscales: (1) Distractibility /Hyperactivity, (2) Adaptability, (3) Reinforcement for Parents, (4) Demandingness, (5) Mood, and (6) Acceptability. The *Parent Domain* has 7 subscales: (1) Competence, (2) Isolation, (3) Attachment, (4) Health, (5) Role Restriction, (6) Depression, and (7) Spouse. A *Life Stressor* score indicates the amount of stress outside the parent-child relationship that the parent is currently experiencing.

Statements such as "My child is not able to do as much as I expected" or "I feel trapped in my responsibilities as a parent" are examples of PSI items. Cronbach's alpha was .92 for stress associated with both the child's and the parents' characteristics, and .95 for the total stress index.

The *Stress Index for Parents of Adolescents*- SIPA (Sheras et al., 1998) is a 112-item questionnaire for parents of adolescents aged 12-18 years. It is possible to calculate the following from the responses:

a)   A stress index for the *adolescent domain (AD)*: measures the level of stress experienced by a parent as a function of the characteristics of his or her adolescent (e.g., mood, behavior problems). There are four Adolescent Domain subscales: moodiness/emotional liability *(MEL)*, social isolation/withdrawal *(ISO)*, delinquency /antisocial *(DEL)*, failure to achieve or persevere *(ACH)*.

b)   Another index for the *parent domain (PD)*: measures the level of stress experienced by a parent as a function of the effect of parenting on other life roles, the relationship with a spouse or partner, social isolation and parenting competence. There are four Parent Domain subscales: life restriction (*LFR*), relationship with spouse/partner (*REL*), social alienation (*SOC*), incompetence/guilt (*INC*).

c)   An index for the *Adolescent-Parent Relationship Domain (APRD)*: measures the perceived quality of the relationship that the parent has with the adolescent, such as the degree of communication and affection between them.

d)   And an index *of Total Parenting Stress (TS):* represents a composite of all the items across all domains and indicates the total stress experienced as a function of parenting a particular adolescent.

Some samples of SIPA items are: "My child often gets in trouble when he or she is with his or her friends", "I often feel guilty after I get angry at my child", and "My child shows affection toward me". Higher scores indicate higher parenting stress. The Cronbach's alpha was .93 for stress associated with both the adolescents' and the parents' characteristics, .90 for stress in the parent-adolescent relationship and .96 for the total stress index.

- The *child rearing styles* of the parents were assessed using a scale (4e–r, Palacios & Sánchez-Sandoval, 2000) that takes into account traditional variables used to define parental styles: affection and communication, demands, and control. Parents answer the 20-item measure using a 5-point Likert scale indicating their degree of agreement with the item. Some examples of the items are: "If I ask my child to do something and s/he does it wrong, I don't ask him/her to try harder because at least s/he has tried" or "A good punishment in time is better than repeated explanations". Cronbach's alpha for the total scale is .79.

- *How parents perceive their similarities or differences with respect to non-adoptive parents* was explored using a series of questions inspired by Kirk (1964) and his conceptualization of the acknowledgment/rejection of differences dimension. Parents were asked if they believed that adoptive children had needs and worries different from those of non-adoptive children, if they thought that in adoptive families there were problems different from those in non-adoptive families, and if child rearing styles and expressions of affection should be different for adopted children. Data analysis showed that these questions were closely interrelated and formed a single factor. Parents who rejected the existence of differences received a score 0, those who strongly insisted on differences scored 4, and those who simply acknowledged some differences had a score somewhere in-between. Cronbach's alpha for this measure was .52.

- *Use of resources and support for adoption.* We developed a questionnaire in which the following resources were presented: the members of the adoption services, other professionals, family members, friends, printed materials, spouse, other adoptive parents, and organizations. Families informed us if they were available to them (yes/no), and the usefulness of these resources was valued on a scale of 1 (very little useful) to 5 (very useful).

RESULTS

Comparison between Adoptive Mothers and Adoptive Fathers

Preliminary analysis concerns similarities and differences in parenting stress between adoptive mothers and adoptive fathers in the current study. Our first question is: Do adoptive fathers and adoptive mothers differ in their experience of parenting stress?

Regarding children younger than 12, mothers and fathers from 104 adoptive families were asked to complete the Parenting Stress Index independently. Finally 104 mothers and 64 fathers answered it. We have analyzed whether the parenting stress of fathers and mothers of the same family are related. Descriptive statistics, correlations and pair-samples t-test appear in Tables 1 and 2. There were significant positive correlations between mother's parenting stress and father's parenting stress in three measures (Total stress, Child Domain and Parent Domain). As indicated in Table 1, correlations were high for all measures, averaging r = .77. The dependent t-test (or paired-samples t-test) compares the means of two related groups to detect whether there are any statistically significant differences between these means. Differences between mothers and fathers were not significant (table 2).

For adolescents, a total of 156 mothers and 107 fathers answered the instrument assessing parental stress (SIPA). The correlations between the scores obtained by the fathers and mothers were very high (.93 in the adolescent domain, .84 in the parent domain and .88 in the total stress score), and no significant differences were found between their scores. T-test analyses indicated no significant differences for mothers versus fathers regarding their parenting stress scores.

Table 1. PSI Mothers and Fathers. Statistical Descriptive and Correlations

Measure		N	Min	Max	*M*	SD	Corr.	Sig.
PSI CD	Mothers	64	1.33	3.43	1.9120	.4710	.786	.000
	Fathers	64	1.26	3.41	1.8771	.4513		
PSI PD	Mothers	64	1.10	3.19	2.0282	.5301	.739	.000
	Fathers	64	1.12	2.73	1.9868	.4920		
PSI TS	Mothers	64	1.23	3.34	1.7987	.4799	.794	.000
	Fathers	64	1.26	2.98	1.7616	.4563		

Table 2. PSI Mothers and Fathers. Paired-samples t-test

	Related differences				
Comparison	M	SD	T	g.l.	Sig.
Pair 1 M-P PSI CD	.0414	.3363	.986	63	.328
Pair 2 M-P PSI PD	.0370	.3391	.874	63	.385
Pair 3 M-P PSI TS	.0349	.2965	.942	63	.350

Since there are no differences between fathers and mothers, and we have more thorough information about a higher number of mothers, it was decided to analyze only the scores of the mothers, which are reported herein.

Comparisons with Non Adoptive Samples

Taking into account PSI data, compared to the normative data (Abidin, 1995), the adoptive mothers of our study do not have a higher-than-average stress level. Quite the contrary, the average total score for the normative data is 222 whereas that of our sample was 186, t(103) = -8.370, p < .001. Average stress scores for the Child Domain in our sample (93) were somewhat lower than the normative sample (98), while average scores for the Parent Domain were significantly lower in our sample (92) than in the normative sample (123), t(103) = -13.827, p<.001 (table 3). The proportion of subjects falling within the clinical range (above the 85th percentile) for the non-parametric chi-square goodness-of-fit test showed that the proportion of mothers in our study within this range is considerably lower than expected for the Parents Domain (1.9%, x2 (1) = 13.949, p<.05) and the Total score (6.7%, x2(1)=5.578, p<.05) but not for the Child Domain (18.3%, p>.05) (see next Figure).

It can therefore be concluded that the adoptive parents taking part in this study have a parenting experience stress score below that the normative data.

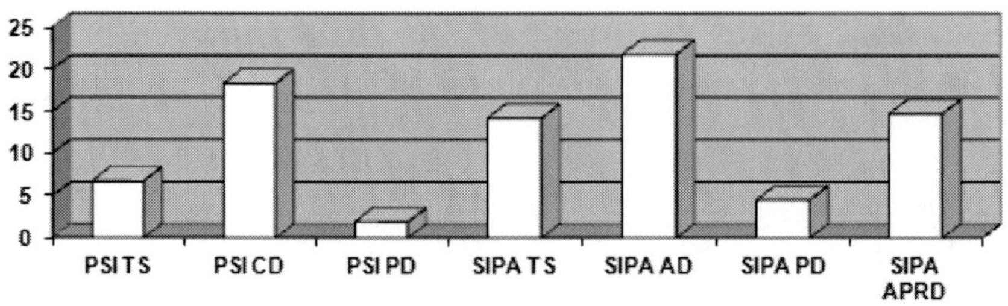

We also compared the stress of adoptive parents of our adolescents with the normative SIPA data (Sheras et al., 1998). If normative data and that obtained from this sample are compared regarding the mean scores, the Total Stress and Parent Domain scores are lower in our sample than in the normative one, with, respectively, $t(155)= -8.46$, $p< .05$, and $t(155)= -10.04$, $p< .001$, but the mean score in the adolescent domain is higher in our sample than in the normative data, with $t(155)= 5.46$, $p< .01$, with no differences in the Parent-Adolescent Relationships Domain ($p= .47$).

Table 3. Parent Stress Index & Stress Index for Parents of Adolescents mean scores (standard deviations) and percentages above the clinical range

	Mean scores (SD)			
	PSI		**SIPA**	
	Normative data[1]	**Adoptive parents[3]**	**Normative data[2]**	**Adoptive parents[3]**
Child /Adolescent Domain	98	93.17 (24.79)	85.2 (25.7)	90.66 (24.97)
Parent Domain	123	92.29 (22.64)	76.5 (19.8)	62.53 (17.35)
Parent-Adolescent Relationships	--	--	33.2 (10.7)	32.56 (11.13)
Total Stress	222	186.21 (43.60)	194.3 (49.7)	185.83 (46.06)

[1] Abidin, 1995. [2] Sheras et al., 1998. [3] Study reported in this chapter. Adapted from Palacios & Sánchez-Sandoval (2006), & Sánchez-Sandoval & Palacios (2012).

When comparing not the mean scores, but the proportion of subjects scoring beyond the "within normal limits" range (up to percentile 85), our scores were similar to those for the normative population in the Parent-Adolescent Relationship Domain (14.7%) and in the Total Stress (14.2%) score, but were higher in the Adolescent Domain, 21.2%, with χ^2 (1)= 5.649, $p< .05$, and lower in the Parent Domain, 4.5%, with χ^2 (1)= 13.522, $p< .001$.

Descriptive Statistics

Table 4 summarizes correlations of child and family demographic variables (e.g., age at adoption) with parenting stress (PSI for children, SIPA for adolescents). In relation to children aged 7-11, most correlations were significant. Children's age, father's age, and years of residing in adoptive homes were positively correlated with parenting stress (total index, parent domain and children domain). The older they are and the longer they have lived together, the greater the parental stress. The correlations between parenting stress and children's age at adoption were not significant (see Table 4 for details). Family's educational level correlated negatively with parenting stress. Parents with lower educational levels perceived greater parental stress.

Table 4. Correlations between demographic variables and family stress (N = 260)

	Children PSI			Adolescents SIPA			
	TS	CD	PD	TS	AD	PD	APRD
Child's AAA (years)	-.029	-.138	.072	.175*	.125	.044	.359**
Child's age (years)	.269**	.196*	.280**	.170*	.120	.083	.299**
Years of residing in adoptive family	.276**	.229*	.263**	.019	.012	.069	-.035
Mother's age	.208*	.185	.190	.070	.007	.060	.174*
Father's age	.254*	.210*	.248*	.120	.087	.074	.191*
Family's education level	-.225*	-.126	-.276**	-.143	-.076	-188*	-.149

Notes. AAA = age at adoption. TS: Total Stress. CD: Child Domain. PD: Parent Domain. AD: Adolescent Domain. APRD: *p<.05 **p < .01.

If we keep paying attention to the stress of families with adopted children of school age (PSI), we see that the correlations with age are greater in the Child Domain. It is interesting to analyze in more detail the correlations with the subscales for each domain (see Table 5). Children's age correlated positively with the subscales Mood, Acceptability and Demandingness (p<.01), and with Distractibility/Hyperactivity and Reinforcement (p<.05). The same scales also positively correlated with the years of residing with their adoptive families (but current age and years of residing in the adoptive homes were highly correlated, p < .001). These subscales correlated negatively with family's education level.

With regards to the Parent Domain, fewer correlations were significant. Children's age correlated positively with parenting stress associated with difficulties with *attachment* to child. Mother's age correlated positively with the subscales *Health* and *Social Isolation*. Father's age correlated positively with the subscales *Spouse* and *Social Isolation*. The lower the parent educational level, the higher the parenting stress related to the partner and to social isolation.

Table 5. Correlations between demographic family variables and family stress

	AAA	Age T2	Time T2	Current age of mother	Current age of father	Family educational level T2
Distractibility/ Hyperactivity	.162	.213[*]	.173	.213[*]	.263[**]	-.214[*]
Reinforces Parent	.100	.250[*]	.225[*]	.126	.118	-.202[*]
Mood	-.011	.270[**]	.272[**]	.138	.216[*]	-.163
Acceptability	.012	.277[**]	.274[**]	.193	.227[*]	-.206[*]
Adaptability	-.015	.167	.171	.095	.131	-.217[*]
Demandingness	.102	.269[**]	.244[*]	.168	.245[*]	-.318[**]
Competence	-.163	.141	.180	.080	.130	.035
Attachment	-.147	.255[**]	.291[**]	.108	.122	-.185
Role Restriction	-.193[*]	.087	.133	.083	.130	-.086
Depression	-.076	.153	.171	.079	.060	-.014
Spouse	-.008	.157	.159	.175	.333[**]	-.123
Isolation	-.001	.145	.145	.232[*]	.232[*]	-.229[*]
Health	-.066	.105	.120	.260[**]	.164	-.182

$*p < .05, **p < .01$.

In relation to stress of parents of adolescents (see Table 5), most correlations were not significant in the scales, Adolescent Domain and Parent Domain. Family's education level correlated negatively with the parent domain (lower level, higher stress). Total stress correlated positively only with children's ages. However, the scale, Adolescent-Parent Relationship Domain (APRD), correlated positively with ages. Mothers of adolescents found increased stress in the relationships with them as their children grew up, and the older they were adopted.

Stress and Other Demographic and Adoption Variables

With regards to families with children aged 7-11 (PSI), we have analyzed parental stress in relation to children's characteristics. Total stress was higher when the adopted were males (t(102)=3.019, p=.003), when they were older in Phase 2 (r=.269, p=.006), and when they had disabilities (t(102)=3.584, p=.001). In the other individual variables, the differences were not significant (age on arrival, individual / siblings adoptions, previous experience of institutionalization and abuse, chronic diseases). In the Child Domain and in the Parent Domain the results were very similar. As shown in Table 6, higher stress was perceived by families with males and with disabled adopted children, on both subscales.

Among mothers of adolescents (SIPA), current adolescent age (r=.170, p=.034) and age at pre-adoption (r=.175, p=.029) were significantly positively correlated to Total Parenting Stress. As can been seen in Table 6, mothers' reports of parenting stress were related with sibling adoption (t(38.263)=2.638, p=.012), with institutionalized children prior adoption (t(154)=2.108, p=.037) and with pre-adoption abuse experiences (t(154)=2.373, p=.019). Thus, mothers who adopted siblings, or children with harder pre-adoption stories, reported higher parenting stress (TS).

Table 6. Relationships between characteristics of the children and parenting stress

	TS			CD			PD		
	M	SD	*P*	*M*	SD	*P*	*M*	SD	*P*
Total									
1. Female	1.7686	.39282	.003	1.8469	.42800	.001	1.6871	.41937	.038
Male	2.0235	.46022		2.1846	.58036		1.8642	.44061	
2. Individual	1.9054	.45607	>.05	2.0291	.55420	>.05	1.7822	.44391	>.05
Sibling	1.8761	.30404		1.9752	.26785		1.7610	.36905	
3. Pre-adoption Residential care	1.8614	.44378	>.05	1.9872	.56380	>.05	1.7345	.43634	>.05
Without pre-adoption Residential care	1.9286	.44956		2.0485	.52685		1.8085	.43962	
4. Maltreatment	2.1378	.67757	>.05	2.3424	.83217	>.05	1.9303	.64415	>.05
Without maltreatment	1.8839	.42101		1.9991	.50490		1.7683	.41851	
5. Chronic illness /disability	2.3589	.57793	.001	2.5935	.67161	.000	2.1281	.57174	.008
Healthy	1.8549	.40463		1.9651	.48975		1.7438	.40773	

The comparison of the subscales mean score (AD, PD and APRD) showed similar results. Mothers who adopted a sibling group, children with pre-adoption maltreatment experiences or with pre-adoptive experiences of residential foster care perceived greater stress on the three subscales. The differences were significant in Adolescent Domain (p<.05) and Adolescent-Parent Relations Domain (p<.05), but not in Parent Domain.

In relation to family characteristics, mothers who adopted a known child (adoptions with whom there was a previous relationship) had a significantly higher (PSI) stress mean score (t(102)=2.353, *p*=.021) than mothers with no previous relationships with their children. Mothers from a low education group showed a higher mean stress (*M* =2.041, DT=.70) than those from the middle education group (*M* =1.838, DT=.75) and than those from a high education group (*M* =1.803, DT=.079) (F(101)=3.131, *p*=.048). There was no significant difference in the severity of stress experienced by mothers of adolescents (SIPA) regarding these variables.

Acknowledgment of Differences

Reports of parenting stress were significantly related with the parents' perception of differences between adoptive and non-adoptive families. The next table summarizes Pearson correlations between variables. Correlations were positive and significant, so that we found that the greater the stress of the mothers, the more these mothers perceived differences between biological families and adoptive ones (see table 7).

And this is a trend that is maintained over time. The correlations were not only significant with the perception that they had at the time of the study (phase 2), but also, the more differences that were perceived by the families in phase 1 of the study, the more stress they perceived in parenthood six years later (phase 2). This is so both in the Total Stress, and in each of the subscales (CD / AD, PD, APRD), in families with school age children, and in families with adolescents.

Table 7. Correlations between perception of differences and family stress

		Children PSI			Adolescents SIPA			
		TS	CD	PD	TS	AD	PD	APRD
Perception of differences T1	Corr.	.265[**]	.257[**]	.225[*]	.237[**]	.181[*]	.151	.329[**]
	Sign.	.007	.009	.023	.003	.027	.066	.000
	N	102	102	102	150	150	150	150
Perception of differences T2	Corr.	.284[**]	.207[*]	.310[**]	.298[**]	.304[**]	.192[*]	.236[**]
	Sign.	.003	.035	.001	.000	.000	.016	.003
	N	104	104	104	156	156	156	156

Notes: TS: Total Stress. CD: Child Domain. PD: Parent Domain. AD: Adolescent Domain. APRD: *p<.05 **p < .01.

Educational Styles

We measured parenting styles through the dimensions implicated in the three principal traditional parenting styles: authoritative, authoritarian, and permissive parenting (Baumrind, 1971; 1973). The table 8 summarizes the descriptive statistics of the three measured subscales: affection and communication, demands and control. Scores can range from 1 to 5.

Table 8. Educational styles' statistical descriptive

	N	Minimum	Maximum	Mean	Typ deviation
Affection & communication	255	2.11	5.00	4.1368	.64130
Demands	255	1.75	5.00	3.7588	.75110
Inductive Control	255	1.75	5.00	3.5078	.75225

These mothers scored medium-high in all three dimensions. Remembering the traditional parenting styles as average, these families could look like authoritative parenting. This style involves not only high demands but also warmth and responsiveness.

To know the possible relationships between parenting stress and parenting styles, we analyzed the correlations between PSI and SIPA scales, and 4er scales. Most correlations were negative and significant (see table 9).

As the Pearson correlations show, the higher the stress is (TS, CD/AD, PD, APRD), the less communicative and affectionate the mothers are. The higher the stress is (TS, CD/AD, PD, APRD), the lower demands the mothers impose on their children or adolescents. And the higher the parenting stress is, the lower the level of inductive control (control characterized by firmness, explanations, and flexibility) the mothers use. These results confirm the intensive relationships between parenting stress and family function.

Table 9. Correlations between educational styles and parenting stress

		Children PSI			Adolescents SIPA			
		TS	CD	PD	TS	AD	PD	APRD
Affection & communication	Corr.	-.454[**]	-.413[**]	-.419[**]	-.578[**]	-.497[**]	-.477[**]	-.550[**]
	Sign.	.000	.000	.000	.000	.000	.000	.000
	N	101	101	101	154	154	154	154
Demands	Corr.	-.260[**]	-.257[**]	-.212[*]	-.276[**]	-.242[**]	-.290[**]	-.168[*]
	Sign.	.009	.009	.033	.001	.003	.000	.037
	N	101	101	101	154	154	154	154
Inductive control	Corr.	-.314[**]	-.256[**]	-.312[**]	-.350[**]	-.354[**]	-.280[**]	-.226[**]
	Sign.	.001	.010	.002	.000	.000	.000	.005
	N	101	101	101	154	154	154	154

$p < .05$, ** $p < .01$, *** $p < .001$.

Resources

In recent years, families have had different resources to cope with the circumstances related with their adoptive parenthood. In the following figure we show the percentage of families that have been provided with specific resources in this process. Undoubtedly, their own partner is the resource most used by these families as regards adoption. On the other hand, almost half of the families say they have been helped by relatives and friends. Of more concern is that one third of families have looked for professional help to respond to some of the challenges that they have found concerning the adoption. About one quarter of the families has resorted to printed material (e.g. books, magazines, etc). A similar proportion has been provided with the help of other adoptive families. There were very few families that were provided with the collaboration of organizations.

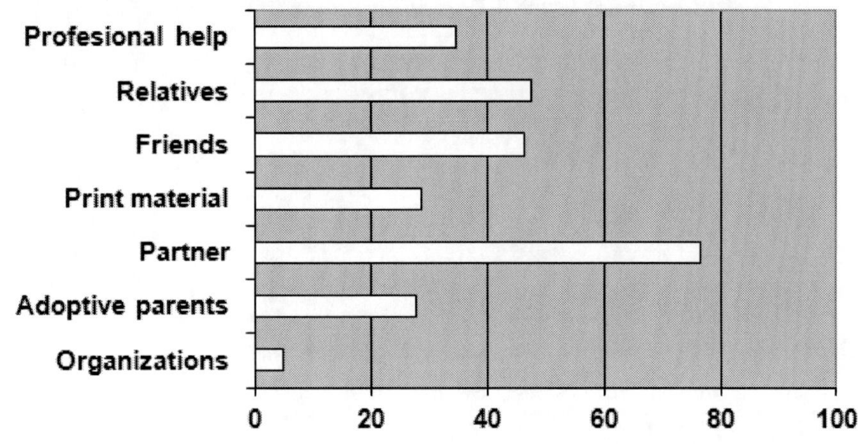

In the case of having used these resources, the families valued their usefulness in relation to the adoption. In general, all resources were evaluated positively, with an average value greater than 3.2 (on a scale of 1 to 5). As shown in table 10, the best valued resources were the spouse (M=4.60), relatives (M=4.05) and friends (M=3.82).

Table 10. Statistical descriptive

	N	Minimum	Maximum	Mean	Typ. deviation
Adoption Service	56	1.00	5.00	3.6964	1.55995
Professional	90	1.00	5.00	3.3111	1.37917
Relatives	120	1.00	5.00	4.0583	1.25220
Friends	120	1.00	5.00	3.8250	1.34516
Printed material	75	1.00	5.00	3.2267	1.34137
Parents	188	1.00	5.00	4.6064	.91591
Other adoptive parents	72	1.00	5.00	3.3611	1.37693
Organizations	13	1.00	5.00	3.6154	1.50214

It would be interesting to know whether parental stress levels are linked to having support and resources with regards to adoptive parenthood. When it comes to public adoption services, their use or not during these recent years is not related, according to the statistical t test comparing the means, with parenting stress with adopted school age children (PSI). However, among adoptive families with adolescents, their use related with higher parenting stress in Adolescent-Parent Relations Domain. Families who used state adoption services reported higher mothering stress regarding their relationship with their adolescent children.

On the other hand, those families that have had some help from specialized professionals (eg. psychologist) show higher levels of stress on all the sub-scales (see figure below). Therefore, for example, the differences were significant in both the total stress of the mothers with school age children (PSI, t(97)=3.782, p=.000) and those with adolescent children (SIPA, t(151)=3.943, p=.000).

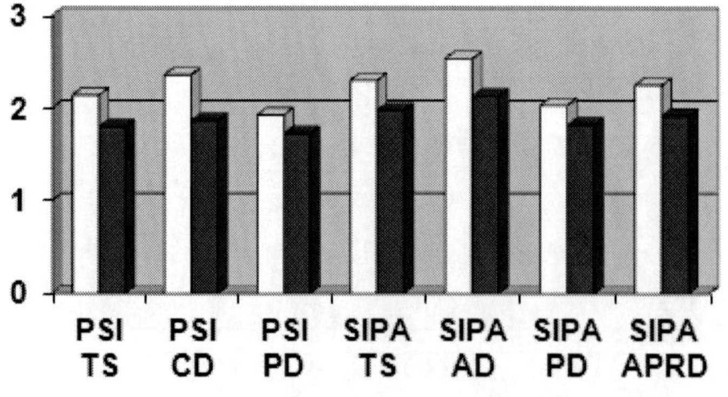

No between-group differences were found in mothers' mean stress (PSI & SIPA) scores according to perceiving the support of friends and relatives (p >.05). So, the families had counted on them independent to their stress level. Similarly, no between-group differences were found in mothers' mean stress (PSI & SIPA) according to other resources (p >.05). Families who had looked for and read printed information, however, did report significantly higher stress in Adolescent Domain than mothers from families without this resource (t(151)=2.315, p=.03.).

Table 11. Correlations between evaluation of resources and parenting stress

		Children PSI			Adolescents SIPA			
		TS	CD	PD	TS	AD	PD	APRD
Adoption team	Corr.	-.617[**]	-.797[**]	-.229	-.084	-.227	.221	-.096
	Sign.	.005	.000	.347	.621	.177	.189	.571
	N	19	19	19	37	37	37	37
Professionals	Corr.	-.242	-.137	-.313	.198	.270[*]	.066	.090
	Sign.	.168	.438	.071	.144	.044	.630	.509
	N	34	34	34	56	56	56	56
Family members	Corr.	-.085	-.117	-.044	.087	.086	.154	-.060
	Sign.	.569	.433	.771	.462	.469	.192	.616
	N	47	47	47	73	73	73	73
Friends	Corr.	-.004	-.019	.017	.055	.077	.023	.016
	Sign.	.978	.896	.907	.653	.531	.854	.897
	N	51	51	51	69	69	69	69
Printed material	Corr.	-.255	-.126	-.330[*]	.004	.208	-.301	.011
	Sign.	.128	.459	.046	.983	.211	.066	.945
	N	37	37	37	38	38	38	38
Partner	Corr.	-.206	-.,167	-.206	-.056	-.049	-.093	.033
	Sign.	.077	.153	.077	.558	.609	.326	.726
	N	75	75	75	113	113	113	113
Other adoptive parents	Corr.	-.048	-.033	-.066	.061	.047	.063	.053
	Sign.	.783	.850	.705	.718	.780	.711	.753
	N	35	35	35	37	37	37	37
Organizations	Corr.	-.965	-.891	-.999[*]	-.336	-.058	-.266	-.641[*]
	Sign.	.168	.300	.024	.343	.873	.458	.046
	N	3	3	3	10	10	10	10

When these families had used these resources, we wanted to know if their satisfaction with them differed depending on the parenting stress levels. As for the parents with school age children (PSI), the negative and significant correlations between parenting stress and the evaluation of the utility of the public adoption teams stand out. The less useful the adoption services are, the higher is their stress. Something similar occurred with the printed material, the less useful, the more stress. In the case of parents with adolescent children, however, the performance of other professionals was assessed more positively as the stress associated with the adolescent's characteristics rose (AD) (see table 11).

Predictors of Parental Stress

A series of hierarchical multiple regression analyses were performed to determine the sources of variation in mothers' assessment of parenting stress. Two hierarchical regressions were carried out to examine the predictive relationship between the preliminary analyzed measures and PSI Total Stress (more details in Palacios & Sánchez-Sandoval, 2006), and SIPA Total Stress (see Sánchez-Sandoval & Palacios, 2012).

Several parent, child and resource variables showed significant relationships with the total score obtained by the mothers in PSI and in SIPA. Two hierarchical regression analyses were carried out, in which the dependent variable was the total stress score and the independent variables were those being shown to relate significantly in the one-to-one comparisons between the variables.

With regards the PSI score, we used a hierarchical method to introduce variables grouped into four clusters: children's characteristics (gender, age at the adoption, current age, special needs, single or sibling adoption), social and demographic characteristics of the parents and type of adoption (adoption where there was a previous relationship); attitudes towards child-rearing and adoption; and finally, the use of resources and support.

Table 12. Summary of Hierarchical Regression Analysis for Variables Predicting Mothers' Total Stress score in Stress Index for Parents of Adolescents

Variable	Model 1			Model 2			Model 3		
	B	SE B	β	B	SE B	β	B	SE B	β
Sibling adoption	.28	.10	.21**	.20	.08	.15*	.20	.07	.15*
Affection and communication				-.38	.05	-.50***	-.39	.04	-.52***
Acceptance/rejection of differences				.09	.03	.19**	.06	.03	.13*
Induction				-.09	.04	-.14*	-.08	.04	-.12*
Professional help							.27	.06	.25***
R^2 (adjusted)	3.8			43.2			49.2		
F	6.989**			29.484***			30.089***		

$p < .05$, ** $p < .01$, *** $p < .001$.
Adapted from Sánchez-Sandoval & Palacios, 2012.

In the regression model on the PSI total stress score (Palacios & Sánchez-Sandoval, 2006) seven variables were entered, in the following order: existence of impairment in the child (B= .30, p>.001), current age (B=.11, n.s.), child's gender (male) (B=.15, p<.05), parent-child relationship previous to adoption (B=.14, p>.05), child-rearing style highlighting affection and communication (B=-.40, p<.001), perception of differences (B=.18, p<.01) and support from organizations (B=.29, p<.05).

These seven predictors together account for 57.5% of the variability observed in total stress in adoptive mothers. Higher levels of stress were then associated with some characteristics of the children (any type of impairment, older current age, male), some characteristics of the parents (child-rearing style entailing less affection and communication, insistence on differences, parent-child relationship before adoption) and with the context of adoption (more frequent use of support services by parents).

For SIPA, as shown in Sánchez-Sandoval & Palacios (2012), the variables were introduced in three blocks: children's characteristics (age on arrival, current age, neglect-abuse and institutionalization experiences before adoption, single or sibling adoption), characteristics of the parents (child-rearing attitudes, acknowledgement-rejection of differences) and, finally, the use of resources and support.

The final lineal regression model included five predictors which together accounted for 49.2% of the variability observed in the stress experienced by adoptive mothers: the level of stress was higher in multiple-adoption cases, when the mothers scored low in affection-communication and in inductive control, when they insisted on the differences or when they had sought help from professionals on adoption related matters. Table 12 shows this data.

CONCLUSION

Adoption is a measure to protect childhood. Despite the complexity of the process, the final objective must be that adoptions are performed with the maximum possible guarantees for success. The data of the adoptions that have taken place in Spain indicate that the degree of family satisfaction with the adoption is very high (León, 2011; Fernández-Molina, Fuentes, & Fernández-Berrocal, 2012; Sánchez-Sandoval, 2011). Even in the case of international adoptions, where a large proportion of children present, at arrival, serious developmental problems (Sánchez-Sandoval, Palacios & León, 2004), the initial adaptation of these children to their new families is described by the families as very positive (Sánchez-Sandoval, León, & Román, 2012). Recent research has brought to light higher parenting stress experienced by parents of children with global delay (Tervo, 2012). After an average of three years living with the adoptive family, the developmental recovery rates of these children are impressive (Palacios, Sánchez-Sandoval, León, & Román, 2010). At the same time, the percentage of adoptions that are interrupted it is very low (Palacios, Sánchez-Sandoval & León, 2005). This data reflects the enormous possibilities adoptive families provide in optimizing the development of these children, as well as the vast quality of the adoptive families within the context of education and development.

We know that there are many variables involved to ensure that an adoption process is carried out successfully. Without underestimating the important differences marked by the initial characteristics of the children being adopted, it is our opinion that much of the success of the entire process depends on the behavior of the adoptive parents. To a large extent, the later adjustment of their children will depend on the actions of the adoptive parents. To interpret and analyze the role of parental behavior in the psycho-social adjustment of children, we took another look at the model proposed by Abidin more than two decades ago. According to this model, the behavior of the parents will be conditioned by the demands of the role as parents. We started with the idea that when parents face the task of educating a child, not all of them do this in the same way. All parents suffer stress at some point in time, with regards to the education of their children; however, they differ in the amount of stress, in the duration, how they interpret the stressful situation, and in the response they give to this search (or not) to adapt to the situation.

In adoptive families, parents have to respond to the demands of parenthood, as well as those of adoptive parenthood. Our initial research question was to understand whether the levels of parenting stress in adoptive families were similar to those of non-adoptive families. Our sample differs from other studies that have analyzed stress in adoptive parenthood, in that it is not a clinical sample but rather it is a broad and representative sample of the domestic adoptions carried out in our region. Our data, with regards to stress in the adoptive parents of children (7 to 11 years old), confirms the results of other studies: it has been found that their stress levels were similar to—and sometimes even lower than—those found in normative samples (Judge, 2003, 2004; Bird et al., 2002; Levy-Shiff et al., 1997). We found that the level of stress related to the children's characteristics (CD) was similar to that in the normative sample; whereas the levels of total stress (TS) and parent domain stress (PD) were lower than in the normative sample. If we bear in mind the percentage of mothers whose stress level exceeds the clinical range, this is much lower among adoptive mothers than that found in the normative data. Only in the case of parenting stress related to the characteristics of the children are the proportions similar between adoptive and non-adoptive. As for the stress of the parents with adolescent children, some differences are found. In comparison with the normative data from non-adoptive families, as in the case of families with younger children, the total stress level and Parent Domain are lower in the adoptive families studied. Only the adolescents ' characteristics (Adolescent Domain in SIPA) are more stressful for their parents, but their own positive perception of parenting (as attested by the parent domain scores in SIPA) brings about a balanced total stress score which is comparable with that of other samples or even lower. However, the proportion of mothers scoring above the clinical cut-off is higher. This probably implies that although, as to general group, adoptive mothers do not experience higher total stress, among the adoptive mothers there is a larger proportion of mothers who are highly stressed, reaching the clinical range.

The first conclusion, therefore, in this sense, is that the mothers of adopted children (7 to 11 years) do not have higher levels of parenting stress. The second conclusion is that parenting stress is greater as the children grow older and are closer to adolescence. We could ask ourselves if this increase the levels of their mothers' stress is contributed by the current age of these children, or the age when they were adopted. It is necessary to remember that, while the school age children (PSI) of our sample were, for the most part, babies (less than 1 year) when they were adopted; the adolescents we interviewed were, on average, three years old at the time of adoption. It is well documented that the age at the time of the adoption appears as a risk factor for later adjustment of the adoptee, with poorer adaptations in older children. The hypothesis could be that the characteristics of the children who are now adolescents were more complicated at the start. However, as the data has shown, during the school years, only the actual age (current age) correlates with all the stress measures, explaining part of the variance in the regression equation. In addition, the initial age of the adolescents does not correlate with the stress sub-scale due to the characteristics of the adolescents (AD), and nor is it a variable that plays a part in the regression equation explaining total parenting stress during adolescence. During adolescence, we also find that the stress level increases because the parent-child relationships become more complicated as children grow (APRD domain). Therefore, as adopted children grow, their mothers find it more difficult to make a correct balance between the demands outlined by the situation and the resources and responses given to adapt to such a situation. Brodzinsky, Smith, & Brodzinsky (1998) had suggested that with adolescence, new tasks appear in the adoptive families. Among the tasks of the adolescents are: integrating adoption into to stable and secure identity, coping with adoption loss, exploring thoughts and feelings about birth family and birth heritage, exploring feelings about the search process, and maintaining open communication with parents about adoption. The adoptive parents of adolescents find they must help the adolescent to cope with ongoing adoption-related loss, fostering positive view of the birth family, supporting the teenager's search interests and plans, helping the adolescent develop realistic expectations regarding searching, and maintaining open communication about adoption. Moreover, we must remember that the differences with non-adoptive families are hardly noticeable; therefore, it is highly possible that we could be talking about demands more related to adolescence than with adoption. In this regard, it would be a good idea to perform more longitudinal studies with adoptive and non-adoptive samples to shed light on this question, and this would enable us to approach the problem from a developmental perspective.

Following the logic of the stress theory, the adults in these families are experiencing their adoptive parenthood with various levels of stress. The way in which adoptive parents carry out successful parenthood, which allows the accomplished integration of their children and appropriate development, will be related to the way in which the stressors that the family encounters are articulated, the resources they have and the significance they attribute to the situation. Remembering the model proposed by Abidin (1995) for the study of the determinant of styles of dysfunctional parenthood, the stressors that a father or a mother experiences would depend on certain characteristics of their children, on certain characteristics of the parents and on certain situational variables. Our data shows that, in the case of mothers, certain characteristics of their children increase the possibilities of more stress, in the way they experience motherhood (among the school age children, having a disability, being older or being a boy; among adolescents: having been adopted along with a biological sibling or having had previous experiences of abuse). These conclusions are extremely relevant when intervening in the adoptive environment. We have been able to identify the strongest stressors linked to the characteristics of adopted children; in other words, it is more probable that when children are adopted with some of these characteristics, the role of the parent becomes more complicated. Since these characteristics put greater demands on the parents, it is essential to bear this in mind for both the training of future adoption applicants and the follow up of these adoptions. In Spain, in the past two decades, major changes have been made regarding the selection and preparation of future adoptive parents, as well as the follow up of these adoptions (León, Sánchez-Sandoval, Palacios, & Román, 2010). Intervention in adoption should try to include the latest discoveries in psychological research.

Among the stress factors related to family dynamics, the data shows a similar tendency to that of the non-adoptive families. The perception of stress is closely correlated with the educational styles of the parents. And this hold true for both adoptive families with school age children and families with adolescent children. The mothers with less affectionate and talkative educational styles show more stress in motherhood. These conclusions coincide with those of León (2011), using the same measures in an international adoption sample, the families with lower stress levels are characterized by the high level of affection and communication expressed to their children, but also by the maintenance of an appropriate level of demands and control. As Tan et al. (2012) indicate, to understand the mechanisms underlying the connection between family stress and child adjustment, many studies have turned to the role of parenting and Baumrind's (1971; 1973) parenting styles. In a study with adopted girls from China, the results showed that adoptive mothers reported relatively mild family stress, frequent authoritative parenting, and few behavior problems in their children. Moreover, family stress and authoritarian and permissive parenting styles positively correlated with children's behavioral problems (Tan et al., 2002). The results conclude that negative parenting mediates the effect of stressful life events on children's psychological symptoms (Grant et al., 2003).

From the model we are analyzing with our data, the balance between stressor events and the resources available to families to confront such stressors constitutes a fundamental aspect. We have explored to what extent the adoptive families have had help in the adoption process, and what relation the use of different resources could have (factor b in the double ACBX model) in their adoptive parenthood experience. Firstly, our data corroborates the importance of personal resources. Thus, families with a lower educational level are experiencing adoptive motherhood with higher stress levels. Secondly, our study corroborates the importance of having social resources. Other research has shown that the more limited the social support, the higher the parenting stress. Our data serves to add certain connotations to this conclusion. Our families, in general, stand out due to the quantity and considerable variety of support sources. In the case of our data, the resources most used by these families are the informal supports (partner, family and friends), these also being those that receive the best evaluation. That is to say, they counted on them and what is more, they have been useful. Furthermore, the families were able to rely on informal support networks independent of whether they had high or low stress levels. The differences were found in the use and evaluation of the formal networks and those specialized in adoption. Some families have also counted on additional support to face the demands of their adoptive parenthood. The women who are experiencing their motherhood with more stress have more often appealed to external resources such as help from organizations, professionals or printed material. At the same time, these services have been perceived as less useful by these families in comparison with informal support. Lastly, the families with high stress levels in parenthood perceived the help of adoption services as less useful, although the action of outside professionals was valued more in those cases of higher levels of stress.

Our conclusion is that since this sample is not clinical, with stress levels similar to non-adoptive families, in most cases informal supports have been enough, as with other families. Only in the cases of high stress levels did families require specialized attention. This specialized attention is not satisfied by the initial, and very general, adoption services, but rather it must be articulated through specialized services, not only in adoption, but in family, child and adolescent development. Moreover, those adoptions that could initially be more complicated (sibling adoption, for instance) should have greater access to support services. Nevertheless, research demonstrates that post-adoption support services are scarce and irregular, with many families failing to gain access to such services (Rushton & Dance, 2002). It is essential to ensure that such resources and help provided is evermore heterogeneous, sophisticated and adapted to the specific needs of the various adoptive family types (Brooks, Allen, and Barth, 2002). Post-adoption services must not perceive the situation as "deficit" (where adopted children are problematic children and adoptive parents are unable to cope with the adoption), but rather, they must be oriented from the recognition that, with enough support, adoptive families can be fully capable of confronting tensions generated by family relationships and the problems derived from past or present experiences (Sánchez-Sandoval & Palacios, 2012).

Our data also sustains the importance of the cognitive processes of attributing significance to situations (factor c in the double ACBX model). The way in which the parents perceive their similarities/differences when compared with non-adoptive families is one of the variables that predicted parenting stress. Our data seems to agree with the finding of Brodzinsky (1990) that an insistence on the differences causes greater adjustment difficulties and family problems for adoptive families. Additionally, being that this research was longitudinal, we were able to confirm how family perceptions are maintained over time; thus, the perception that families had six years ago is related with the current parenting stress—the greater the perception of differences, the higher the stress. This perception is probably fruit, in part, of their own experience as adoptive parents, so that the more complicated adoptions at first could be linked with a worse subsequent adjustment of the adopted children. However, it is noteworthy to mention that in the regression equation that explains the stress in the parenthood of the parents of adolescents, once the effect of the individual variables of the children has been taken into consideration, the perception of differences continues to explain part of the variance of the stress. In the same line, Viana and Welsh (2010) showed that pre-adoption family expectations were significantly related with post-adoption parenting stress. Our data emphasizes the importance of parental belief systems. Again, this data has major repercussions on the practical level. The preparation and education phase of potential adopters is an ideal point for professionals to work on the adjustment of the parents' expectations regarding the adoption.

In conclusion, this data validates the model of parenting stress proposed for the analysis of the adjustment of the adoptive families. The data again reflects that adoption is, at the same time, a normal and a specific circumstance, bringing parents some sources of strain which are common to any other form of parenthood, together with certain others which are specifically linked to adoption. As our data and those of other authors appear to substantiate, although adoptive families find it more complicated to educate some children than others, depending on their characteristics at the start, other family and contextual variables can compensate or complicate this reality even more.

ACKNOWLEDGMENTS

The research reported in this chapter was funded by the Andalusian Department of Social Affairs in Andalusia, Spain. Our most sincere thanks go to all the families who unselfishly participated in this study. My appreciation goes Professor J. Palacios for encouraging me to write this chapter.

REFERENCES

Abidin, R. (1990). *Parenting Stress Index/short form manual.* Los Angeles, CA: Western Psychological Services.

Abidin, R. (1992). The determinants of parenting behavior. *Journal of Clinical Child Psychology, 19,* 298–301.

Abidin, R. (1995). *Parenting Stress Index (3rd edn).* Odessa, FL: Psychological Assessment Resources, Inc.

Anthony, L. G., Anthony, B. J., Glanville, D. N., Naiman, D. Q., Waanders, C., & Shaffer, S. (2005). The relationships between parenting stress, parenting behaviour and preschoolers' social competence and behaviour problems in the classroom. *Infant Child Development, 14,* 133–154. doi: 10.1002/icd.385.

Baker, B. L., Blacher, J., & Olsson, M. B. (2005). Preschool children with and without: behaviour problems, parents' optimism and well-being. *J Intellect Disabil Res., 49,* 575-590.

Baumrind, D. (1971). Current patterns of parental authority. *Developmental Psychology, 4* (1), 1-103.

Baumrind, D. (1973). The development of instrumental competence through socialization. In A. D. Pick (Ed.), *Minnesota symposium on child psychology* (pp. 3-46). Minneapolis, MN: University of Minnesota Press.

Beckman, P. J., & Pokorni, J. L. (1988). A longitudinal study of families of preterm infants: Changes in stress and support over the first two years. *The Journal of Special Education, 22,* 55–65.

Bejenaru, A. & Roth, M. (2012). Romanian adoptive families: Stressors, coping strategies and resources. *Children and Youth Services Review, 34* (7), 1317-1324.

Berástegui, A. (2007). La adaptación familiar en adopción internacional: un proceso de estrés y afrontamiento. *Anuario de Psicología, 38(2),* 209-224.

Bird, G., Peterson, R., & Miller, S. H. (2002). Factors associated with distress among support-seeking adoptive parents. *Family Relations, 51,* 215-220.

Brodzinsky, D. M. (1987). Adjustment to adoption: A psychosocial perspective. *Clinical Psychology Review, 7,* 25-47.

Brodzinsky, D. (1990). A stress and coping model of adoption adjustment. In D.M. Brodzinsky & M. D. Schechter (Eds.), *The psychology of adoption* (pp. 3-24). New York: Oxford University Press.

Brodzinsky, D. M., Smith, D. W. & Brodzinsky, A. B. (1998). *Children's adjustment to adoption.* (Vol. 38). London: SAGE.

Brooks, D., Allen, J., & Barth, R. P. (2002). Adoption service use, helpfulness, and need: A comparison of public and private agency and independent adoptive families. *Children and Youth Services Review, 24,* 213-238.

Ceballo, R., Lansford, J. E., Abbey, A., & Stewart, A. J. (2004). Gaining a Child: Comparing the Experiences of Biological Parents, Adoptive Parents, and Stepparents. *Family Relations, 53* (1), 38-48.

Cohen, N. J., Duvall, J., & Coyne, J. C. (1994). *Characteristics of Post-adoptive families presenting for mental health service.* Newmarket, Ontario: Children's Aid Society of York Region.

Cohen, J. J. & Westhues, A. (1990). *Well-functioning families for adoptive and foster children*. Toronto: University of Toronto Press.

Deater-Deckard, K. (1998). Parenting stress and child adjustment: Some old hypotheses and new questions. *Clinical Psychology: Science and Practice, 5,* 314-332.

Deater-Deckard. K. (2004). *Parenting stress.* Yale University Press.

Estes, A., Munson, J., Dawson, G., Koehler, E., Zhou, X. H., & Abbott, R. (2009). Parenting stress and psychological functioning among mothers of preschool children with autism and developmental delay. *Autism, 13*(4), 375–387.

Fernández-Molina, M., Fuentes, M. J. & Fernández-Berrocal, P. (2012). Parental satisfaction predictors in families with adopted adolescents. *Revista mexicana de Psicología, 29* (1), 49-56.

Gagnon-Oosterwaal, N., Cossette, L., Smolla, N., Pomerleau, A., Malcuit, G., Chicoine, J.F., Céline Belhumeur, C., Jéliu, G., Bégin, J. & Séguin, R. (2012). Pre-adoption adversity, maternal stress, and behavior problems at school-age in international adoptees. *Journal of Applied Developmental Psychology, (in press,* available online 15 July 2012.

Grant, K., Compas, B., Stuhlmacher, A., Thurm, A., McMahon, S., & Halpert, J. (2003). Stressors and child and adolescent psychopathology: Moving from markers to mechanisms of risk. *Psychological Bulletin, 129*(3), 447–466.

Grant, K. E., Compas, B. E., Thurm, A. E., McMahon, S. D., & Gipson, P. (2004). Stressors and child and adolescent psychopathology: Measurement issues and prospective effects. *Journal of Clinical Child and Adolescent Psychology, 33,* 412-425.

Groothues, C., Beckett, C., & O'Connor, T. (1998). The outcome of adoptions from Romania. *Adoption & Fostering, 22*(4), 30-39.

Groze, V. (1994). Clinical and nonclinical adoptive families of special-needs children. *Families in Society, Feb,* 90-104.

Hassall, R., Rose, J., & McDonald, J. (2005). Parenting stress in mothers of children with an intellectual disability: the effects of parental cognitions in relation to child characteristics and family support. *J Intellect Disabil Res., 49,* 405-418.

Havighurst, R. J. (1972). *Developmental tasks and education.* New York: McKay.

Hidalgo, M. V. (1994). *El proceso de convertirse en padre y madre. Análisis ecológico desde la psicología evolutiva.* Unpublished Doctoral Dissertation. Universidad de Sevilla.

Hill, R. (1958). Generic features of families under stress. *Social Casework, 49*(2), 139-150.

Judge, S. L. (2003). Determinants of parental stress in families adopting children from Eastern Europe. *Family Relations, 52,* 241-248.

Judge, S. L. (2004). The impact of early institutionalization on child and family outcomes. *Adoption Quarterly, 7,* 31-48.

Karras, J., VanDeventer, M., & Braungart-Riker, J. (2003). Predicting shared parent-child book reading in infancy. *Journal of Family Psychology, 17,* 134-146.

Katz, L. (1986). Parental stress and factors for success in older-child adoption. *Child Welfare, LXV,* 569-578.

Kaye, K. (1990). Acknowledgment or Rejection or Differences? In D. M. Brodzinsky & M. D. Schechter (Eds.), *The psychology of adoption* (pp. 121-143). New York: Oxford University Press.

Kirk, H. D. (1964). *Shared fate.* New York: Free Press.

Kirk, H. D. (1985). *Adoptive kinship. A modern institution in need of reform.* Port Angeles: Ben-Simon Publications.

Leigh, B. & Milgrom, J. (2008). Risk factors for antenatal depression, postnatal depression and parenting stress. *BMC Psychiatry 2008, 8*(24).

León, E. (2011). *Desarrollo, adaptación y ajuste psicológico de los niños y niñas adoptados internacionalmente.* Unpublished Doctoral Dissertation. University of Seville.

León, E., Sánchez Sandoval, Y., Palacios, J., & Román, M. (2010). Programa de Formación para la Adopción en Andalucía. *Papeles del Psicólogo, 31* (1), 3-13.

Levy-Shiff, R., Zoran, N., & Shulman, S. (1997). International and domestic adoption: child, parents, and family adjustment. *International Journal of Behavioral Development, 20,* 109-129.

Mainemer, H., Gilman, L. C., & Ames, E. W. (1998). Parenting stress in families adopting children from Romanian orphanages. *Journal of Family Issues, 19,* 164-180.

McCubbin, H. I., & Patterson, J. M. (1983). The family stress process: The double ABCX model of adjustment and adaptation. *Marriage and Family Review, 6,* 7-37.

McGlone, K., Santos, L., Kazama, L., Fong, R., & Mueller, C. (2002). Psychological stress in adoptive parents of special-needs children. *Child Welfare, 81,* 151-171.

McMahon, C.A. & Meins, E. (2012). Mind-mindedness, parenting stress, and emotional availability in mothers of preschoolers. *Early Childhood Research Quarterly, 27* (2), 245–252.

Neece, C. L., Green, S. A. & Baker, B. L. (2012). Parenting Stress and Child Behavior Problems: A Transactional Relationship Across Time. *American Journal on Intellectual and Developmental Disabilities, 117* (1), 48-66.

Östberg, M. & Hagekull, B. (2000). A Structural Modeling Approach to the Understanding of Parenting Stress. *Journal of Clinical Child Psychology , 29* (4), 615-625.

Palacios, J. (1997). Familias adoptivas. In M. J. Rodrigo & J. Palacios (Eds.), *Familia y desarrollo humano .* Madrid: Alianza.

Palacios J., & Sánchez-Sandoval, Y. (2000). Escala revisada de Evaluación de Estilos Educativos (4e-r) [Revised scale for the Evaluation of Child Rearing Styles(4e-r)] University of Sevilla. Unpublished manuscript.

Palacios, J. & Sánchez-Sandoval, Y. (2006). Stress in parents of adopted children. *International Journal of Behavioral Development,* 30 (6), 481-487.

Palacios, J., Sánchez Sandoval, Y., & León, E. (2005). Intercountry adoption disruptions in Spain. *Adoption Quarterly,* 9(1), 35-55.

Palacios, J., Sánchez-Sandoval, Y., & Sánchez-Espinosa, E. (1996). La adopción en Andalucía. *Apuntes de Psicología, 48,* 9-29.

Palacios, J., Sánchez-Sandoval, Y., León, E. & Román, M. (2010). Adopción: recuperación tras la adversidad inicial. In A. Almeida & N. Fernandes (Ed.), *Intervenção psicosocial com crianças, jovens e famílias* (pp. 273-286). Coimbra: Almedina.

Patterson, G. R. (1988). Stress: A change agent for family process. In N. Garmezy & M. Rutter (Eds.), *Stress, coping, and development in children* (pp. 235-264). Baltimore: John Hopkins University Press.

Pinderhughes, E. E. (1996). Toward understanding family readjustment following older child adoptions: The interplay between theory generation and empirical research. *Children and Youth Services Review, 18,* 115-138.

Pozo, P., Sarriá, E., & Méndez, L. (2006). Estrés en madres de personas con trastornos del espectro autista. *Psicothema, 18* (3), 342-347.

Rijk, C., Hoksbergen, R. A. C., ter Laak, J.,van Dijkum, C., & Robbroeckx, L. (2006). Parent who adopt deprived children have a difficult task. *Adoption Quarterly, 9,* 37–61.

Rosenthal, J. A. & Groze, V. K. (1992). *Special needs adoption: a study of intact families.* New York: Praeger.

Rushton, A. & Dance, C. (2002). *Adoption support services for families in difficulty: A literature review and survey of UK practice.* London: BAAF.

Sánchez-Sandoval, Y. (2011). Satisfacción con la adopción y con sus repercusiones en la vida familiar (Adoptive parents' satisfaction with the adoption experience and with its impact on family life). *Psicothema, 23* (4), 630-635.

Sánchez-Sandoval, Y. & Palacios, J. (2012). Stress in adoptive parents of adolescents. *Children and Youth Services Review, 34* (7), 1283-1289.

Sánchez Sandoval, Y., León, E., & Román, M. (2012). Adaptación familiar de niños y niñas adoptados internacionalmente. *Anales de Psicología, 28* (2), 558-566.

Sánchez Sandoval, Y., Palacios, J., & León, E. (2004). Características de los niños y niñas procedentes de adopciones internacionales: historia previa y nivel de desarrollo. *Portularia,* 269-276.

Se, S. & Moon, H. (2012). Do korean young children's daily routines and their mothers' parenting stress differ according to socioeconomic status? *Social, Behavior and Personality, 40* (3), 481-500.

Sheras, P. L., Abidin, R. R., & Konold, T. R. (1998). *Stress index for parents of adolescents.* Odessa, FL: Psychological Assessment Resources, Inc.

Silva, L. M. T., & Schalock, M. (2012). Autism parenting stress index: Initial psychometric evidence. *Journal of Autism and Developmental Disorders, 42,* 566-574.

Tan, T. X., Camras, L. A., Deng, H., Zhang, M. & Lu, Z. (2012). Family stress, parenting styles, and behavioral adjustment in preschool-age adopted Chinese girls. *Early Childhood Research Quarterly, 27*(1), 128–136.

Tervo, R. C. (2012). Developmental and Behavior Problems Predict Parenting Stress in Young Children With Global Delay. *Journal of Child Neurology, 27*(3) 291-296.

Viana, A.G., & Welsh, J.A. (2010). Correlates and predictors of parenting stress among internationally adopting mothers: A longitudinal investigation. *International Journal of Behavioral Development, 34*(4), 363-373.

Visconti, K.J. (2005). Parental stress and child behavioral adjustment in children with congenital heart disease. In K.V. Oxington (Ed.), *Stress and health : New research.* (pp. 1–42). NY: Nova Science Publishers.

Webster, R. I., Majnemer, A., Platt, R. W., & Shevell, M. I. (2008). Child health and parental stress in school-age children with a preschool diagnosis of developmental delay. *J Child Neurol, 23,* 32-38.

Chapter 4

DIFFERENT SENSITIVITY TO CHRONIC STRESS INDUCED COGNITIVE DEFICIT AND IMMUNE ALTERATION IN BALB/C AND C57BL/6 INBRED MICE: INVOLVEMENT OF HIPPOCAMPAL NO PRODUCTION AND TH1/TH2 BALANCE

María Laura Palumbo and Ana María Genaro
CEFYBO-CONICET, 1ª. Cátedra de Farmacología, Facultad de Medicina, UBA,
Buenos Aires, Argentina

ABSTRACT

Stress is defined as any situation capable of perturbing the physiological or psychological homeostasis. While response to stress is a necessary survival mechanism, prolonged stress can have several repercussions affecting behavioral, endocrine and immunological parameters. Two genetically different inbred murine strains C57BL/6 and BALB/c, show distinct behavioral and immunological responses. In this chapter we show a comparative study on the effect of chronic mild stress upon learning and memory and immunity in BALB/c and C57BL/6 mice. Stressed BALB/c showed poor learning performance related to structural and neurochemical changes observed in the hippocampus, such as a decrease of neurogenesis, a decrease of neural nitric oxide synthase (nNOS) activity and an increase in reactive oxygen species (ROS) levels. These alterations were not found in C57BL/6 mice subjected to CMS. In vivo administration of a nNOS inhibitor induced behavioral alterations in both strains. Moreover, in vitro treatment with a nNOS inhibitor induced an increase in ROS levels. Respect to immune response, CMS BALB/c mice showed a decrease in the T-lymphocyte and an increase of B-lymphocyte mitogen-stimulated proliferation, and an imbalance towards Th2 cytokines. In addition, CMS BALB/c mice had poor antibody production after in vivo immunization with a T-cell depending antigen. On the contrary, CMS C57BL/6 animals showed an increase in the reactivity of T-lymphocytes without changes in the B-lymphocytes reactivity, no changes in humoral response after immunization and an imbalance towards Th1 cytokines. Concerning the participation of the classically stress-associated hormones (catecholamines and corticosterone) in the above mentioned findings, the results indicate that there was not a temporal coincidence between the increase of corticosterone and catecholamines and the behavioral and immune alterations. Taking into account, our results suggest a different vulnerability to cognitive deficit and immune alterations after chronic stress exposure in BALB/c and C57BL/6 mice. These different responses could be related to a differential regulation of hippocampal NO production and peripheral Th1/Th2 cytokine balance. In addition, the relationship between these effects is also analyzed.

INTRODUCTION

In the last decades, stress has become an important aspect of modern life. Exposure to adverse situations affects virtually all people in the whole world. Every day, we are challenged by a considerable number of stressors, as varied as divorce, an exam, a relative' serious illness, an accident, a natural disaster, being unemployed, moving house and so on. Stress is defined as any situation capable of perturbing the physiological or psychological homeostasis. While response to stress is a necessary survival mechanism, prolonged stress can have several repercussions affecting behavioral, endocrine and immunological parameters (McEwen, 1998). Recognition of these effects has led McEwen to develop a new terminology to link the protective and damaging effect of the biologic response to stressors, namely, allostasis and allostatic overload (McEwen, 2008). These two terms allow for a more restricted and precise definition of the overused word "stress", and provide a view of how the essential protective and adaptive effects of the physiological mediators that maintain homeostasis are also involved in the cumulative effects of daily life when they are mismanaged or overused. Allostasis refers to the adaptive processes that maintain homeostasis through the production of mediators such as adrenalin, cortisol and cytokines. These mediators of the stress response promote adaptation in the aftermath of acute stress, but they also contribute to allostatic overload, the wear and tear on the body and brain that result from being "stressed out" (McEwen, 2008).

On the other hand, it has been observed that C57BL/6 and BALB/c, two genetically different inbred strains of mice, differ one from another in several behavioral responses and in neurodevelopment and neurochemistry parameters. Thus, BALB/c is considered an emotive and anxious strain with a low basal locomotor activity and increased stress reactivity; whereas C57BL/6 is considered a non-emotive, non-anxious and active strain in different experimental situations, such as the open-field test or the elevated plus-maze test (Belzung and Griebel, 2001; Tang *et al.*, 2002). Concerning the neurochemical studies, BALB/c mice show approximately two fold lower levels of serotonin in the forebrain than C57BL/6 strain (Zhang *et al.*, 2004). The concentration of 17-OH-pregnenolone, a neurosteroid related to behavior, e.g. aggression, adaptation to stress or learning in mice, is significantly higher in the whole brain of C57BL/6 than in BALB/c animals (Tagawa *et al.*, 2006). Moreover, significantly less maternal care and elevated stress-induced corticosterone levels were observed in BALB/c as compared to C57BL/6J mice (Priebe *et al.*, 2005). Also, genetic control of the Th1/Th2 balance has been related to differences in both innate (Watanabe *et al.*, 2004) and acquired immunity (Guiñazú *et al.*, 2004).

Deregulation of cytokines induced by stress exposure (Th1 versus Th2) has been reported to be involved in the pathogenesis of many human illnesses such as autoimmune diseases, sleep disturbance, major depression and other disorders (Kaufmann *et al.*, 2007; Schwarz *et al.*, 2001).

Stress is a key factor in the development of several pathologies, including psychiatric diseases such as anxiety and major depression, disruption of neuroendocrine systems, alterations of the immune response and even cancer (McEwen, 2007, 2008; Glaser and Kiecolt-Glaser, 2005; Reiche *et al.*, 2004). Therefore, a lot of interest has been given to the understanding of causes and effects of responses of the organism to stressors. The main mediators in the adaptive response to stressors involve glucocorticoids, catecholamines and the balance between pro-inflammatory (Th1) versus anti-inflammatory (Th2) cytokines (McEwen, 2008).

In this context, we show a comparative study on the effect of stress exposure upon learning and memory and immunity in Th1-biased C57BL/6 versus Th2-biased BALB/c mice. We show previous and new results and we discuss the correlation between peripheral mediators with brain and cognitive alterations. This integrated study could help understanding of causes and effects of the responses of the organism to stressors and could be useful to generate new strategies to the treatment of the adverse consequences of stress.

MATERIALS AND METHODS
ANIMALS

Inbred female BALB/c and C57BL/6 mice were purchased from Veterinary School of the University of Buenos Aires. Sixty-day-old mice weighing between 23 and 25 g at the beginning of the experiments were used. Mice were housed and maintained on an 8:00 AM to 8:00 PM light/dark cycle under controlled temperatures (18-22°C). Except as indicated below, food and water were freely available. Animal care was in accordance with the principles and guidelines of the Guide for the Care and Use of Laboratory Animals, US National Research Council, 1996. Two weeks before the beginning of the experiments, phases of the estrous cycle were monitored daily in order to verify that all mice have a synchronized estrous cycle.

CHRONIC MILD STRESS MODEL

The stress scheme was slightly modified from those previously used in rats (Willner *et al.*, 1992) and mice (Monleon *et al.*, 1995). Animals were housed singly and exposed to: one 16-h period of water deprivation; two periods of continuous overnight illumination; two periods (7 and 17 h) of 45° cage tilt; one 17-h period in a soiled cage (100 ml water in sawdust bedding); one period (8 h) of food deprivation; one 17-h period of paired housing (animals were always housed in the same pairs, but host cages were alternated between each member of the pair). All individual stressors used had been classified as "mild" according to the Animals Scientific Procedures Act of 1986 (UK legislation). The stressors were scheduled throughout nine weeks in a similar manner to that previously described (see CMS scheme in Palumbo *et al.*, 2007). Animals were left undisturbed in their home cages 24h prior to sacrifice.

BEHAVIORAL TESTS

Open Field

Open-field habituation was performed using a rectangular chamber (42 cm x 35 cm x 15 cm) made of gray polyvinylchloride (PVC) (Frisch *et al.*, 2005). The floor of the open field was uniformly divided into 30 squares of 7 x 7 cm. A low-level loudspeaker provided a broad spectrum masking noise. The apparatus was cleaned with water containing 0.1% acetic acid after each trial. Mice were acclimated to the testing room for at least 20 min prior to testing. On the first day animals were placed in the open field (first exposure) and locomotor activity was evaluated. Behavioral parameters recorded during 5-min sessions were: (1) crossings (horizontal activity): the number of horizontal lines crossed; (2) rearing (vertical activity): the number of times a mouse stood on its hind legs with forelegs in the air or against the wall; and (3) corner time: the time spent in any corner. After 24 h mice were re-exposed to the open field to evaluate changes in behavioral parameters. The open field test was performed between 5:00 and 7:00 pm. Sessions were recorded using a video camera (Sony DCB-DVD810). Because mice demonstrate less exploratory activity in a familiar environment, this simple test assesses the ability of the mouse to learn and remember the open-field chamber. Habituation was estimated as the relative decrease in activity between the first exposure and re-exposures to the open field (Frisch *et al.*, 2005).

Y-Maze Spontaneous Alternation

Spontaneous alternation behavior in a Y-maze task was recorded and evaluated as a spatial memory task. The apparatus consisted of three identical black plexiglass arms (l × w × h, 28 × 10 × 20 cm). Mice were acclimated to the testing room for at least 20 min prior to testing. At the beginning of the session, mice were placed at the end of one fixed arm of the Y-maze and allowed to explore freely for 6 min. The sequence of arm entries was recorded using a video camera (Sony DCB-DVD810). An alternation refers to three successive visits to the three separate arms of the maze. The alternation percentage was calculated as the number of alternations divided by the total arm entries minus 2, multiplied by 100 (Dillon *et al.*, 2008; Kim *et al.*, 2008).

Passive Avoidance

The step-through passive avoidance response was examined between 10:00 AM and 2:00 PM every day. The apparatus consisted of two compartments; one was illuminated with a 60 W lamp and the other was dark. The compartments were separated by a guillotine door (20 x 20 mm). Before the first trial, each mouse was allowed to explore both the illuminated and dark compartments freely for 180 s, and the time spent in the dark and light compartment was measured (light-dark distribution test). On the first day, mice were placed into the illuminated compartment. When all four paws were on the grid of the dark compartment, the mouse received a shock of 0.5 mA for 3 s. Mice could escape from the shock only by stepping back into the safe illuminated compartment. Mice were then returned to their home cages. One hour and 24 h after training, mice were tested and the response latency for entering the dark compartment was measured. The latency of mice that did not move into the dark compartment for more than 5 min was taken as 300 s.

EVALUATION OF ADULT NEUROGENESIS

Administration of 5-Bromo-2'-Deoxyuridine and Tissue Preparation

Mice received intraperitoneal injections of 5-bromo-2'-deoxyuridine (BrdU, Sigma-Aldrich, St. Louis, MO, USA) 50 mg/kg every 12 hours for 5 consecutive days. Four weeks after the last BrdU injection, mice were anesthetized (100 µg ketamine + 10 µg xylazine g^{-1}, i.m.) and perfused intracardially with PBS and then with 4% paraformaldehyde (PFA). Housing, treatments, surgery and euthanasia were carried out according to NIH guidelines, and all experiments were performed following guidelines laid by the Leloir Institute animal welfare committee. Brains were removed and sectioned (40 µm) using a sliding microtome (Leica, Wetzlar, Germany).

Immunohistochemistry

For BrdU immunostaining, free-floating coronal sections (40-µm thick) were washed with Tris-buffered saline (TBS) and incubated for 2 hours in 50% formamide solution at 65°C and then in 2N HCl at 37°C. Sections were washed with TBS, blocked for 1 hour with TBS containing 3% donkey serum and 0.25% Triton X-100, and incubated for 72 hours with the primary antibodies in blocking solution. Primary antibodies were: rat anti-BrdU (1:200; Boehringer Manheim, Roche, Basel, Switzerland) and mouse anti-neuron-specific nuclear protein (anti-NeuN; 1:50, kindly provided by F.H. Gage), included in some sections to corroborate the neuronal phenotype. Secondary antibodies were donkey anti-rat Cy-3 and donkey anti-mouse Cy-5 (1:250; Jackson ImmunoResearch, West Grove, Pennsylvania, United States).

Cell Counting

For immunohistochemical analysis of adult hippocampal neurogenesis, 1 every 12 coronal sections spanning the entire dentate gyrus were taken for each mouse. Neurogenesis was assessed counting $BrdU^+$ cells using fluorescence microscopy (Zeiss Axiovert 135M) with a 10x objective and a DDC camera (Hamamatsu ORCA C474295). Only $BrdU^+$ cells located in the granule cell layer and subgranular zone of the dentate gyrus (DG) were counted. The total number of labeled cells per dentate gyrus was then obtained for each mouse by multiplying the number of $BrdU^+$ cells x 12. It is well known that, four weeks after of the last BrdU injection the majority of $BrdU^+$ cells in the dentate gyrus are mature neurons (Kempermann *et al.*, 2003). The phenotype $BrdU^+$ cell was corroborated by NeuN labeling.

Confocal images were taken using a Zeiss Pascal confocal microscope (Zeiss, Jena, Germany) with a 1-μm pinhole. Co-localization was analyzed in single optical planes taken through the entire z-axis of each cell using Zeiss LSM Image Browser Software.

DETERMINATION OF THE OXIDATION STATE IN HIPPOCAMPUS

NOS Activity

Nitric oxide synyhase activity was determined by measuring conversion of [^{14}C] L-arginine (300 mCi/mmol, Perkin Elmer Inc., Waltham, MA, USA) to [^{14}C] L-citrulline as described by Bredt and Snyder (1990).

In brief, the hippocampi were pre-incubated in 50 mM HEPES buffer, pH 7.4 pre-warmed and equilibrated with 5% CO_2 in O_2.

Then tissues were homogenized by sonication in 1 mL of medium containing 20 mM HEPES (pH 7.4), 1mM dithiothreytol (DTT), 1 μM leupeptin, 0.45 mM $CaCl_2$ and 0.2 mM phenylmethanesulphonyl fluoride (PMSF) at 37°C for 30 min 5% CO_2 in O_2 in the presence of [^{14}C] L-arginine (0.5 μCi).

The reaction was stopped by quick ice cooling and the samples were centrifuged at 20,000 x g for 10 min at 4°C. Supernatants were passed through 2 mL Dowex AG 50 WX-8 (sodium form) (Bio-Rad, Hercules, CA, USA) columns. [^{14}C] L-citruline was eluted with 2 mL of water and quantified by liquid scintillation counting.

As expected the presence of a broad-spectrum NOS inhibitor L-NAME (Sigma-Aldrich, St. Louis, MO, USA), completely inhibit NOS activity in all groups of animals (data not shown). Results are expressed as pmoles of [^{14}C] L-citruline produced by g of tissue weight in 30 minutes. In some experiments, an eNOS inhibitor L-N5-1-Iminoethyl-ornithine hydrochloride (L-NIO, 0.8 μmol/L) or nNOS inhibitor 7-NI (10 μmol/L) (Sigma-Aldrich, St. Louis, MO, USA) was added.

Analysis of Reactive Oxygen Species

Determination of reactive oxygen species (ROS) was based on the method previously described (Keston and Brand, 1965; LeBel *et al.*, 1989). The method relies on oxidation of the non-fluorescent probe, 2,7-dichlorofluorescin diacetate (DCFH, Sigma-Aldrich, St. Louis, MO, USA), by reactive oxygen species, to form the highly fluorescent 2,7-dichloro-fluorescein (DCF).

Briefly, after sacrifice, the whole brain was immediately removed and, the hippocampus was dissected on ice and homogenized in ice-cold Locke´s buffer (NaCl 154 mmol/L, KCl 5.6 mmol/L, NaHCO3 3.6 mmol/L, CaCl2 2.3 mmol/L, glucosa 5.6 mmol/L, HEPES 5 mmol/L). Then, the homogenate was diluted in ice-cold Locke´s buffer to obtain a concentration of 0.5 mg tissue/mL. Aliquots of the homogenate were incubated with 2,7-dichlorofluorescin diacetate (final concentration 5 μmol/L) at 37° C for 15 min. Results were expressed as pmol/mg tissue/min.

Catalase Activity Measurement

Catalase activity, as measured by the loss of absorbance at 240 nm, was assayed according to the method of Beers (1952). Briefly, 10% w/v tissue homogenates were made in 50 mM phosphate buffer and therefore were centrifuged at 42000 × g for 15 min. A supernatant aliquot was incubated with 0.036% (w/w) hydrogen peroxide solution (H_2O_2). The time required to decrease the absorbance at 240 nm from 0.45 to 0.40 absorbance units was registered. One unit will decompose 1.0 μmol of H_2O_2/min at pH 7 at 25 °C. Results were calculated as catalase (CAT) units/mg tissue and expressed as mean ± SEM.

Superoxide Dismutase (SOD) Activity Measurement

SOD activity was determinated by the procedure of McCord and Fridovich (1969). Briefly, the tissues were homogenized at 10% w/v in a 216 mM, pH 7.8 phosphate buffer solution and were centrifuged at 900 × g at 4°C for 10 min. A supernatant aliquot was mixed with 216 mM, pH 7.8 phosphate buffer, 10.7 mM EDTA, 1.1 mM C cytochrome and 0.108 mM xanthine at 25 °C. Reaction started with the addition of 0.1 ml of xanthine oxidase (XO) enzyme solution (2 U/ml) (Sigma-Aldrich, St. Louis, MO, USA). The increase in the absorbance at 550 nm for 5 min was registered.

One unit of SOD is defined as the amount that inhibits the rate of reduction of cytochrome c by 50% in a coupled system, using xanthine and xanthine oxidase at pH 7.8 at 25 °C in a 3 ml reaction volume. Results were calculated as SOD units/mg tissue and expressed as mean ± SEM.

Determination of Glutathione

Determination of reduced glutathione (GSH) was performed by the GSH reductase recycling assay according to Tietze (1969). It based on the principle that GSH can be measured by an enzymatic recycling procedure in which it is sequentially oxidised by 5,5'-dithiobis-(2-nitrobenzoic acid; DTNB, Sigma-Aldrich, St. Louis, MO, USA) and reduced by NADPH in the presence of glutathione reductase. The rate of formation of 2-nitro-5-thiobenzoic acid (TNB) can be followed using a spectrophotometer and GSH quantified by reference to a standard curve. Briefly, the hippocampi were sonicated in 100 mM sodium phosphate buffer, pH 7.5 with 1mM EDTA. Trichloroacetic acid (TCA, 5%) was added to precipitated proteins and homogenates were centrifuged to 3700 rpm at 4°C for 10 min. Total and oxidized glutathione (GSSG) was determined in each sample. Homogenate was incubated 1 h with 1M 3-vinil pyridine (Sigma-Aldrich, St. Louis, MO, USA) a scavenger of GSH, for quantifying GSSG. Then, the reaction mixture (1 mM DTNB, 200 U/ml glutathione reductase (GR), 1mM NADPH and 100 mM sodium phosphate buffer pH 7.5 with 1mM EDTA) was added. Then, the absorbance at 405 nm was measured in an ELISA plate reader (Bio-Rad, Hercules, CA, USA). The GSH was calculated as the difference between the total glutathione and GSSG.

DETERMINATION OF LYMPHOCYTE ACTIVITY *IN VITRO*

Cell Suspensions and Culture Conditions

Lymphoid cell suspensions from control and CMS mice were obtained as previously described (Edgar *et al.*, 2002). Briefly, mice were sacrificed by decapitation and lymph nodes (axilary, inguinal and mesenteric) were removed and disrupted through a 1 mm metal mesh, and the cell suspension was filtered through a 10 μm nylon mesh. The suspension was depleted of red blood and dead cells by centrifugation over Ficoll/ Hypaque (density 1.084 from Sigma-Aldrich, St. Louis, MO, USA). After three washes in RPMI-1640 medium, cells were re-suspended in RPMI 1640 supplemented with 10% of batched-tested non-stimulatory fetal calf serum, 2 mM glutamine, 100 U/ml of penicillin, 100 μg/ml of streptomycin, and 50 μM beta-mercaptoethanol. Cell viability was estimated according to the Trypan blue exclusion criteria and was higher than 90%.

Mitogen Assay

Proliferation was determined by culturing 2×10^5 cells per well in 96-well plates in 100 μl triplicated aliquots in supplemented medium. Aliquots of 100 μl of mitogens were added to each microculture to yield the appropiate concentration: Concanavalin A (Con A; Sigma Aldrich, St. Louis, MO, USA) (0.5, 1 and 2 μg/ml) was used as a T-cell selective mitogens, and lipopolysaccharide (LPS; Sigma Aldrich, St. Louis, MO, USA) (30 μg/ml) as a B-cell selective mitogens, to induce proliferation. In control cultures, stimulants were replaced by 100 μl of culture medium. Then cells were cultured at 37 °C in a 5% CO_2 atmosphere for different periods. Mitogenic activity was measured by adding 1 μCi [^{3}H]-thymidine (20 Ci/mmol, Perkin Elmer Inc., Waltham, MA, USA) per well for the last 18-h period of culture. The thymidine incorporation was measured by scintillation counting after retention over GF/C glass-fiber filters (Whatman, Brentford, UK) of the acid insoluble macromolecular fraction.

The means of the triplicated determinations were calculated for each mitogen concentration. Mitogen-stimulated cells displayed the expected kinetic proliferation, with a peak of proliferation at the third day of culture. Results are expressed as stimulation index (S.I.) calculated as the rate between dpm values obtained from experimental cultures and those obtained from unstimulated cells.

Mitogen-stimulated cells displayed the expected kinetic proliferation, with a peak of proliferation at the 3rd day of culture.

Cytokine Release

To stimulate cytokines production lymphoid cells (1×10^6/ml) were incubated with Con A (1 μg/ml) for 24 h at 37 °C in a 5% CO_2 atmosphere in a Falcon 24-well plate, as previously described (Palumbo *et al.*, 2010; Takeno *et al.*, 2004). After incubation, culture supernatants were harvested and their IFN-γ and IL-10 levels were determined by ELISA kits (Amersham

Biosciences, Little Chalfont, Buckinghamshire, UK). It is important to note that 1 μg/ml of Con A is the optimal concentration that stimulated T cells proliferation giving a peak of proliferation at the third day of culture.

ANTIBODY PRODUCTION

Inmunization

Sheep red blood cells (SRBC) were used as immunogen to evaluate T-cell-dependent humoral response and lipopolysaccharide (LPS, Sigma-Aldrich, St. Louis, MO, USA) was used to determinate T-cell-independent humoral response.

For SRBC response, mice (n = 12) were intraperitoneally (i.p.) immunized on day 0 and boosted on day 11 with 0.2 ml of 4% SBRC in saline. Blood samples were collected for antibody determination on day 10 (primary response) and on day 18 (secondary response). For LPS, each mouse (n = 12) received an i.p. injection of 10 Ag LPS in 0.1 ml saline and blood samples were collected on day 10. Mice injected with vehicle were used as controls.

Antibody Titers

Serum obtained from retroorbital blood samples was stored at -20 °C until assayed. Quantitative enzyme-linked immunoadsorbent assay (ELISA) was performed to determine SRBC-specific antibodies. Briefly, 96 well plates (Greiner bio-one) were coated overnight with SRBC membranes (10 μg/ml) or LPS (2 μg/ml).

Dilutions of sera were added and incubated 2 h at room temperature, plates were washed, and samples were incubated with a goat IgG anti-mouse IgG phosphatase alkaline conjugated (Sigma-Aldrich, St. Louis, MO, USA) and p-nitrophenylphosphatase (Sigma-Aldrich, St. Louis, MO, USA) as substrate for developing coloration that was read at 405 nm. Reactions were considered positive when optical density (O.D.) values were above the mean value plus 2 S.D. of normal sera (sera from non-immunized vehicle injected mice that gave non-statistical differences among them).

HORMONE EVALUATION

Corticosterone Determination

To avoid fluctuations on plasma corticosterone levels due to circadian rhythms, animals were bled at 12:00 PM on the day of sacrifice. Blood from animals under different experimental conditions was collected on ice in 0.25 M EDTA and phases were separated in a refrigerated centrifuge. Plasma was stored at -80°C until the assay was performed. Corticosterone levels were determined by high-pressure liquid chromatography (HPLC) as a protocol slightly modified from that previously used in rats by Sargent (1985).

Catecholamines Assay

Catecholamines concentrations were determinated in spleen samples by a fluorometric assay (Laverty and Taylor, 1968). Briefly, spleens were homogenized in 12.5% sodium sulfite, 10% EDTA in 0.4 N percloric acid. After 24 h at 4ªC the homogenate was centrifugated at 5000 rpm for 10 min. The supernatants were brought to pH 8.2 and seeded in pre-washed alumina columns.

The eluate was oxidized with iodine in an alkaline medium. The fluorescence was recorded at 375 nm in a spectrofluorometer using an excitation source of 325nm.

STATISTICAL ANALYSIS

Data were analyzed using two-way ANOVA to examine significance of main effects and interactions. When interaction was significant, simple effects analysis (F) was made. When interaction was not significant, the Bonferroni's (t) post-hoc test was applied. Passive avoidance and antibody production data were not normally distributed; hence the non-parametric Mann-Whitney U-test was performed. Open field habituation data in animals treated with L-NAME were analyzed by two-way ANOVA for repeated measures (F) followed by Bonferroni (t). Student's t-test (T) was used to evaluate open field exploratory activity during the first exposure between two groups. Corticosterone data were analyzed with the non-parametric Friedman T^2-test. Differences between means were considered significant if $p < 0.05$.

RESULTS

Differential Effect of Chronic Stress on the Learning and Memory in BALB/c and C57BL/6 Mice

The effect of stress on learning and memory has been well documented in a diverse array of species from fish to human (Kim and Yoon 1998; McEwen 2000). To investigate the effect of stress on learning and memory performance, we used three different tasks. The Open Field task was performed to determine the ability to habituate to a novel environment; the Y-maze to evaluate spatial memory by measuring the rate of spontaneous alternation among arms and the passive avoidance to evaluate memory retention of aversive stimulus. Table 1 summarized the performance in different tests for control and stressed animals. For Open Field task, control BALB/c mice displayed habituation to the environment after repeated exposure, as indicated by the decrease in crossing (52%) and in rearing activity (55%) and by the increase in the time that mice stayed in the corner squares (82%). In addition, CMS exposure induced a significant lower habituation respect to control (crossing: $p < 0.001$; rearing: $p < 0.01$; corner time: $p < 0.05$). On the contrary, both control and CMS C57BL/6 mice showed habituation capacity 24 hs post-training indicated by the decrease in the number of crossings (45% and of 52%, respectively) and in the number of rearing (44% and 43%, respectively), and by the increase in the time remained in the corner of the cage (239% and 633%, respectively).

Table 1. Performace in open field, Y-maze and Passive Avoidance for control and CMS BALB/c and C57BL/6 mice

Strain		BALB/c		C57BL/6	
Condition		N	CMS	N	CMS
Open field [a]	**Croosing** decrease respect to training (%)	52 ± 5	3.98 ± 0.4 ***	45 ± 7	42 ± 5
	Rearing decrease respect to training (%)	55 ± 6	28 ± 3 **	44 ± 9	43 ± 7
	Corner time increase respect to training (%)	82 ± 6	55 ± 10 *	239 ± 80	633 ± 271
Y maze [b] spontaneous alternation (%)		68 ± 4	38 ± 4 ***	62 ± 3	57 ± 3
Passive avoidance [c] mice with maximal latency to escape (%)		70	20 *	40	67

a) Number of crossing, corner time and number of rearing are shown. Results are expressed as percentages respect to the first exposure and represent the mean ± SEM of 12 mice of each group. b) The percentage of spontaneous alternation was evaluated according to material and methods. Results represent the mean ± SEM of 8 mice of each group. c) The latency of scape 24 h post-training was determined for each group of mice. Results are shown as the percentage of mice with maximal latency to escape for 9 or 10 mice of each group. $*p < 0.05$, $**p < 0.01$, $***p < 0.001$ respect to corresponding control.

Similarly, BALB/c but not C57Bl/6 mice showed a decrease in the alternation of spontaneous behavior examined in a Y-maze task. Two-way ANOVA showed significant changes in the percentage of spontaneous alternation that depend on condition (control or CMS) and the strains of mice [interaction: strain x condition, $F(3,33) = 11.71$, $p < 0.01$]. As described in Table 1, simple effects analysis showed a significant decreased in CMS-BALB/c mice as compared to control [$F(1,33) = 35.26$, $p < 0.001$]. Non-significant differences were found in the percentage of spontaneous alternation between CMS and control C57BL/6 animals [$F(1,33) = 0.97$, NS].

Finally, in the passive avoidance task, both BALB/c and C57BL/6 mice showed a similar latency to enter to the dark compartment during the training phase (data not shown). Twenty four hours after the foot shock of 0.5 mA the latency to escape to the dark compartment was measured (Table 1).

The percentage of CMS BALB/c mice that showed high latency to escape to the dark compartment was significantly lower than control BALB/c mice (20 and 77%, $U = 21$, p< 0.05). On the contrary, the percentage of CMS C57BL/6 mice that showed low latency to escape to the dark compartment was non-significant higher than control C57BL/6 mice (67 and 40%, $U = 44$, ns) (Table 1).

Alteration of Neurogenesis by Stress Exposure in BALB/c but not in C57Bl/6 Mice

A decrease in the rate of adult hippocampal neurogenesis has been described after CMS (Lee *et al.*, 2006; Guo *et al.*, 2009; Dagytė *et al.*, 2011), which could be one of the mechanisms underlying the memory deficits described above.

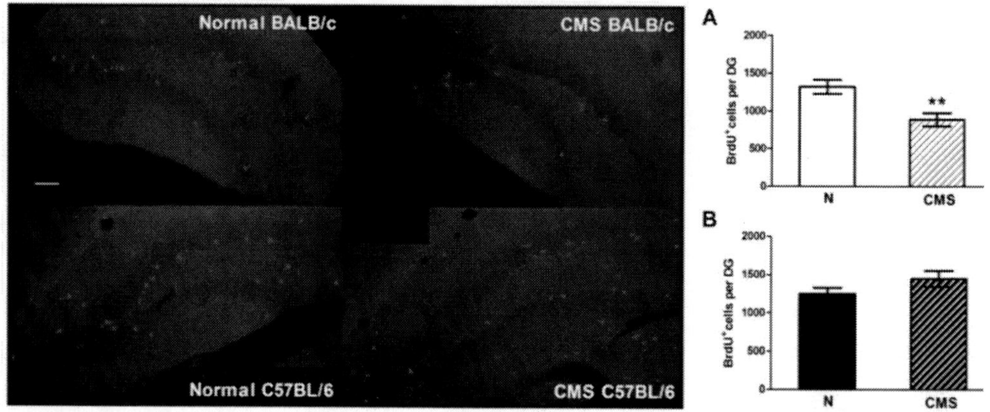

Representative images of the dentate gyrus in mice belonging to each of the groups are shown. BrdU immunofluorescence is indicated in red. Calibration bar: 100 μm. Quantification of BrdU$^+$ cells in the dentate gyrus (DG) monitored 28 days after the last BrdU injection in control (N) and CMS in BALB/c (A) and C57BL/6 (B) mice. Data are mean ± SEM for 6 mice in each group. ** $p < 0.01$ with respect to control.

Figure 1. Adult hippocampal neurogenesis.

To address this question we monitored the correlation of adult neurogenesis with the impaired memory after CMS exposure. Control and stressed mice received two daily injections of BrdU 50 mg/kg during five consecutive days, four weeks before sacrifice. Adult neurogenesis was assessed by counting BrdU$^+$ cells in the dentate gyrus of the hippocampus. Four weeks after labeling, most newborn cells within the granule cell layer were neurons (Kempermann *et al.*, 2003) (data non-shown). Two-way ANOVA indicated significant changes in the number of BrdU$^+$ cells depending on strain (BALB/c or C57BL/6) and condition (control or CMS)[interaction: strain x condition; $F (3,20) = 11.90, p < 0.01$]. As can be seen in Figure 1 A, CMS-BALB/c mice exhibited a significant decrease (about 30%) in the number of BrdU$^+$ cells respect to control mice (simple effects analysis; $F (1,20) = 11.041; p < 0.01$). However, stress exposure did not have effect on neurogenesis in C57Bl/6 mice $F (1,20) = 2.42$; NS) (Figure 1B). Figure 1 depicts representative images of BrdU$^+$ cells in the dentate gyrus using fluorescence microscopy in BALB/c and C57BL6 mice exposed or not to stress.

Determination of the Oxidation State in Hippocampus of BALB/c and C57BL/6 Mice Induced by Chronic Stress

To evaluate if the chronic stress affect the oxidation state in the hippocampus of BALB/C and C57BL/6 mice, we studied the activity of the nitric oxide synthase (NOS), the levels of reactive oxygen species (ROS) and antioxidant defences like catalase (CAT), superoxide dismutase (SOD) and reduced glutathione (GSH) levels.

Table 2 summarized the results obtained for control and stressed BALB/c and C57Bl/6 mice. Two-way ANOVA indicated significant changes in the total NOS activity depending on strain (BALB/c or C57BL/6) and condition (control or CMS) [interaction: strain x condition; F (3,28) = 43.55, $p < 0.001$]. Simple effects analysis showed that total NOS activity was significantly different between hippocampal homogenates of CMS and control BALB/c mice (F (1,28) = 63.36, $p < 0.001$).

In addition, preincubation with 7-NI or L-NIO (nNOS and eNOs inhibitors, respectively) indicated that this decrease was due to a reduce nNOS activity (table 2). Thus, two-way ANOVA showed significant changes in nNOS activity depending on strain and condition [interaction: strain x condition; F (3,28) = 55.14, $p < 0.001$]. Simple effects analysis showed a significant decrease in nNOS activity in stressed BALB/c mice respect to control (F (1,28) = 88.14, $p < 0.001$). However, in CMS C57BL/6 mice a non-significative difference in NOS activity or nNOS activity was observed respect to control (F (1,28) = 1.88, NS; F (1,28) = 1.24, NS) (table 2).

**Table 2. Oxidative state in hippocampus of BALB/c and C57BL/6 mice
induced by chronic stress**

Strain	BALB/c		C57BL/6	
Condition	N	CMS	N	CMS
NOS total activity (pmol [^{14}C] L-citruline/ g tissue/30 min)	320 ± 16	110 ± 8 ***	543 ± 41	580 ± 29
nNOS total activity (pmol [^{14}C] L-citruline/ g tissue/30 min)	290 ± 15	95 ± 10 ***	362 ± 14	387 ± 16
ROS (pmol/mg/min)	4.88 ± 0.13	6.32 ± 0.18 ***	5.57 ± 0.17	6.20 ± 0.24
Units of catalase/mg of tissue	9.03 ± 0.64	7.74 ± 0.33	11.01 ± 0.71	11.75 ± 3.21
Units of SOD /mg of tissue	198 ± 10	162 ± 18	163 ± 5	164 ± 3
pmol of GSH	339 ± 45	367 ± 25	367 ± 28	350 ± 55

Total NOS activity, nNOS activity, ROS production, and the catalase (CAT), superoxide dismutase (SOD) and reducide glutathione (GSH) levels were determined in hippocampus from BALB/c and C57BL/6 in control (N) and CMS mice. Results represent the mean ± SEM of: 8 mice of each group for NOS activity and 2 independent experiments performed in duplicate with 3 mice of each group. ***$p < 0.001$ respect to corresponding control.

Respect to ROS production, two-way ANOVA revealed a significant interaction in ROS productions depending on strain and condition [interaction: strain x condition; $F (3,23) = 4.43, p < 0.05$]. Simple effects analysis showed significant differences in ROS production in the hippocampus from CMS BALB/c mice regarding control [$F (1,20) = 28.00, p < 0.001$] but, non-significant differences were found between control and CMS C57BL/6 mice [$F (1,20) = 3.98$, NS] (table 2).

Concerning antioxidant defenses, two-way ANOVA indicated that chronic stress did not induce significant changes in the CAT, SOD and GSH levels neither in BALB/C nor C57BL/6 mice [between condition (control and CMS), CAT: $F (1,23) = 0.64$, NS; SOD: $F (1,23) = 1.03$, NS; GSH: $F (1,23) = 0.17$, NS] (table 2).

Effects of *In Vivo* Treatment with L-NAME in BALB/c and C57BL/6 Mice

As described above, stressed BALB/c, but not C57Bl/6 mice, showed poor learning performance in several behavioral tasks. Moreover, in BALB/c mice the magnitude of oxidative stress was increased in hippocampus of CMS mice together with a marked decrease in NO production, however no changes were observed in C57BL/6 mice. On the other hand, it was suggested that NO directly acts as an antioxidant (Miranda *et al.*, 2000). Taking into account these findings, we investigate if nNOS inhibition is involved in behavioral alterations observed in CMS animals. To investigate if nNOS inhibition is able to modify the behavior of BALB/c and C57BL/6 mice, the effect of oral administration of 7-NI to animals was studied for 4 weeks.

Figure 2 shows that the administration of the nNOS inhibitor in control BALB/c mice induced an increase in locomotor activity [crossing $F (3,23) = 19.883, p < 0.001$; rearing $F (3,23) = 9.104, p < 0.001$ and corner time $F (3,23) = 28.978, p < 0.001$]. Thus, after 1 week of 7-NI administration, animals showed an increase in horizontal ($t = 6.155, p < 0.001$) and vertical ($t = 4.637, p < 0.001$) activity. Accordingly, a decrease in the time spent in the corner ($t = 6.524, p < 0.001$) was found. Moreover, poor memory retention was observed in 7-NI-treated animals after 2 weeks. Thus, control animals showed a decrease in locomotor activity when re-exposed to open field 24 h after the inicial trial (crossing $t = 6.73, p < 0.001$; rearing $t = 7.67, p < 0.001$; corner time $t = 7.08, p < 0.001$). But, only a significant decrease was observed in rearing for animals treated with 7-NI for 2 weeks (crossing $t = 0.80$, NS; rearing $t = 2.05, p < 0.05$; corner time $t =1.20$, NS). Similar results were observed after 4 weeks of treatment (data not shown).

In addition, in control C57BL/6 mice the inhibition of nNOS by 7-NI induced changes in locomotor activity [crossing $F (3,23) = 12.55, p < 0.001$; rearing $F (3,23) = 13.89, p < 0.001$ and corner time $F (3,23) = 9.36, p < 0.001$]. Thus, after two weeks of treatment a significant decrease was observed in locomotor horizontal activity ($t = 5.35, p < 0.001$), and in the number of rearing ($t = 5.91, p < 0.001$) and an increase in the corner time ($t = 4.75, p < 0.001$).

Moreover, control animals showed a decrease in locomotor activity when re-exposed to open field 24 h after the inicial trial (crossing $t = 13.46, p < 0.001$; rearing $t = 1.420$, NS; corner time $t = 10.32, p < 0.001$). But, non-significant decreases were observed for animals treated with 7-NI after 1 week of treatment.

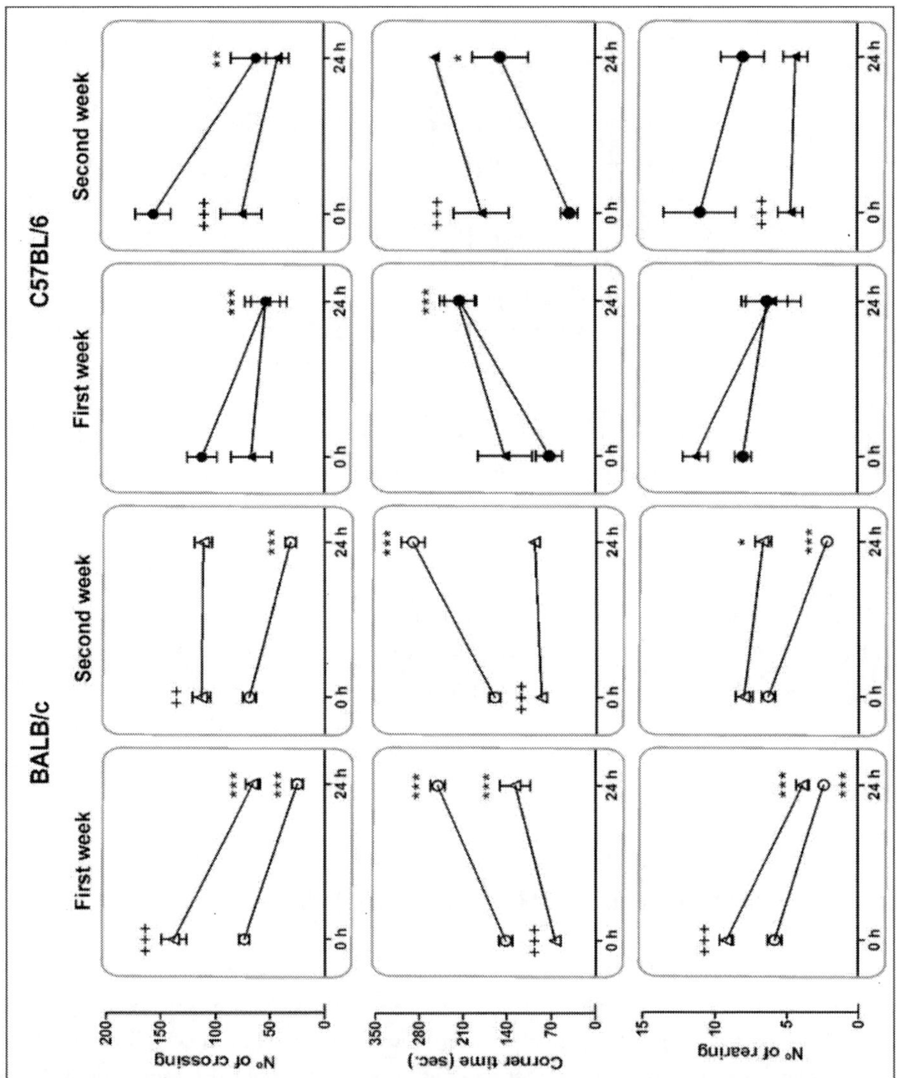

Crossing , corner time and rearing in the first and second week of 7-NI treatment in BALB/c (Δ) and C57BL/6 (▲) and in the control untreated BALB/c (○) and C57BL/6 (●). Results represent the mean ± SEM of 6 mice for each group. ++p < 0.01, +++p < 0.001 versus corresponding control; *p < 0.05, **p < 0.01, ***p < 0.001 versus training.

Figure 2. Mouse behavior in the open field after chronic nNOS inhibitor treatment (7-NI).

ROS Production in the Presence of 7-NI, a Specific nNOS Inhibitor, in the Hippocampus of BALB/c and C57BL/6 Mice

To study the participation of NOS in ROS production, ROS levels were determined in the presence of 7-NI, a specific nNOS inhibitor, in the hippocampus of BALB/C and C57BL/6.

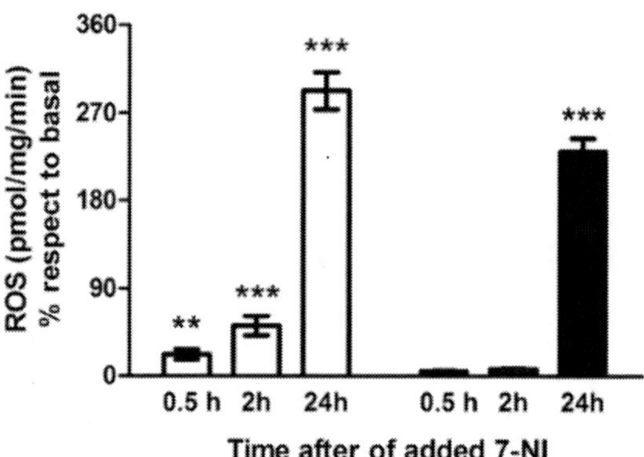

ROS production in the presence of 7-NI (10μmol/L) (NOS inhibitor) in hippocampus of control BALB/c (white bars) and C57BL/6 (black bars) to different times after adding 7-NI (0.5 h, 2 h and 24 h). Results represent the mean ± SEM of 2 independent experiments performed in duplicate with three animals of each group. **$p < 0.01$, ***$p < 0.001$ respect to corresponding control.

Figure 3. ROS levels in the presence of 7-NI.

As shown in Figure 3, the nNOS inhibition produced a time-dependent increase in ROS levels in BALB/c mice [two-way ANOVA repeat measured, 30 min: t (3,30) = 3.29; $p < 0.01$; 2 h: t (3,30) = 6.84; $p < 0.001$; 24 h: t (3,30) = 66.99; $p < 0.001$]. Respect to C57BL/6 mice, high ROS levels was observed only at 24 hours after 7-NI addition [two-way ANOVA repeat measured, 30 min: t (3,30) = 0.44; NS; 2 h: t (3,30) = 0.81; NS; 24 h: t (3,30) = 61.21; $p < 0.001$] (Figure 3).

Immunological Response in BABL/c and C57BL/6 Mice

To investigate whether chronic stress exposure was associated with changes in immune response, we analized the in vitro lymphocyte reactivity and the antibody production in BALB/c and C57BL/6 mice. To study in vitro lymphocyte reactivity cell were stimulated with the optimal T or B mitogens concentrations. Due to the well-known lymphoid profile, lymph nodes cell suspensions were used for Con A-induced T selective mitogen proliferation, while spleen lymphocyte suspensions were used to evaluate lipopolysaccharides (LPS) (B-cell mitogen) effect. Thymidine uptake of unstimulated control lymphocytes was similar for both strains (see legend table 3). Two-way ANOVA revealed that T- and B-cell proliferations were significantly different depending on both strain and condition [interaction: strain x condition, T-cell: F (3,44) = 59.09, $p < 0.001$ and B-cell: F (3,44) = 5.81, $p < 0.05$; respectively]. Simple effects analysis revealed that lymphoid cells from CMS BALB/c animals had a lower T cell response to the mitogen Con A [F (1,44) = 59.00, $p < 0.001$] and a higher B cell response to LPS [F (1,44) = 24.39, $p < 0.001$] than cells from control mice. On the contrary, T cells from CMS C57Bl/6 mice [F (1,44) = 13.25, $p < 0.001$] give a higher proliferative response than normal T cells. However, no differences were found between control and CMS B cell proliferation [F (1,44) = 2.30, NS] (table 3). To investigate whether chronic stress exposure was associated with changes in antibody production BALB/c and C57BL/6 mice were inoculated with, T-dependent, SRBC, and T-independent, LPS, antigens and IgM and IgG levels were determined by ELISA.

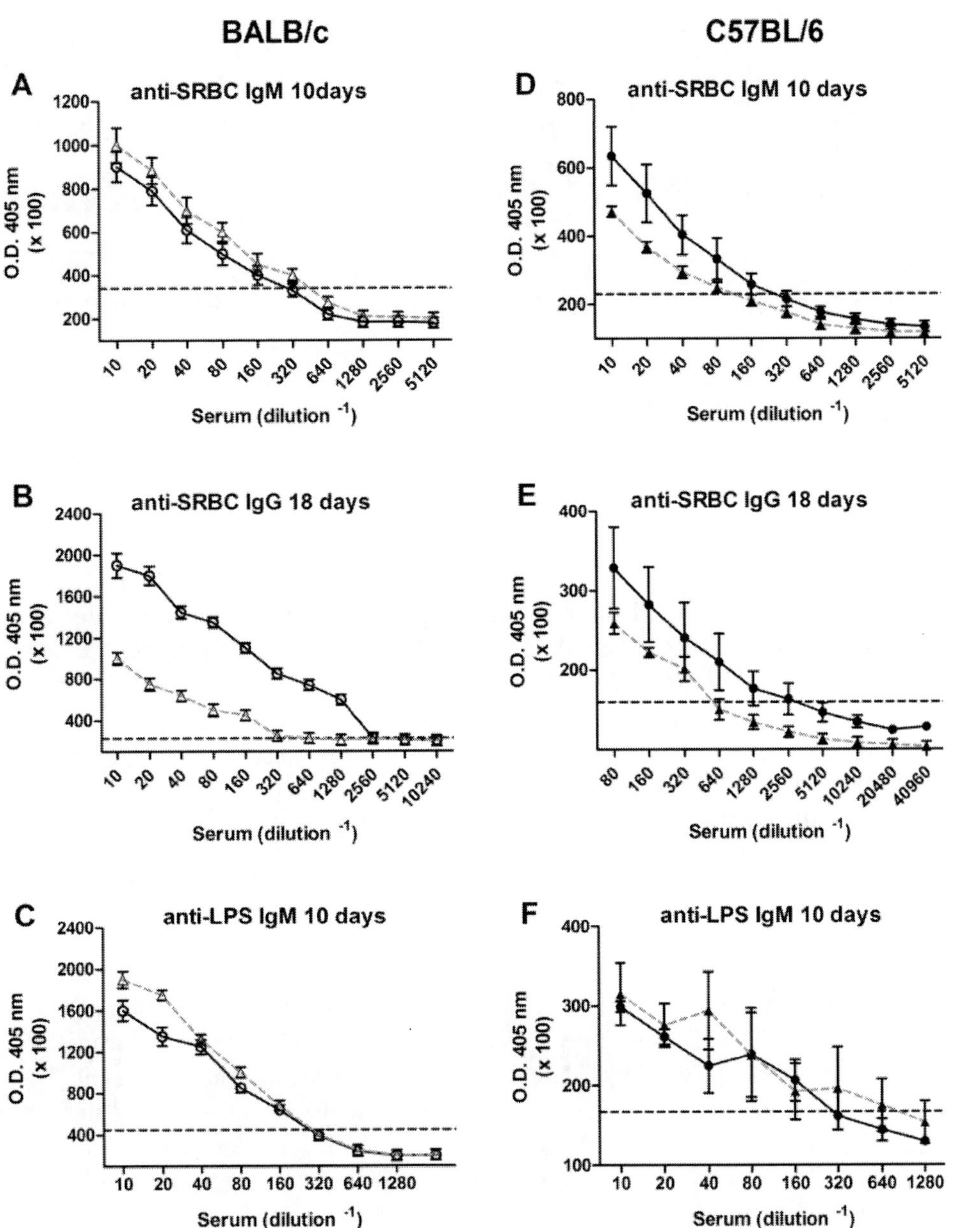

Antibody titers following SRBC and LPS immunization in control (○) and CMS (△) BALB/c mice and in control (●) and CMS (▲) C57BL/6 mice; were immunized with SRBC, 4% in saline (panels A and D), and boosted on day 11 with 4% of SRBC in saline (panels B and E) or immunized with LPS (10 μg in saline) (panel C and F). Serum was collected on day 10 or on day 18 and assayed for the presence of IgM (panels A, C, D and F) or IgG (panels B and E) by ELISA. The curves shown are representative of 2 independent experiments with 4 mice of each group. Each experiment was performed with one or two sera of each experimental condition. Dotted line represents the OD values + 2 S.D. of normal sera (without immunization).

Figure 4. Antibody production.

Table 3. Lymphocyte proliferation

Stimulation index (SI)	BALB/c		C57BL/6	
	N	CMS	N	CMS
T-lymphocytes	27.07 ± 2.77	6.79 ± 1.01 ***	15.53 ± 2.12	28.09 ± 2.61 ***
B-lymphocytes	5.49 ± 0.58	10.88 ± 1.04 ***	3.14 ± 0.34	4.21 ± 0.41

Proliferation of B and T-lymphocytes were determined by [^{3}H]-thymidine uptake from BALB/c and C57BL/6 in control (N) and CMS mice. Results are expressed as stimulation index (SI) and represent the mean ± SEM of 4 independent experiments with three animals for each group. ***p < 0.001 respect to the corresponding control. [^{3}H]-thymidine uptake for non-stimulated cells was: BALB/c, control: 2195 ±442 and CMS: 2677 ± 547 and C57BL/6, control: 3515 ± 742 and CMS: 3251 ± 546.

As can be seen in Figure 4 the anti-SRBC IgM titers were non-significantly different between control and CMS BALB/c mice [$U = 26$; NS; Figure 4A]. On the contrary, the IgG antibodies production was affected in CMS BALB/c mice after second immunization [$U = 3$; $p < 0.001$; Figure 4B]. The anti-LPS IgM titers was non-significant different in CMS respect to control BALB/c mice [$U = 21.5$; NS; Figure 4C]. On the other hand, the anti-SRBC and anti-LPS IgM titers were not affected in stressed C57BL/6 mice [$U = 27$; NS; Figure 4D; $U = 16$; NS; Figure 4E and $U = 23$; NS; Figure 4F, respectively].

Th1/Th2 Balance

To evaluate the effect of stress in Th1/Th2 balance in both strains of mice, INF-γ (Th1 cytokines) and IL-10 (Th2 cytokines) were determined in supernatants from Con A-stimulated lymphocytes. Two-way ANOVA revealed that significant changes in Th1/Th2 balance were observed depending on the strain of mice and the condition [interaction: strain x condition, $F (3,43) = 393.07$, $p < 0.001$]. As can be seen in figure 5, simple effects analysis showed that a significant decrease in TH1/TH2 balance in CMS BALB/c mice [$F (1,43) = 98.50$, $p < 0.001$] regarding control. However, a significant increase was observed in CMS C57BL/6 mice [$F (1,43) = 248.00$, $p < 0.001$] respect to control C57BL/6 mice.

Correlation Analysis between Behavior and Th1/Th2 Balance

To ascertain if the memory impairment observed in stressed BALB/c mice could be associated to cytokine profile, the correlation coefficient was determined. As shown in figure 6, the Pearson's correlation test showed a positive correlation between the percentage of decrease crossings respect to training (in percentage) and the relation Th1/Th2 (defined as

IFN-γ/IL-10 ratio) in BALB/c mice taking both control and CMS ($r = 0.9363$, $p < 0.0001$). However, no correlation was found in C57BL/6 mice ($r = 0.0600$, NS).

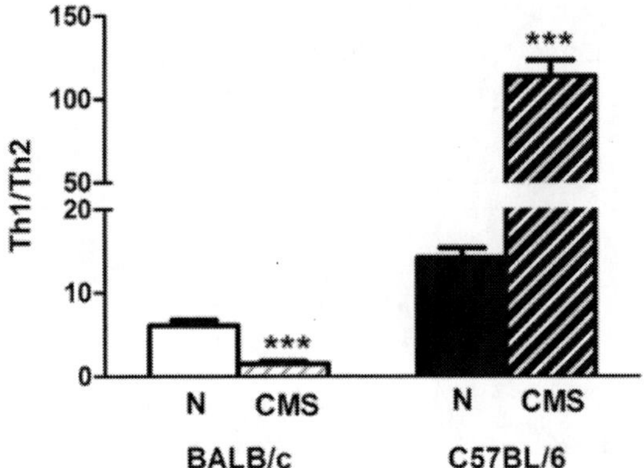

This ratio was defined as IFN-γ/IL-10 ratio in control (N) and CMS, BALB/c and C57BL/6 mice. Results represent the mean ± SEM 2 independent experiment with 6 mice for each group. ***$p < 0.001$.

Figure 5. Th1/Th2 balance.

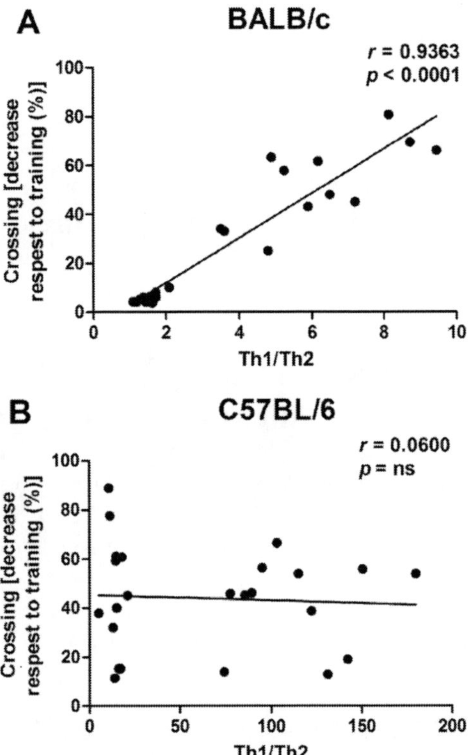

Correlation analysis between the crossing decrease percentage respect to training and the Th1/Th2 balance in BALB/c (A), $r = 0.9363$, $p < 0.0001$ and C57BL/6 (B) mice, $r = 0.0600$, $p = $ ns. Twelve mice in each group were used for this analysis.

Figure 6. Correlation between behavior and Th1/Th2 balance.

Classical Stress Hormones Levels

It is well known that stress involves activation of the HPA axis and SNS. For this reason, two classical stress hormones, corticosterone and norepinephrine, were determined in BALB/c and C57BL/6 mice during CMS exposure (Figure 7 A y B, respectively).

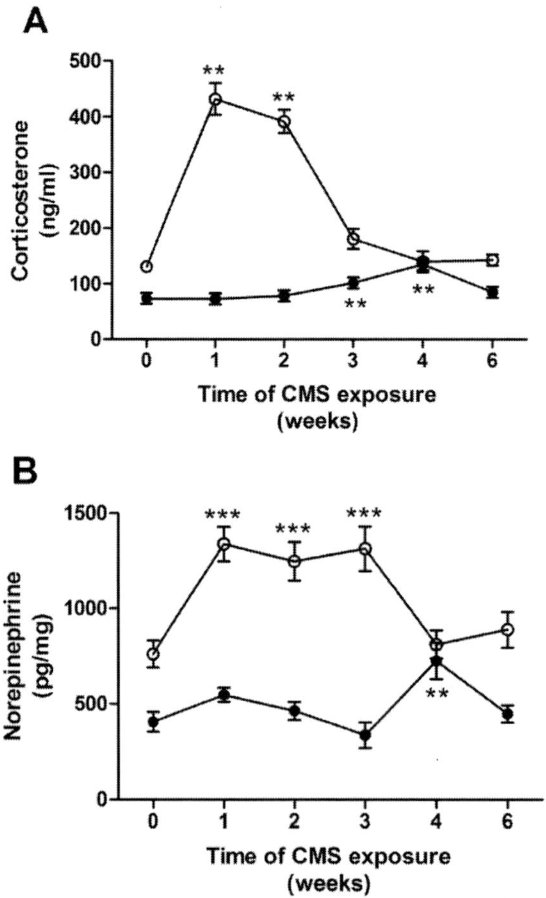

Catecholamines and corticosterone analyses were performed in control (non-exposed) and 1-6 weeks CMS-exposed in both BALB/c (○) and C57BL/6 (●) mice. Results represent the mean ± SEM of the three independent experiments with three mice of each group. $**p < 0.01$, $***p < 0.001$ respect to control.

Figure 7. Catecholamine concentrations in spleen samples and serum corticosterone levels from control and CMS-exposed mice.

For corticosterone, Friedman analyses revealed significant differences in the corticosterone levels of BALB/c ($T^2 = 18.20$, $p < 0.001$) and C57BL/6 mice ($T^2 = 5.90$, $p < 0.001$). BALB/c animals subjected to the CMS procedure showed a significant increase in hormone levels during the first 2 weeks of exposure (CMS vs control, $p < 0.01$ for 1 and 2 weeks of CMS exposure). After 3 weeks of stress, serum corticosterone levels returned to basal values and did not show any statistically significant differences when compared to controls (after 6 weeks, NS). Corticosterone of C57BL/6 mice exposed to the CMS model showed an increase in the 3rd and 4th weeks of CMS exposure ($p < 0.01$), returning to basal levels after 6 weeks of CMS (CMS vs control, NS) (Figure 7A).

For catecholamine, two-way ANOVA revealed a significant interaction between the strains and the different weeks of CMS exposure [$F (11,83) = 7.01, p < 0.001$]. As shown in figure 7B, splenic norepinephrine (NE) concentrations showed a pattern similar to serum corticosterone levels in both strains. Simple effects analysis showed that BALB/c mice presented an early increase of NE, which was lost after 3 weeks of CMS exposure [1st, 2nd and 3rd weeks of CMS vs control; $p < 0.001$]. However, C57BL/6 mice showed an increase of NE only on 4th week ($p < 0.01$), which was lost after 6 weeks of CMS exposure (Figure 7B).

DISCUSSION

Here we showed an integrated study about the effects of stress in learning and memory, immune and endocrine system using two genetically different inbred strains of mice, namely C57BL/6 and BALB/c. To perform this study we exposed animals to the chronic stress model described by Willner *et al.* (1992) in rats and Monleon *et al.* (1995) in mice, as previously detailed (Palumbo *et al.*, 2007). This is a heterotypic model that implies a chronic low-grade stress offering a reasonable approximation to the diverse stresses of daily life offering a realistic simulation of the biological effects of chronic stress.

The effect of stress on learning and memory has been well documented in a diverse array of species from fish to human (Kim and Yoon, 1998). A growing body of work suggests that stress could act in many ways to affect the processes that underlie learning and memory. Memory researchers have identified the hippocampus as a crucial brain structure involved in key aspects of memory formation. In particular, structural alterations in the hippocampal formation and reduction of neurogenesis in the adult dentate gyrus have been observed in different animal models of chronic stress (McEwen *et al.*, 2001). According to our previous results (Palumbo *et al.*, 2009) here we show that exposure to chronic stress was able to induce a deficit in learning and memory in BALB/c mice but not in C57Bl/6 mice. A decrease in the rate of adult hippocampal neurogenesis has been described after CMS (Lee *et al.*, 2006; Guo et al., 2009; Dagyté et al., 2011), which could be one of the mechanisms underlying memory deficits described above. To address this question we monitored the correlation of adult neurogenesis with the impaired memory after CMS exposure. As previously reported, CMS exposure induced a decrease in neurogenesis in BALB/c mice (Palumbo *et al.*, 2012), but no changes were found in C57Bl/6 mice.

Oxidative stress has been related to the pathogenesis of many neurodegenerative and neurological disorders. Under normal conditions, these toxic species are produced by celular metabolism and neutralized by endogenous antioxidant defences. However, in adverse conditions, celular defences might result insufficient leading to increased vulnerability and eventually to cell death (Ischiropoulos and Beckman 2003). We found that oxidative state is not altered in stressed C57Bl/6 mice. Interestingly, in BALB/c mice exposure to chronic stress induced an increase in ROS production that was not related to a decrease in antioxidant defences but to a decrease in NO production. Moreover, in vivo administration of a nNOS inhibitor induced behavioral alterations in both strains. In addition, in vitro nNOS inhibition led to an increase in ROS production. Together, these results suggest an important role for

NO as a protection against insults that trigger the tissue toxicity as suggested by Winks and collaborators (Wink *et al.*, 1996; Wink and Michell, 1998; Thomas *et al.*, 2008).

Studies on brain-immune interactions have revealed bidirectional connections between the neural and neuroendocrine systems and the immune system (Sternberg, 2000). The immune system can signal the central nerve system through the action of cytokines (Eskandari *et al.*, 2003). Deregulation of cytokines (Th1 versus Th2) has been reported to be involved in the pathogenesis of many human illnesses such as autoimmune diseases, sleep disturbance, major depression and other disorders (Kaufmann *et al.*, 2007; Schwarz *et al.*, 2001). Therefore, we evaluated the effect of stress on immune functions by the ability of lymphoid cells to proliferate and produce Th1 and Th2 cytokines. According to our previous results (Palumbo *et al.*, 2010), mitogen-induced T-cell proliferation is decreased, whereas B-cell proliferation is increased, in BALB/c exposed to stress. In addition, an alteration in T-cell dependent antibody production after immunization was observed in these mice. On the contrary, an increase in the proliferative response of T-cell without changes in B-cell proliferation and in antibody production was noted in CMS C57BL/6. Furthermore, as previously reported (Palumbo *et al.*, 2010) stress induced a Th2 response in BALB/c and a Th1 response in C57BL/6 mice. Finally, a correlation between poor memory performance and the increase of the Th2/Th1 balance was found. These results suggest that vulnerability to cognitive deficit associated with stress exposure could be related to a differential regulation of Th1/Th2 cytokine balance, suggesting a better learning performance for individuals that produce Th1 type cytokine after stress exposure.

It was demonstrated that stress involves the activation of the hypothalamic-pituitary-adrenal (HPA) axis and the sympathetic nervous system (SNS) which, in turn, modulate the immune response. Moreover, it was reported that corticosterone administration induces neuronal atrophy in the hippocampal CA3 subfield which, in turn, induces memory impairment (McEwen, 2001). In this context, the participation of activation of HPA and SNS systems in immunological and behavioral effects induced by CMS exposure was investigated. Results of BALB/c mice subjected to CMS showed a moderate increment of corticosterone and catecholamine levels by the first three weeks, returning to basal levels after 4 weeks of stress exposure. However, deficit in T-cell response and memory impairment appear after 4 weeks of CMS exposure (Silberman *et al.*, 2002; Palumbo *et al.*, 2007). It is important to note that it is not possible to rule out that the early hormone increase could be inducing late changes in immune and behavioral parameters. In addition, results of C57BL/6 mice subjected to CMS showed an increase of corticosterone and catecholamine levels but not memory impairment or deficit in T-cell response. These findings support the hypothesis that there is no correlation between hormone increase and immune or behavior alterations.

CONCLUSION

These results show that BALB/c mice are more vulnerable to the effects of stress than C57BL/6 mice depending on a differential regulation of the Th1/Th2 cytokine balance. In C57BL/6 mice, stress induces a Th1 response with an increase of IFN-γ production that in turn could be a protective mechanism against the neurodegenerative processes. On the other hand, an increase in Th2 cytokines and a decrease in IFN-γ correlate with a poor memory performance in CMS BALB/c mice. In fact, C57Bl/6 mice showed no significant ROS production or changes in the rate of adult neurogenesis. On the contrary, tissue toxicity together with increases in oxidative stress and neuronal decrease were induced in CMS BALB/c mice. On the other hand, our results suggest an important role for decreased NO production in memory impairment under stress conditions. Further studies are needed to determine the relationship between NO production and Th1/Th2 balance.

Finally, the present results could be useful to generate new strategies for the treatment of adverse consequences of stress and ageing memory impairments taking into account cytokines mediated actions.

CONFLICTS OF INTEREST

The authors declare that there are no conflicts of interest.

ACKNOWLEDGMENTS

The authors thank María Rosa Gonzalez Murano for the technical assistance, Daniel Gonzalez for his valuable help in the animal stress model, and Noemí Cappano and Patricia Fernandez for the secretarial assistance. This work was supported by grants from CONICET (PIP 00281) and from the University of Buenos Aires (UBACyT 2002010010633) to AMG.

REFERENCES

Beers R.F. Jr., Sizer I.W. (1952). A spectrophotometric method for measuring the breakdown of hydrogen peroxide by catalase. *J. Biol. Chem.,*195: 133-140.

Belzung C.,Griebel,G. (2001). Measuring normal and pathological anxiety-like behaviour in mice: a review. *Behav. Brain Res.*, 125: 141-149.

Bredt D.S., Snyder S.H. (1990). Isolation of nitric oxide synthetase, a calmodulin-requiring enzyme. *Proc. Natl. Acad. Sci. USA*, 87: 682-685.

Dagytė G., Crescente I., Postema F., Seguin L., Gabriel C., Mocaër E., Boer J.A., Koolhaas J.M. (2011). Agomelatine reverses the decrease in hippocampal cell survival induced by chronic mild stress. *Behav. Brain. Res.*, 218: 121-128.

Dillon G.M., Qu X., Marcus J.N., Dodart J.C. (2008). Excitotoxic lesions restricted to the dorsal CA1 field of the hippocampus impair spatial memory and extinction learning in C57BL/6 mice. *Neurobiol. Learn. Mem.*, 90: 426-433.

Edgar V.A., Cremaschi G.A., Sterin-Borda L., Genaro A.M. (2002). Altered expression of autonomic neurotransmitter receptors and proliferative responses in lymphocytes from a chronic mild stress model of depression: effects of fluoxetine. *Brain Behav Immun.*, 16: 333-350.

Eskandari F., Webster J.I., Sternberg E.M. (2003). Neural immune pathways and their connection to inflammatory diseases. *Arthritis Res. Ther.*, 5: 251-265.

Frisch C., De Souza-Silva M., Söhl G., Güldenagel M., Willecke K., Huston J.P., Dere E. (2005). Stimulus complexity dependent memory impairment and changes in motor performance after deletion of the neuronal gap junction protein connexin36 in mice. *Behav. Brain Res.,* 157: 177-185.

Glaser R.; Kiecolt-Glaser J.K. (2005). Stress-induced immune dysfunction: implications for health. *Nat. Rev. Immunol.,* 5: 243-251.

Guiñazú N., Pellegrini A., Giordanengo L., Aoki M.P., Rivarola H.W., Cano R., Rodrigues M.M., Gea S. (2004). Immune response to a major Trypanosoma cruzi antigen, cruzipain, is differentially modulated in C57BL/6 and BALB/c mice. *Microbes Infect.,* 6: 1250-1258.

Guo Y.J., Zhang Z.J., Wang S.H., Sui Y.X., Sun Y. (2009). Notch1 signaling, hippocampal neurogenesis and behavioral responses to chronic unpredicted mild stress in adult ischemic rats. *Prog. Neuropsychopharmacol. Biol. Psychiatry,* 33: 688-694.

Ischiropoulos H., Beckman J.S. (2003). Oxidative stress and nitration in neurodegeneration: cause, effect, or association? *J. Clin. Invest.,* 111: 163-169.

Kaufmann I., Eisner C., Richter P., Huge V., Beyer A., Chouker A., Schelling G., Thiel M. (2007). Lymphocyte subsets and the role of TH1/TH2 balance in stressed chronic pain patients. *Neuroimmunomodulation,* 14: 272-280.

Kempermann G., Gast D., Kronenberg G., Yamaguchi M., Gage F.H. (2003). Early determination and long-term persistence of adult-generated new neurons in the hippocampus of mice. *Development,* 130: 391-399.

Keston A.S., Brand T.R. (1965). The fluorometric analysis of ultramicro quantities of hydrogen peroxide. *Anal. Biochem.,* 11: 1-5.

Kim J. J. and Yoon K. S. (1998) Stress: metaplastic effects in the hippocampus. *Trends Neurosci.,* 21: 505-509.

Kim M.J., Choi S.J., Lim S.T., Kim H.K., Kim Y.J., Yoon H.G., Shin D.H. (2008). Zeatin supplement improves scopolamine-induced memory impairment in mice. *Biosci. Biotechnol. Biochem.* 72: 577-581.

Laverty R., Taylor K.M. (1968). The fluorometric assay of catecholamines and related compounds: improvements and extensions to the hydroxyindole technique. *Anal. Biochem.,* 22: 269-279.

LeBel, C.P., Odunze, I.N., Adams, J.D. Jr, Bondy, S.C. (1989). Perturbations in cerebral oxygen radical formation and membrane order following vitamin E deficiency. *Biochem. Biophys. Res. Commun.,* 163: 860-866.

Lee K.J., Kim S.J., Kim S.W., Choi S.H., Shin Y.C., Park S.H., Moon B.H., Cho E., Lee M.S., Choi S.H., Chun B.G., Shin K.H. (2006). Chronic mild stress decreases survival, but not proliferation, of new-born cells in adult rat hippocampus. *Exp. Mol. Med.,* 38: 44-54.

McCord J.M. and Fridovich I. (1969). Superoxide dismutase. An enzymic function for erythrocuprein (hemocuprein). *J. Biol. Chem.,* 244: 6049-6055.

McEwen B. S. (2000) Effects of adverse experiences for brain structure and function. *Biol. Psychiatry,* 48: 721-731.

McEwen B.S. (1998). Protective and damaging effects of stress mediators: allostasis and allostatic load. *N. Engl. J. Med.,* 338: 171-179.

McEwen B.S. (2001). Plasticity of the hippocampus: Adaptation to chronic stress and allostatic load. *Ann. NY Acad. Sci.,* 933: 265-277.

McEwen B.S. (2008). Central effects of stress hormones in health and disease: understanding the protective and damaging effects of stress and stress mediators. *Eur. J. Pharmacol.*, 583: 174-185.

McEwen BS. (2007). Physiology and neurobiology of stress and adaptation: central role of the brain. *Physiol. Rev.*, 87: 873-904.

Miranda K.M., Espey M.G., Wink D.A. (2000). A discussion of the chemistry of oxidative and nitrosative stress in cytotoxicity. *J. Inorg. Biochem.*, 79: 237-240.

Monleon S., Aquila P., Parra A., Simon V.M., Brain P.F., Willner P. (1995). Attenuation of sucrose consumption in mice by chronic mild stress and its restoration by imipramine. *Psychopharmacology*, 117: 453-457.

Palumbo M.L., Canzobre M.C., Pascuan C.G., Ríos H., Wald M., Genaro A.M. (2010). Stress induced cognitive deficit is differentially modulated in BALB/c and C57Bl/6 mice: correlation with Th1/Th2 balance after stress exposure. *J. Neuroimmunol.*, 218: 12-20.

Palumbo M.L., Fosser N.S., Ríos H., Zorrilla Zubilete M.A., Guelman L.R., Cremaschi G.A., Genaro A.M. (2007). Loss of hippocampal neuronal nitric oxide synthase contributes to the stress-related deficit in learning and memory. *J. Neurochem.*, 102: 261-274.

Palumbo M.L., Zorrilla-Zubilete M.A., Cremaschi G.A., Genaro A.M. (2009). Different effect of chronic stress on learning and memory in BALB/c and C57BL/6 inbred mice: Involvement of hippocampal NO production and PKC activity. *Stress*, 4: 350-361.

Palumbo ML, Trinchero MF, Zorrilla-Zubilete MA, Schinder AF, Genaro AM. (2012). Glatiramer acetate reverts stress-induced alterations on adult neurogenesis and behavior. Involvement of Th1/Th2 balance. *Brain. Behav. Immun.*, 26: 429-438.

Priebe K., Romeo R.D., Francis D.D., Sisti H.M., Mueller A., McEwen B.S., Brake W.G. (2005). Maternal influences on adult stress and anxiety-like behavior in C57BL/6J and BALB/cJ mice: a cross-fostering study. *Dev. Psychobiol.*, 48: 95-96.

Reiche EM, Nunes SO, Morimoto, HK. (2004). Stress, depression, the immune system, and cancer. *Lancet Oncol.*, 5: 617-625.

Sargent R.N. (1985). Determination of corticosterone in rat plasma by HPLC. *J. Anal. Toxicol.*, 9: 20-23.

Schwarz M.J., Chiang S., Müller N., Ackenheil M. (2001). T-helper-1 and T-helper-2 responses in psychiatric disorders. *Brain Behav. Immun.*, 15: 340-370.

Silberman D.M., Wald M., Genaro A.M. (2002). Effects of chronic mild stress on lymphocyte proliferative response. Participation of serum thyroid hormones and corticosterone. *Int. Immunopharmacol.*, 2: 487-497.

Sternberg E.M. (2000). Interactions between the immune and neuroendocrine systems. *Prog. Brain Res.*, 122: 35-42.

Tagawa N., Sugimoto Y., Yamada J., Kobayashi Y. (2006). Strain differences of neurosteroid levels in mouse brain. *Steroids*, 71: 776-784.

Takeno M., Yoshikawa H., Kurokawa M., Takeba Y., Kashiwakura J.I., Sakaguchi M., Yasueda H., Suzuki N. (2004). Th1-dominant shift of T cell cytokine production, and subsequent reduction of serum immunoglobulin E response by administration in vivo of plasmid expressing Txk/Rlk, a member of Tec family tyrosine kinases, in a mouse model. *Clin. Exp. Allergy*, 34: 965-970.

Tang X., Orchard S.M., Sanford L.D. (2002). Home cage activity and behavioral performance in inbred and hybrid mice. *Behav. Brain Res.*, 136: 555-569.

Thomas D.D., Ridnour L.A., Isenberg J.S., Flores-Santana W., Switzer C.H., Donzelli S., Hussain P., Vecoli C., Paolocci N., Ambs S., Colton C.A., Harris C.C., Roberts D.D., Wink D.A. (2008). The chemical biology of nitric oxide: implications in cellular signaling. *Free Radic. Biol. Med.*, 45: 18-31.

Tietze F. (1969). Enzymic Method for Quantitative Determination of Nanogram Amounts of total and Oxidized Glutathione. *Analytical Biochemistry,* 27: 502-522.

Watanabe H., Numata K., Ito T., Takagi K.,Matsukawa A. (2004). Innate immune response in Th1- and Th2-dominant mouse strains. *Shock,* 22: 460-466.

Willner P., Muscat R., Papp M. (1992). Chronic mild stress-induced anhedonia: a realistic animal model of depression. *Neurosci Biobehav. Rev.,* 16: 525-534.

Wink D.A., Hanbauer I., Grisham M.B., Laval F., Nims R.W., Laval J., Cook J., Pacelli R., Liebmann J., Krishna M., Ford P.C., Mitchell J.B. (1996). Chemical biology of nitric oxide: regulation and protective and toxic mechanisms. *Curr. Top Cell Regul.,* 34: 159-187.

Wink D.A., Mitchell J.B. (1998). The chemical biology of nitric oxide: Insights into regulatory, cytotoxic and cytoprotective mechanisms of nitric oxide. *Free Rad. Biol. Med.*, 25: 434-456.

Zhang X., Beaulieu J.M., Sotnikova T.D., Gainetdinov R.R., Caron M.G. (2004). Tryptophan hydroxylase-2 controls brain serotonin synthesis. *Science*, 305: 217.

In: Psychology of Stress
Editors: Leandro Cavalcanti and Sofia Azevedo

ISBN: 978-1-62417-109-3
© 2013 Nova Science Publishers, Inc.

Chapter 5

STRESS AND HOMOSEXUALITY

*Charbonnier Elodie[1] and
Graziani Pierluigi[2]*
[1]Unimes/Aix-Marseille Univ, Aix-en-Provence, France
[2]Unimes, Nîmes, France

ABSTRACT

Homosexuals are one of the most stressed groups of individuals (Lewis, Derlega, Griffin & Krowinski, 2003). The various stressful experiences which they face have been grouped under the term "minority stress" (Meyer, 1995). This model takes account of the excess amount of stress experienced by individuals belonging to these stigmatised social categories, in particular sexual minorities. Homosexuals are faced with numerous stressors such as family reactions, the attitudes of society (D'Augelli, 2002; Meyer, 2003) and the revelation of their homosexuality ((Robohm, Litzenberger & Pearlman, 2003). This revelation is often a stressful experience, and the stress is accentuated by the possibility that it may lead to rejection. At the same time, this announcement is a liberating experience conducive to the construction of identity (Rosario, Schrimshaw & Hunter, 2004) and the improvement of quality of life (Halpin & Allen, 2004; Savin-Williams, 2001).

The use or abuse of substances are coping strategies widely used by homosexuals to cope with the stress they are feeling (McCabe, Bostwick, Hughes, West & Boyd, 2010). These strategies are particularly favoured in adolescence and early adulthood, as capacities to cope with stressful events are still being developed (Compas, Conner-Smith, Saltzman, Thomsen & Wadsworth, 2001). Although adolescence is a period characterised by the presence of numerous stressors (emotional, physical, social, identity-related, affective...), young homosexuals are confronted with additional stressors (non-compliance with the norm, discrimination, revelation of their sexual orientation...). The ineffectiveness of coping strategies and the significant number of stressors are elements which may contribute to the suffering of young homosexuals amongst whom the incidences of consumption or abuse of substances (Cochran, Ackerman, Mays & Ross, 2004; Wilsnack et al., 2008), suicidal behaviour (Silenzio, Peña, Duberstein, Cerel & Knox, 2007; Suicide Prevention Resource Center, 2008) and psychiatric disorders (Kitts, 2005) are higher than amongst young heterosexuals.

According to the transactional stress model (Lazarus & Folkman, 1984) it is the interpretation of the situation which generates stress, stress therefore depending on the cognitive evaluation made by the subject and the resources they think they have to cope with it. Based on this model, we have sought to evaluate the manner in which young homosexuals cope with the stress they feel when revealing their homosexuality. For this purpose, 400 young homosexuals replied to a questionnaire evaluating the risks encountered during this situation (primary evaluation), their options for action and the coping strategies which they had put in place (secondary evaluation). Two groups were created, the first being questioned on which revelation of their homosexuality had been the most stressful during their life (group 1), and the second on which situation during their life had been the most stressful for them (group 2); we excluded those who replied the announcement of their homosexuality.

Our results demonstrate that the announcement of one's homosexuality is judged more "risky" than other stressful situations, the main fears being linked to the possibility of hurting someone as a result of this announcement. The respondents reported fewer possibilities for action during the revelation of their homosexuality than when faced with another stressful situation. During the announcement of their homosexuality, the most commonly used strategies related to personal growth and a positive re-evaluation of the situation. The announcement of one's homosexuality does not therefore necessarily constitute a negative stressor (Iwasaki & Ristock, 2007). This data supports the "stress-related growth" (SRG) model which argues that stressors do not systematically lead to negative consequences but that they can also induce positive changes. This data led to the creation of the term "coming-out growth" (COG), applying this model to the announcement of homosexuality.

INTRODUCTION

Homosexuals are one of the most stressed groups of individuals (Lewis, Derlega, Griffin & Krowinski, 2003). 58% of teenage homosexuals (12-17 years of age), think that their sexual orientation will be a source of difficulties in their life, and this proportion is even higher amongst young men (Padilla, Crisp & Rew, 2010). Minorities experience specific stressors in addition to those encountered by the general population (Meyer & Northridge, 2007), diverse stressful experiences which are grouped under the term "minority stress" (Meyer, 1995). This model takes account of the stress experienced by individuals belonging to stigmatised social categories. According to Meyer (1995), there is a continuum between distal and proximal stressors. Distal stressors are related to external, objective events, which do not depend on the individual. Homophobia, for example, is a distal stressor specific to homosexuals. Proximal stressors are more subjective, and are linked to the characteristics of the individual. The construction of their homosexual identity can constitute a proximal stressor, as the realisation of their non-compliance with the norm can generate stress. The revelation of their homosexuality can be considered as both a proximal and distal stressor, as it represents both an internal and external stress. Indeed, the declaration in itself is considered as a stressful experience, as it involves defining oneself as different, that's to say as gay, lesbian or bisexual (Bonet, Wells & Parsons, 2007), and this stress is accentuated by the possibility that it may lead to rejection (D'Augelli, 2002; Meyer, 2003).

STRESS AND THE REVELATION OF HOMOSEXUALITY

The revelation of their homosexuality is the main stressor encountered by young homosexuals (Robohm, Litzenberger & Pearlman, 2003). Declaring that you are homosexual is often a difficult and stressful occasion (Savin-Williams, 2001; Willoughby, Malik & Lindahl, 2006) but one that is not necessarily a negative stressor (Iwasaki & Ristock, 2007). This revelation is an important moment, one which promotes personal development and the construction of a homosexual identity (Coursaud, 2002). It generates a transformation of personal and social identity (Morris, 1997) and may promote a more ready acceptance of one's sexual orientation (Rosario, Schrimshaw & Hunter, 2004). Each revelation will be an opportunity for the construction or reconstruction of homosexual identity (Mellini, 2009).

By not revealing their sexual orientation, some homosexuals find themselves in an uncomfortable position and in an anxious state of mind, dominated by the fear that their family and friends will discover their sexual identity, this state persisting until they come out of the closet (Savin-Williams, 1998). Many homosexuals hide their sexual orientation out of fear of being rejected by others, feeling ashamed and harbouring negative emotions about themselves (CSAT, 2001). The fear of rejection can lead some homosexuals to shrink from making this declaration. Only 33% of young homosexuals (12-17 years of age) have revealed their sexual orientation to their mother and 22% to their father (Padilla et al., 2010). Their anxieties are even more numerous when they live with their parents, depend on them financially or belong to another minority group (Savin-Williams & Esterberg, 2000). Religious belief in particular is considered as one of the main barriers to this revelation. However, this declaration may promote an increase in well-being, an improvement in quality of life (Halpin & Allen, 2004; Savin-Williams, 2001) and engender various positive emotions such as feelings of relief and release. It may also have an impact on resilience and coping strategies (Monroe, 2001). Five different areas may be affected by this declaration: "growth in honesty/authenticity", "identity growth" "growth in mental health/resilience", "social /relational growth" and "advocacy / generativity" (Vaughan, 2007).

However, the revelation of homosexuality also creates suffering. With regards to their non-compliance with the "norm" that is heterosexuality, homosexuals have to cope with a certain number of rejections, whether from within the family or from their academic environment (Grov, Bimbi, Nanin & Parsons, 2006). When they reveal their homosexuality they face negative attitudes and scorn from their friends, and parents are often unsupportive in the face of these difficulties (Hefez, 2003). Homosexuals who have revealed their homosexuality are said to run a four times greater risk of attempting suicide than those who haven't done so (D'Augelli, Hershberger & Pilkington, 1998). The risk of an actual attempt being made is even higher when the declaration is made early, as younger homosexuals don't have sufficient resources to cope with any rejection that may occur (Remafedi, Farrow & Deisher, 1991). Moreover, homosexuals who have declared their homosexuality to their family have worse family relationships than those who stay in the closet (D'Augelli, Grossman, Starks & Sinclair, 2010). This declaration often arouses negative reactions. More than half of homosexuals experience a negative reaction from their parents, sadness, denial and anger being the most frequently observed attitudes displayed by the latter (Savin-Williams & Ream, 2003; Willoughby et al., 2006). However, over time, an improvement in parental attitudes may be observed (Charbonnier & Graziani, 2011; D'Augelli et al., 2010).

This revelation can have dramatic consequences, and young people may find themselves living on the street or in hostels (Mallon, Aledort & Ferrera, 2002), excluded from the family home by their family or preferring to leave in order to escape a disharmonious family environment (Beck, Firdion, Legleye & Schiltz, 2010).

This data can be linked to "stress related growth" (SRG) which supports the idea that stressors do not automatically lead to negative consequences but can also generate positive changes. This idea is found in Taylor's cognitive adaptation theory (Taylor, 1983) and is linked to the positive psychology movement (Seligman & Csikszentmihalyi, 2000). Homosexuals also perceive the revelation of their homosexuality as an SRG, that's to say a stressful event from which they emerge having grown (LaSala, 2000; Oswald, 2000), which has led to the creation of the term "coming-out growth" (COG). For Vaughan and Waehler (2010), COG is not simply an experience of SRG, but is rather considered as a unique process as it includes experiences which are not tackled in the literature on SRG. Declaring one's homosexuality is therefore a complex experience, one that is both liberating and calming, yet at the same time stressful and able to generate significant suffering. The stress related to this particular situation is induced both by the fact of making the declaration but also by the anticipation of reactions of rejection, particularly by the family.

STRESS AND FAMILY ATTITUDES

Lesbians, gays and bisexuals seem to communicate less with their parents than heterosexuals (Espelage, Aragon, Birkett & Koenig, 2008). 68% of gays and 55% of lesbians experience negative reaction from their parents to the declaration of their homosexuality (Willoughby et al., 2006). Around 30% of lesbians, gays or bisexuals (15-21 years of age) are said to have been subjected to verbal abuse from their family in relation to their sexual orientation and 10% have been attacked physically (Pilkington & D'Augelli, 1995). 33% of these displays of rejection are said to come from the mother, 29% from the father and 19% from siblings (SOS Homophobie, 2004). Yet, parental attitudes of rejection may be linked to relationship and attachment disorders, academic problems, substance abuse and depression (Hale, Van der Valk, Engles & Meeus, 2005; Pedersen, 1994; Piko, 2000). Conversely, positive parental attitudes to the homosexuality of their child are associated with the development of harmonious social behaviours (Rohner, Khaleque & Cournoyer, 2003) and well-being (Floyd, Stein, Harter, Allison & Nye, 1999) amongst young homosexuals. These positive attitudes are also negatively correlated with the risk of attempting suicide (Eisenberg & Resnick, 2006), of developing internalised homophobia (Nungesser, 1983; Savin-Williams, 1989), and of engaging in risky sexual behaviour (Vincke, Bolton, Mak & Blank, 1993).

All parents have a certain number of expectations with regard to their child and its development. Children who, once they are adults, develop in line with parental expectations generate a feeling of security and accomplishment in their parents. And so, parents who assess the personal and social development of their children positively display greater well-being, higher self-esteem and a greater sense of being in control of their environment (Ryff, Lee, Essex & Schmutte, 1994). Conversely, a child who does not comply with parental expectations, as may be the case with homosexual children, can disturb the parents' well-being (Julien, 2000). Generally speaking, parental positions undergo a positive change over time (Charbonnier & Graziani, 2011), as parents with homosexual children have to progress through various stages in order to adapt to the sexual orientation of their child (Robinson, Walter & Skeen, 1989). These stages may be associated with those of grief (shock, denial, guilt, anger and acceptance) (Kübler-Ross, 1975). The consciousness of homosexuals also changes over time, as the construction of their sexual identity is progressive and frequently stress-generating.

STRESS AND THE CONSTRUCTION OF HOMOSEXUAL IDENTITY

Defining yourself as a homosexual involves the adoption of a non-traditional identity, the restructuring of the conception you have of yourself, and changing the relationships you maintain with society (Reynolds & Hanjorgiris, 2000). The first model to account for the different stages which homosexuals go through in order to live lives which fully express their sexual orientation is a six-stage one (Cass, 1979):

- "Identity Confusion": the person realises that they are different.
- "Identity Comparison": the young person makes the supposition that they could be homosexual and experiments with heterosexual and/or homosexual behaviour.
- "Identity Tolerance": an awareness of their homosexuality begins to emerge.
- "Identity Acceptance": this includes first contacts with the homosexual community.
- "Identity Pride": the stage when the subject integrates into the homosexual community.
- "Identity Synthesis": the individual accepts themselves and others.

In 1996, a new model was developed, concerning lesbians initially (McCarn & Fassinger, 1996), and then adapted for gays (Fassinger & Miller, 1996). It reflects the development of sexual identity from an individual and group point of view and considers the construction of sexual identity as a continuous and interactive process, with the term "phases" replacing "stages". The first phase begins with an attraction to an individual of the same sex, an attraction which is not necessarily understood. Then comes a time of exploration and curiosity which can involve various feelings such as fear, sadness and excitement. Subsequently, the individual is likely to attempt to get to know the homosexual community, and will then become aware of the discriminations which homosexuals can encounter. The last phase of the process is a feeling of comfort and acceptance of one's homosexuality.

And so, the construction of one's homosexual identity involves a period of negotiation, whether it concern relationships with oneself, with others or with society. This construction involves a period of crisis characterised by questioning, discomfort and indecision. So, each "stage" or "phase" may generate stress. This stress is increased by homophobia and heterosexism, all the more so as homosexuals are more attentive and sensitive to these phenomena during this process (Reynolds & Hanjorgiris, 2000). This stress can lead homosexuals to put strategies in place in an attempt to reduce it, as for example the use and abuse of substances.

STRESS AND CONSUMPTION OF SUBSTANCES

Lesbians, gays and bisexuals consume more alcohol and drugs than the general population, are less often able to abstain from consumption and more frequently continue their consumption into adult life (CSAT, 2001). In the USA, disorders linked to the use of substances are prevalent amongst this group (Cochran, Ackerman, Mays & Ross, 2004; Cochran, Sullivan & Mays, 2003; Wilsnack et al., 2008). The proportion of smokers for example is higher amongst lesbians and gays than amongst heterosexuals (Burgard, Cochran & Mays, 2005; Greenwood et al., 2005; Mays, Yancey, Cochran, Weber & Fielding, 2002). Exposure to severe or chronic stress may induce or reinforce the use or abuse of substances (Décamps, 2010; Sinha, 2008). According to the transactional approach to stress (Lazarus & Folkman, 1984; Lazarus & Folkman, 1987), the use of substances can be considered as a coping strategy, that's to say an attempt to adjust to stress, a behaviour aiming to face up to and adapt to situations judged to be stressful and to calm the emotional tension which they generate. However, over time the consumption itself can become a source of stress by generating new constraints (Battaglia, 2010), leading the consumers to devise new adjustment strategies such as, for example, compensatory behaviour involving cross-addiction or poly-addictive behaviour.

The use and/or abuse of substances can be considered as strategies employed by homosexuals to cope with their shame, stress and social difficulties, but also to facilitate the expression of their emotions or engagement in new forms of behaviour, particularly in the sexual domain (Cabaj, 2000). During adolescence, the use of substances is favoured, as capacities to cope with stressful events are still being established (Compas, Conner-Smith, Saltzman, Thomsen & Wadsworth, 2001). Yet, while adolescence is a period characterised by numerous stressors (emotional, physical, social, identity-related or affective), adolescent homosexuals have to cope with additional stressors (non-compliance with the norm, discrimination, revelation of their sexual orientation…). The addition of these two dimensions (weakness of coping strategies and significant stressors) may contribute to initiating and/or reinforcing their addictive behaviours.

The over-consumption observed in this group is also linked to the stress generated by the experience of discrimination (Meyer, 1995; Meyer, 2003), the exposure to instances of heterosexism (Bobbe, 2002) and internalised homophobia (Amadio & Chung, 2004; Cabaj, 2000; CSAT, 2001; Jaffe, Clance, Nichols & Emshoff, 2000). The use of alcohol and drugs is a strategy which may be particularly employed by homosexuals to temporarily conceal the various negative emotions generated by internalised homophobia (Weber, 2008). According to McCabe and al. (2010) it may be the accumulation of several experiences of discrimination (racial/ethnic discrimination, gender discrimination ...) which encourages consumption amongst homosexuals. Their over-consumption can therefore be considered as the result of environmental factors characterised by stigmatisation and marginalisation (McCabe et al. 2010). Conversely, the support of the immediate group can have a protective role, which has a limiting effect on the use of products. And so, parental acceptance may play a protective role, all the more so when the young homosexual finds himself in a context of stress (Padilla et al., 2010). Consequently, treatment of addictions amongst homosexuals involves taking into consideration experiences of homophobia, heterosexism and internalised homophobia, as well as the stressful situations specific to homosexuals, such as the revelation of their homosexuality, as these can be occasions when substances are taken and/or abused or risky behaviour engaged in (Charbonnier, 2012).

STUDY OF THE STRESS ASSOCIATED WITH A DECLARATION OF HOMOSEXUALITY

In order to better understand the stress associated with making a declaration of homosexuality, we carried out a study of 400 French subjects reporting themselves to be homosexuals (145 women and 255 men), between 16 and 28 years of age (M = 21.8; SD = 2.6). Our aim was to highlight the characteristics of the stress associated with a declaration of homosexuality, as compared with other stressful events which young homosexuals may encounter. This study is based on the transactional model of stress (Lazarus & Folkman, 1984) which places the emphasis on the way in which the subject interprets the stressful transaction. In this model, it is not the event which is considered as a stressor, but rather the cognitive assessment made by the subject. So, the assessment of the stressful situation is said to take place in two stages. First of all, a rapid, automatic, preliminary assessment, which allows the subject to determine whether the situation represents a threat or not, a danger or a challenge. Then a secondary assessment, during which the subject assesses their resources and summons the efforts necessary to cope with the stressful situation (coping strategies).

Two subject groups were formed, each one given a different brief:

Brief 1 (group 1): "recall the declaration of your homosexuality which was the most stressful in your life and reply to the following questions" (N = 252 subjects)

Brief 2 (group 2): "recall the most stressful event you have experienced in your life and reply to the following questions" (N = 148 subjects) (we excluded those who gave the declaration of their homosexuality as an answer).

Through our questionnaire, we assessed different variables such as:

- *The characteristics of the situation:* The respondents assessed their level of preparation and initiative, and the number of times the stressful situation had been repeated. They also specified the people involved in the situation.
- *The risks incurred (preliminary assessment):* They evaluated the presence of 14 risks to them during the stressful situation on a scale from 0 ("not at all") to 4 ("very great").
- *Their options for action (secondary assessment):* they assessed the relevance of four possible courses of action: ("change the situation or do something", "accept it", "find out more before taking action", "refrain from doing what they wanted to do") on a similar scale.
- *Taking of substances or engaging in risky behaviour:* they were asked to specify if they had resorted to the use of substances or engaged in risky or addictive behaviours in order to feel better in the chosen stressful situation on a scale from 0 ("not at all") to 3 ("greatly").

‒ *Risk of suicide:* the presence of suicidal ideas and behaviour during the situation was assessed, as was the risk of suicide at the time the questionnaire was being administered, using the Suicide Behaviors Questionnaire-Revised (SBQ-Revised) (Osman et al., 2001).

The declaration of homosexuality which proved to be the most stressful (group 1) was largely that made to parents and/or to other members of the family (71.4%). Conversely, amongst the participants in group 2 (another stressful situation), the results were much more mixed, where the situation might involve, for example, their parents (15.5%), their partner (10.1%) or their friends (8.7%). On average, the revelation of homosexuality which was the most stressful took place around the age of majority, gays making the declaration earlier than lesbians (F = 0.7; p < 0.05). More than one declaration was found to be stressful as 42.9% of respondents in group 1 declared that they had found "more than three declarations to be stressful" and 32.9% had experienced "one or two stressful declarations". This was not the case for the other stressful situations, 73% of the participants in group 2 declaring that they had never encountered stressful situations of the same type. A repetitive or even chronic stressful situation can test an individual's feelings of being in control, even more so if they have to cope with a situation which they don't succeed in managing.

A revelation of homosexuality involved a great deal more preparation than the other stressful situations, the means in the two groups being significantly different (F = 22.3; p< 0.0001). Indeed, 25.8% of respondents in group 1 had "planned" the declaration of their homosexuality completely, as against 12% of those in group 2. The predictable nature of a stressful confrontation allows the subject to prepare themselves better to confront the situation. Moreover, on average, the participants in group 1 were more active in instigating the stressful situation than the participants in group 2 (F = 32.8; p< 0.0001), 37.7% of the individuals in group 1 being "totally responsible" for initiating the situation as against 18.9% of those in group 2. A stressful situation which the subject has created increases their feeling of being in control, unlike one which is imposed on them.

Table 1, Means (and standard deviations) of options for action (on a scale from 0 to 4), for the two subject groups, and comparison of means (ANOVA)

	Group 1		Group 2			
	Means	Standard deviation	Means	Standard deviation	F	p
CHANGE/DO SOMETHING	0.9	1.2	1.5	1,5	20.9	0.0001
ACCEPT	3	1.2	2.8	1.4	2.4	0.12
FIND OUT MORE	1.2	1.3	1.7	1.6	13.4	0.0001
REFRAIN	1.3	1.5	1.7	1.6	9.3	0.002

The four most common risks encountered during a revelation of homosexuality were all linked to other people and the possibility of hurting them ("Losing the affection of someone important to you", "Causing pain to a loved one", "Losing the approval or respect of someone important to you", "Disrupting the customary habits of a loved one"). Conversely, during other stressful situations, the most significant risks were essentially linked to the individual.

The risk with the highest mean in group 2 was the following: "Damaging your own health, safety or well-being". For the two subject groups, the favoured course of action was "acceptance". However options for action were significantly fewer during a declaration of homosexuality than during other stressful situations (see table 1).

Table 2. Sample numbers for each answer by group, and means comparison (ANOVA)

Behaviour adopted in order to feel better	Terms of response	Group 1 (N=252)	Group 2 (N=148)	F	p
Eating more	"Not at all"	185	111	0.2	0.8
	"A little"	31	17		
	"to a moderate extent"	20	11		
	"a lot"	16	9		
Drinking alcohol	"Not at all"	170	96	0.03	0.7
	"A little"	28	19		
	"to a moderate extent"	30	19		
	"a lot"	24	14		
Smoking	"Not at all"	152	89	2.5	0.5
	"A little"	27	13		
	"to a moderate extent"	34	15		
	"a lot"	39	31		
Taking drugs	"Not at all"	185	97	5	0.1
	"A little"	24	19		
	"to a moderate extent"	20	12		
	"a lot"	23	20		
Risky behaviour	"Not at all"	176	99	3.3	0.3
	"A little"	26	12		
	"to a moderate extent"	23	17		
	"a lot"	27	20		

At the time when the questionnaire was administered, the subjects in group 1 presented a mean score on the suicide risk assessment scale of 7.2 (SD = 3.6), which was 7.7 (SD = 3.7) for those in group 2. There were no significant differences between the two groups (F = 1.6; p = 0.2). According to the authors (Osman et al., 2001) the risk of suicide is considered as higher when the score is 7 or higher. So the participants in our sample present a high suicide risk. As regards the presence of suicidal behaviours, 24.2% of the subjects in group 1 and 19.6% of those in group 2 stated that they had "attempted to kill themselves" during the stressful situation, although the difference between the groups was not significant (F = 0.6 ; p = 0.4). Moreover, 39.7% of the respondents in group 1 and 35.8% of the subjects in group 2 stated that they "at least thought of ending it all" during the stressful situation. Here also, there were no significant differences between the groups (F = 1.1; p = 0.3). Consequently, during the declaration of homosexuality which was the most stressful, the risk of exhibiting suicidal ideas or behaviours was not greater than during another extremely stressful situation. However, it is important to note the high prevalence of suicidal ideas and acts amongst young homosexuals when they are confronted with the most stressful situation of their life, whatever the situation. We can draw the same conclusion for recourse to the use of substances or engagement in risky behaviour. No significant differences were noted between the two groups but these behaviours seem to be strategies much used to cope with stress (see table 2). Out of the overall sample, 39.8% had used cigarettes "a little, at least", in order to feel better, 33.5% alcohol, 31.2% had engaged in risky behaviour, 29.5% had taken drugs and 26% had eaten more than usual.

In addition to the normal problems and difficulties associated with adolescence and early adulthood, young homosexuals face specific stresses which heterosexuals do not encounter, such as homophobia or the declaration of their homosexuality. They often find themselves defenceless against this situation, judging it to be more risky and feeling less able to cope with it than with other stressful situations encountered during their life. The perception of a heightened threat and the poor options for action explain the highly stressful nature of this situation. Consequently, for young homosexuals who find the declaration of their homosexuality difficult, it seems to us important to offer them space to reflect on this declaration, to prepare for it, to explore the opportunities and consequences of their revelation but also to develop techniques for stress management. Our data takes account of the links existing amongst young homosexuals between stress, suicidal ideas and/or behaviours and the use of dysfunctional strategies (consumption of substances ...). Consequently, stress management is a course of action to be preferred in order to prevent suicide and the use or abuse of substances amongst this group. But in order for this support to be possible, it is essential that professionals reflect on their own prejudices and beliefs with regard to homosexuality and become aware of the specific difficulties and stressors which homosexuals are faced with.

REFERENCES

Amadio, D. M., & Chung, B. Y. (2004). Internalized homophobia and substance use among lesbian, gay, and bisexual persons. *Journal of Gay and Lesbian Social Services: Issues in Practice, Policy, and Research,* 17, 83-101.

Battaglia, N., Bruchon-Schweitzer, M., Décampsc, G. (2010). Introduction. Esquisse d'une approche intégrative du concept d'addiction : regards croisés. *Psychologie française,* 55, 261-277.

Beck, F., Firdion, J. M., Legleye, S., & Schiltz, M. A. (2010). *Les minorités sexuelles face au risque suicidaire. Acquis des sciences sociales et perspectives.* Saint Denis INPES.

Bobbe, J. (2002). Treatment with lesbian alcoholics: Healing shame and internalized homophobia for ongoing sobriety. *Health and Social Work,* 27, 218-222.

Bonet, L., Wells, B. E., & Parsons, J. T. (2007). A positive look at a difficult time: A strength based examination of coming out for lesbian and bisexual women. *Journal of LGBT Health Research,* 3, 7-14.

Burgard, S. A., Cochran, S. D., & Mays, V. M. (2005). Alcohol and tobacco use patterns among heterosexually and homosexually experienced California women. *Drug and Alcohol Dependence,* 77, 61-70.

Cabaj, R. P. (2000). Substance abuse, internalized homophobia, and gay men and lesbians: Psychodynamic issues and clinical implications. In J. R. Guss & J. Drescher (Eds.), *Addictions in the gay and lesbian community* (pp. 5-24). Binghamton, NY: The Haworth Press.

Cass, V. C. (1979). Homosexual identity formation: A theoretical model. *Journal of Homosexuality*(4), 219-235.

Charbonnier, E., & Graziani, P. (2011*). La perception de jeunes lesbiennes et gais concernant l'attitude de leurs parents à l'égard de leur homosexualité. Revue canadienne de santé mentale communautaire*, 30, 31-46.

Charbonnier, E., Graziani, P. (2012). Les stratégies de coping que les jeunes homosexuels mettent en place lors de la divulgation de leur homosexualité. *Journal de thérapie comportementale et cognitive*, 22, 24-31

Cochran, S. D., Ackerman, D., Mays, V. M., & Ross, M. W. (2004). Prevalence of non-medical drug use and dependence among homosexually active men and women in the US population. *Addiction*, 99, 989-998.

Cochran, S. D., Sullivan, J. G., & Mays, V. M. (2003). Prevalence of mental disorders, psychological distress, and mental health services use among lesbian, gay, and bisexual adults in the United States. *Journal of Consulting and Clinical Psychology*, 71, 53-61.

Compas, B. E., Conner-Smith, J. K., Saltzman, H., Thomsen, A. H., & Wadsworth, M. E. (2001). *Coping with stress during childhood and adolescence: problems, progress, and potential in theory and research. psychological bulletin*, 127, 87-127.

Coursaud, J. B. (2002). *L'homosexualité entre préjugés et réalités*. Toulouse: Milan.

CSAT. (2001). *A provider's introduction to substance abuse treatment for lesbian, gay, bisexual, and transgender individuals*. Rockville, MD: Center for substance abuse treatment.

D'Augelli, A., Grossman, A., Starks, M., & Sinclair, K. (2010). Factors Associated with Parents' Knowledge of Gay, Lesbian, and Bisexual Youths' Sexual Orientation. *J GLBT Fam Stud*, 6(2), 178-198.

D'Augelli, A. R., Hershberger, S. L., & Pilkington, N. W. (1998). Lesbian, gay, and bisexual youth and their families: disclosure of sexual orientation and its consequences. *Am J Orthopsychiatry*, 68(3), 361-375.

D'Augelli, A. R. (2002). Mental Health Problems among Lesbian, Gay, and Bisexual Youths Ages 14 to 21. *Clin Child Psychol Psychiatry*, 7(3), 433-456

Décamps, G., Idier, L., Koleck, M. (2010). Conduites addictives avec ou sans substance. Etude de leurs déterminants psychologiques. *Alcoologie et Addictologie*, 32(4), 269-278.

Décamps, G., Scroccaro, N., Battaglia, N. (2009). Stratégies de coping et activités compensatoires chez les alcooliques abstinents. *Annales Médico-Psychologiques*, 167, 491-496.

Eisenberg, M. E., & Resnick, M. D. (2006). Suicidality among gay, lesbian and bisexual youth: The role of protective factors. *Journal of adolescent health*, 39, 662-668.

Espelage, D., Aragon, S., Birkett, M., & Koenig, B. (2008). Homophobic teasing, psychological outcomes, and sexual orientation among high school students: what influence do parents and school have? *School Psych Rev*, 37(2), 202-216.

Fassinger, R. E., & Miller, B. A. (1996). Validation of an inclusive model of homosexual identity formation in a sample of gay men. *Journal of Homosexuality*, 32, 53-78.

Floyd, F. J., Stein, T. S., Harter, K. S. M., Allison, A., & Nye, C. L. (1999). Gay, lesbian, and bisexual youths: separation-individuation, parental attitudes, identity consolidation, and well-being. *Journal of youth and adolescence*, 28, 719-739.

Greenwood, G. L., Paul, J. P., Pollack, L. M., Binson, D., Catania, J. A., Chang, J., et al. (2005). Tobacco use and cessation among a household-based sample of US urban men who have sex with men. *American Journal of Public Health*, 95, 145-151.

Grov, C., Bimbi, D. S., Nanin, J. E., & Parsons, J. T. (2006). Race, ethnicity, gender, and generational factors associated with the coming-out process among lesbian, and bisexual individuals. *J Sex Res*, 43(2), 115-121.

Hale, W. W., Van der Valk, I., Engles, R., & Meeus, W. (2005). Does perceived parental rejection make adolescents sad and mad? The association of perceived parental rejection with adolescent depression and aggression. *Journal of adolescent health*, 36, 466-474.

Halpin, S. A., & Allen, M. W. (2004). Changes in the psychosocial well-being during stages of gay identity development. *Journal of Homosexuality*, 47, 109-126.

Hefez, S. (2003). Adolescence et homophobie. In C. Broqua, F. Lert & Y. Souteryrand (Eds.), *Homosexualités au temps du sida* (pp. 147-168). Paris: ANRS.

Iwasaki, Y., & Ristock, J. L. (2007). The nature of stress experienced by lesbians and gay men. *Anxiety Stress Coping*, 20(3), 299-319.

Jaffe, C., Clance, P. R., Nichols, M. F., & Emshoff, J. G. (2000). The prevalence of alcoholism and feelings of alienation in lesbian and heterosexual women. In J. R. Guss & J. Drescher (Eds.), *Addictions in the gay and lesbian community* (pp. 25-35). Harrington Park, NJ: The Haworth Press.

Julien, D. (2000). Famille d'origine et homosexualité. In M. Simard & J. Alary (Eds.), *Comprendre la famille : actes du 5e symposium québécois de recherche sur la famille* (pp. 210-222). Québec: Presse Universitaire du Québec.

Kübler-Ross, E. (1975). Les derniers instants de la vie. Genève: Labor et Fides.

LaSala, M. C. (2000). Gay male couples: The importance of coming out and being out to parents. *Journal of Homosexuality*, 39, 47-71.

Lazarus, R. S., & Folkman, S. (1984*). Stress, Appraisal and Coping*. New York: Springer Publishing.

Lazarus, R. S., & Folkman, S. (1987). Transactional theory and research on emotions and coping. *Eur J Pers*, 1(3), 141–169.

Lewis, R. J., Derlega, V. J., Griffin, J. L., & Krowinski, A. C. (2003). Stressors for Gay Men and Lesbians: Life Stress, Gay-Related Stress, Stigma Consciousness, and Depressive Symptoms. *J Soc Clin Psychol*, 22(6), 716-729.

Mallon, G. P., Aledort, N., & Ferrera, M. (2002). There's no place like home: achieving safety, permanency, and well-being for lesbian and gay adolescents in out-of-home care settings. *Child Welfare*, 81(2), 407-439.

Mays, V. M., Yancey, A. K., Cochran, S. D., Weber, M., & Fielding, J. E. (2002). Heterogenity of health disparities among African American, Hispanic and Asian American Women: Unrecognized influences of sexual orientation. *American Journal of Public Health,* 92, 632-639.

McCabe, E. S., Bostwick, W. B., Hughes, T. L., West, B. T., & Boyd, C. J. (2010). The Relationship Between Discrimination and Substance Use Disorders Among Lesbian, Gay, and Bisexual Adults in the United States. *American Journal of Public Health*, 100, 1949-1952.

McCarn, S. R., & Fassinger, R. E. (1996). Revisioning sexual minority identity formation: A new model of lesbian identity and its implications for counseling and research. *The Counseling Psychologist*, 24, 508-534.

Mellini, L. (2009). Entre normalisation et hétéronormativité : la construction de l'identité homosexuelle. *Déviance et société*(33), 3-26.

Meyer, I. H. (1995). Minority stress and mental health in gay men. *J Health Soc Behav*, 36(1), 38-56.

Meyer, I. H. (2003). Prejudice, social stress, and mental health in lesbian, gay, and bisexual populations: conceptual issues and research evidence. *Psychol Bull,* 129(5), 674-697.

Meyer, I. H., & Northridge, M. E. (2007). *The Health of Sexual Minorities: Public Health Perspectives of Lesbian, Gay, Bisexual and Transgender Populations.* New York: Springer.

Monroe, E. J. (2001). *Drawing upon the experiences of those who are out: A qualitative study of the coming-out process of gays and lesbians.* The University of Iowa, Doctoral dissertation.

Morris, J. F. (1997). Lesbian coming out as a multidimensional processes. *Journal of Homosexuality*, 33, 1-22.

Nungesser, L. G. (1983). *Homosexual acts, actors, and identities.* New York: Praeger.

Osman, A., Bagge, C. L., Gutierrez, P. M., Konick, L. C., Kopper, B. A., & Barrios, F. X. (2001). *The Suicidal Behaviors Questionnaire-Revised (SBQ-R): validation with clinical and nonclinical samples. Assessment,* 8(4), 443-454.

Oswald, R. (2000). Family and friendship relationships after young women come out as bisexual or lesbian. *Journal of Homosexuality*, 38, 65-83.

Padilla, Y. C., Crisp, C., & Rew, D. L. (2010). Parental Acceptance and Illegal Drug Use among Gay, Lesbian, and Bisexual Adolescents: Results from a National Survey. *Social Work*, 55, 265-275.

Pedersen, W. (1994). Parental relations, mental health, and delinquency in adolescents. *Adolescence*, 29, 975-990.

Piko, B. (2000). Perceived social support from parents and peers: which is the stronger predictor of adolescent substance use? *Substance use & misuse*(35), 617-630.

Pilkington, N. W., & D'Augelli, A. R. (1995). Victimization of lesbian, gay, and bisexual youth in community settings. *J Community Psychol*, 23(1), 34-56.

Remafedi, G., Farrow, J. A., & Deisher, R. W. (1991). Risk factors for attempted suicide in gay and bisexual youth. *Pediatrics*, 87(6), 869-875.

Reynolds, A. L., & Hanjorgiris, W. F. (2000). Coming out: Lesbian, gay, and bisexual identity development. In R. M. Perez, D. K. A. & K. J. Bieschke (Eds.), *Handbook of counseling and psychotherapy with lesbian, gay, and bisexual clients* (pp. 35-55). Washington, DC: American Psychological Association.

Robinson, B. E., Walter, L. H., & Skeen, P. (1989). Response of parents to learning that their child is homosexual and concern over AIDS: a national study. *Journal of Homosexuality*, 18(1-2), 59-80.

Robohm, J. S., Litzenberger, B. W., & Pearlman, L. A. (2003). Sexual abuse in lesbian and bisexual young women: Associations with emotional/behavioral difficulties, feelings about sexuality, and the "coming out" process. *J Lesbian Stud,* 7(4), 31-47.

Rohner, R. P., Khaleque, A., & Cournoyer, D. E. (2003). Cross-national perspectives on parental acceptance-rejection theory. *Marriage and family review,* 35, 85-105.

Rosario, M., Schrimshaw, E. W., & Hunter, J. (2004). Gay-related stress and emotional distress among gay, lesbian, and bisexual youths: A longitudinal examination. *Journal of Consulting and Clinical Psychology*, 70, 967-975.

Ryff, C. D., Lee, Y. H., Essex, M. J., & Schmutte, P. S. (1994). My children and me :mid-life evaluations of grown children and self. *Psychology and Aging,* 9(2), 195-205.

Savin-Williams, R., & Ream, G. (2003). Sex variations in the disclosure to parents of same-sex attractions. *J Fam Psychol*, 17(3), 429–438.

Savin-Williams, R. C. (1989). Coming out to parents and self-esteem among gay and lesbian youths. *J Homosex*, 18(1-2), 1-35.

Savin-Williams, R. C. (1998). The disclosure to families of same-sex attractions by lesbian, gay, and bisexual youths. *Journal of Research on Adolescence,* 8, 49-68.

Savin-Williams, R. C. (2001*). Mom, Dad, I'm gay: How families negotiate coming out.* Washington, DC: American Psychological Association.

Savin-Williams, R. C., & Esterberg, K. G. (2000). Lesbian, gay, and bisexual families. In D. H. Demo, K. R. Allen & M. A. Fine (Eds.), *Handbook of family diversity* (pp. 197-215). New York: Oxford University Press.

Seligman, M. E. P., & Csikszentmihalyi, M. (2000). Positive psychology: An introduction. *American Psychologist*, 55, 5-14.

Sinha, R. (2008). Chronic stress, drug use, and vulnerability to addiction. Annals of the New York Academy of Sciences, 1141, 105-130.

SOS Homophobie. (2004). *Rapport 2004 sur l'homophobie. Paris: SOS Homophobie.*

Taylor, S. E. (1983). Adjustment to threatening events: A theory of cognitive adaptation. *American Psychologist*, 38, 1161-1173.

Vaughan, M. (2007). *Coming out growth: Conceptualizing and assessing experiences of stress-related growth associated with coming out as lesbian or gay.* The University of Akron, Doctoral Dissertation.

Vaughan, M. D., & Waehler, C. A. (2010). Coming Out Growth: Conceptualizing and Measuring Stress-Related Growth Associated with Coming Out to Others as a Sexual Minority. *Journal of Adult Development*, 17, 94–109.

Vincke, J., Bolton, R., Mak, R., & Blank, S. (1993). Coming out and AIDS-related high-risk sexual behavior. Archives of sexual behavior, 22, 559-586.

Weber, G. N. (2008). Using to Numb the Pain: Substance Use and Abuse Among Lesbian, Gay, and Bisexual Individuals. *Journal of Mental Health Counseling,* 30, 31-48.

Willoughby, B. L. B., Malik, N. M., & Lindahl, K. M. (2006). Parental Reactions to Their Sons' Sexual Orientation Disclosures: The Roles of Family Cohesion, Adaptability, and Parenting Style. *Psychol Men Masc*, 7(1), 14-26.

Wilsnack, S. C., Hughes, T. L., Johnson, T. P., Bostwick, W. B., Szalacha, L. A., Benson, P., et al. (2008). Drinking and drinking-related problems among heterosexual and sexual minority women. *Journal of Studies on Alcohol and Drugs,* 129-139.

In: Psychology of Stress
Editors: Leandro Cavalcanti and Sofia Azevedo

ISBN: 978-1-62417-109-3
© 2013 Nova Science Publishers, Inc.

Chapter 6

PSYCHOLOGICAL FACTORS INFLUENCING INTER-INDIVIDUAL VARIATION IN CARBON DIOXIDE-INDUCED STRESS RESPONSE

Kristin Vickers[*]
Institute for Stress and Wellbeing Research
and Department of Psychology, Ryerson University,
Toronto, Ontario, Canada

ABSTRACT

People vary markedly in their response to the same stressor. Possibly, psychological factors hold promise in advancing our understanding of this inter-individual variation in stress responsivity. Indeed, the psychology underlying stress reactivity is an active and important focus of extensive ongoing scientific investigation. Researchers interested in the psychology of stress have increasingly turned their attention towards laboratory stress provocation paradigms. This approach enables a controlled experimental environment in which to measure stress response before, during, and after the stressful provocation. It also affords the opportunity to manipulate putative causal factors implicated in individual stress response. Recently, use of 35% carbon dioxide (CO_2)-enriched air (the 35% CO_2 challenge) has emerged as a particularly promising laboratory stress provocation paradigm (e.g., Vickers et al., 2012). The purpose of this chapter is to overview new findings about the psychology of stress that have been illuminated through 35% CO_2 provocation of the human stress response. The chapter focuses especially on the research conducted in the years since Zvolensky and Eifert (2001)'s seminal review of the psychology underlying the CO_2 response. Particular attention is spent on description of the psychological factors (e.g., anxiety sensitivity; Telch et al., 2011) that could aggravate stress responsivity. Emphasis is also placed on the need for research into factors promoting resilience in the face of the CO_2 stressor. Ultimately, clarifying how psychological factors influence individual differences in stress responsivity could yield targets for intervention in the treatment of extreme stress responses.

---

[*] Correspondence to Kristin Vickers, PhD, Department of Psychology, Ryerson University, 350 Victoria St., Toronto, ON M5B2K3, Canada. Fax: 416-979-5273; Email: kvickers@ryerson.ca; Tel: 416-979-5000 ext. 7727.

INTRODUCTION

Recently, researchers have increasingly turned their attention to the reasons accounting for variability across persons in their response to a common stressor. Psychological differences have emerged as a particularly promising avenue to pursue in this research trajectory. The purpose of this chapter is to overview established findings about the psychological characteristics that affect individual response to one specific stressor, the 35% carbon dioxide (CO_2) challenge.

Striking inter-individual variability characterizes how people respond to the same stressor, as lay wisdom and psychological science both suggest. Indeed, the commonsense opinion that one person's thrilling roller coaster ride is another's terrifying ordeal is amply bolstered by empirical evidence indicating that someone's reaction to particular situations (e.g., a new job) or stimuli (e.g., a thunderstorm) often depends on the specific individual in question (Blonna, 2007). Furthermore, in many cases, whether a possibly stress-inducing situation or stimulus is even a stressor at all arguably depends on a certain person's perception that the state of affairs represents a threat with which that person cannot cope (e.g., Lazarus, 1966). (It should be noted that in other cases, the stimulus or situation itself is widely accepted as traumatic (American Psychiatric Association [APA], 1994) and thus universally stress-provoking, for example, an assault). As such, determining how people respond to a potential or universal stressor necessitates examining individual responses to a common situation or stimulus across the studied population.

Ethical and moral concerns obviously make administration of a universal stressor to a sample unacceptable. Accordingly, two other approaches are customarily used to study how people react to stressors. In one, persons' reactions to naturally occurring stressors (e.g., a hurricane) are observed. In the other, a very mild potentially stress-inducing stimulus is administered in a laboratory environment, and participants' responses are assessed. Taking each approach in turn, the naturalistic approach has indisputably afforded researchers a wealth of valuable insight concerning risk factors increasing the likelihood of stress reactions. To illustrate, prior history of psychopathology (Brewin et al., 2000) or another trauma (Rosenberg and Kosslyn, 2011) augments the probability of a stress reaction occurring after a subsequent stressor. Indeed, with this finding in mind, some researchers posit that previously suffering from trauma in childhood in particular can engender a kind of "scar" upon an individual's mental well-being that subsequent stressors, in turn, may aggravate (Nolen-Hoeksema and Rector, 2011). (It should be emphasized that some catastrophic stressors imbue stress reactions in almost all victims, regardless of the victims' prior exposure to trauma; for example, over 90% of rape victims suffer stress reaction symptoms in the week following the attack; Foa and Riggs, 1995). More generally, although the approach of observing individual reactions after a naturally occurring stressor can impart useful probative knowledge, this naturalistic observation method also has its limitations. Specifically, in this method, researchers cannot manipulate putative risk (or protective) factors prior to the stressor. As such, causality is difficult to deduce from naturalistic observation.

Experimental methods using the controlled laboratory environment to administer a mild potentially stress-inducing stimulus do indeed afford inferences about causality and are thus widely used with this goal in mind. For example, participants might listen to different kinds of music or no music at all (as manipulated by the researchers) and be told that they will have to give a speech. Then, whether certain types of music (if any) significantly affect one's response to expecting to having to give a speech can be measured. (Often in this type of paradigm, no speech is really given; the deception is justified ethically by the knowledge accrued from observing how participants truly react when believing that they will give a speech; see Sandstrom and Russo, 2010, p. 139). Along these lines, research at Ryerson University (home of the Institute for Stress and Wellbeing Research) has revealed that positively valenced but low arousal music significantly improves the physiological recovery from a speech-threat stressor better than does white noise (Sandstrom and Russo, 2010). Notably, although useful information can certainly result from this experimental approach, it too has its limitations; questions about the ecological validity—or dearth therefore—of the stimulus used to provoke mild stress in the lab setting inevitably emerge. Consequently, findings about individual factors predicting stress responsivity gleaned from both naturalistic and experimental methods are often jointly considered in the interest of advancing psychological knowledge.

In line with the goal of further understanding factors involved in individual stress responsivity, this chapter will focus on a particular experimental method used to provoke the human stress response, the 35% CO_2 challenge. Recently, use of this specific experimental approach has emerged as a particularly promising laboratory stress provocation paradigm (e.g., Kaye et al., 2004). The advantages of utilizing the 35% carbon dioxide challenge to engender a mild stress reaction have been discussed elsewhere (e.g., Kaye et al., 2004; Wetherell et al., 2006); how the challenge is administered and its effects on the body also have received extensive attention in a recent review paper (Vickers et al., 2012) and will not be repeated here. Briefly, to set the stage for the findings on stress reactivity using this stress provocation method, the 35% carbon dioxide challenge requires participants to take a full (e.g., vital capacity) breath of a gas mixture containing 35% carbon dioxide (the rest is room air). The immediate effects of inhaling this gaseous mixture are activation in both the sympathetic nervous system (increased blood pressure) and the parasympathetic nervous system (lowered heart rate), as well as increased cortisol and breathlessness, and mild anxiety in normal participants. The challenge has shown good test-retest reliability (Kaye et al., 2004), and its ability to stimulate many bodily systems simultaneously has led to the proposal that it may be a useful noninvasive physiological stressor to assess the human stress response (Wetherell et al., 2006).

TYPES OF FACTORS INFLUENCING RESPONSE TO THE CO_2 CHALLENGE

Use of the 35% CO_2 challenge has helped to clarify the factors that may influence likelihood of a more intense emotional reaction (consistent with greater stress) post-challenge. Several different (yet often overlapping) categories of putative causal factors have received considerable investigative attention and subsequently substantial empirical support. These include one's prior history of learning and/or mental distress (see the aforementioned reference to Brewin et al., 2000), biological factors, and cognitive psychological processes, among others.

PRIOR LEARNING OR MENTAL DISTRESS IN RESPONSE TO THE CHALLENGE AND STRESSORS GENERALLY

Considering each type of possible causal factor in turn, one's prior history of learning or mental distress has been shown to influence reactivity after the 35% CO_2 challenge. Perhaps the best example of this point in human research comes from seminal research by Battaglia and colleagues (e.g., Battaglia et al, 2007; Ogliari et al., 2010), which indicates that childhood parental loss (along with other stressful events) increases emotional responding to the 35% CO_2 challenge in adulthood. More generally, as applied to stress reactivity to a variety of stressors, the influence of one's prior learning (in the behaviorist sense of the word) is perhaps most clearly shown in animal research, in which any effects are more difficult to ascribe to cognition and are thus frequently interpreted purely at the level of behavior. Along these lines, Cook and Mineka's (1989) seminal research in rhesus monkeys cleverly revealed that monkeys will learn to fear a toy snake if they observe a videotape of another monkey manifesting extreme fear in the presence of that toy snake. Indeed, numerous findings along these lines amply indicate that a novel stressful reaction to a stimulus (e.g., a toy snake; Cook and Mineka, 1989) can be learned via modeling or via classical conditioning (for an example in humans, see Ohman et al., 1975). With a specific focus on the 35% CO_2 challenge in mind, it is interesting to note that although stressors are often conceptualized as external (e.g., outside one's own body) situations or stimuli, McNally and Lukach (1992) have revealed that panic attacks themselves--short-lived paroxysms of terror accompanied by physiological and cognitive symptoms (APA, 1994)--are in some cases traumatic stressors. Specifically, 17% of the participants met lifetime criteria for posttraumatic stress disorder (PTSD) following their most frightening panic attack. This finding potentially relates to learning explanations (among others) of stress reactivity; indeed, the influential modern learning theory of panic disorder (Bouton et al., 2001) posits that unexpected bodily symptoms (regardless of external stressors) may, via learning, become conditioned stimuli provoking intense terror (e.g., a panic attack). Perhaps not surprisingly, those who have a history of panic attacks prior to the challenge are more likely to have an intense emotional reaction consistent with stress to the 35% CO_2 challenge (e.g., Perna et al., 1995), possibly partly because of this learning history (along with other reasons).

BIOLOGICAL FACTORS INFLUENCING RESPONSE TO THE CHALLENGE AND STRESSORS GENERALLY

The role of biological factors in stress responsivity has also been clarified via research on animals. More specifically, animal studies have elucidated the importance of keeping in mind the organism's biological reality when positing hypotheses about stress reactivity. To illustrate, in Cook and Mineka's (1989) research, rhesus monkeys could never learn to fear a flower—even if they repeatedly watched a videotape (artificially created) in which another monkey appeared to respond fearfully in the presence of a flower. Indeed, biology constrains to some extent the learning that can occur across all species. Importantly, this biological constraint is often difficult to alter, just as one's prior history of mental distress or learning cannot be changed. (Of course, current mental distress can certainly be treated, and extinction paradigms can attenuate the effects of prior learning, but these past experiences are, by definition, a part of an organism's history that must be taken into account when considering individual stress responses). Thus, knowledge about how biological factors promote stress reactions is important, to be sure, but the practical implications of such information are sometimes less immediate. This is arguably the case with respect to biological factors influencing reactivity to the 35% CO_2 test as well. Here, a polymorphism in the 5-HTT gene (the serotonin transporter gene) predicts more intense fear after the 35% CO_2 challenge in normal participants (e.g., Schmidt et al., 2000; Schruers et al., 2011). Specifically, the LL (two long alleles) genotype is associated with greater emotional responding, relative to the SS (two short alleles) and SL genotypes. (Schruers and colleagues (2011) also identified a tri-alleleic genotype predicting more fear to CO_2; these researchers used two breaths of 17.5% enriched air to approximate a single breath of 35% CO_2). As Schruers and colleagues (2011) note, these and related findings may eventually pave the way for new efficacious pharmacological treatments.

PSYCHOLOGICAL FACTORS INFLUENCING RESPONSE TO THE CHALLENGE AND STRESSORS GENERALLY

In the meantime, another category of causal factor in stress reactivity--cognitive psychological factors--arguably continues to merits empirical attention. Indeed, the idea that certain personality or dispositional traits may influence one's characteristic response to stressors has long captured researchers' attention, with numerous ground-breaking contributions along the way (e.g., Friedman and Rosenman, 1974; Millon, 1996). To illustrate, greater hostility has been linked to increased cardiac reactivity to stressors (e.g., Margiotta et al., 1990), whereas more a "laid back" (Blonna, 2007, p. 41) disposition predicts less frustration and daily stressors (e.g., Lyness, 1993). Importantly, cognitive psychological factors can often be altered through therapy and/or lifestyle changes, resulting in reduced stress reactivity (e.g., Davison et al., 1991).

The rest of this chapter overviews selective literature on the psychological factors influencing individual stress response to the 35% CO_2 challenge. Over a decade ago, a seminal review in this general area of carbon dioxide reactivity was published (Zvolensky and Eifert, 2001). The current chapter is designed to complement and extend the previous outstanding review by updating the findings and focusing specifically on the 35% CO_2 test, the physiological effects of which are markedly different than those of carbon dioxide inhalations using lower concentration of CO_2 for longer time periods (Vickers et al., 2012).

The research using the 35% CO_2 challenge as a probe of the human stress response (e.g., Kaye et al., 2004; Loft et al., 2007; Shufflebotham et al., 2009; Wetherell et al., 2006) is relatively new, and undoubtedly much will be learned in the ongoing and upcoming investigations. But stress research is not the first approach to use the 35% carbon dioxide challenge. Quite to the contrary, numerous studies over decades of research have utilized this same 35% carbon dioxide challenge for a different purpose, namely to provoke panic attacks in those with the psychiatric condition of panic disorder. This psychological literature has thoroughly explored individual differences in reactivity to this provocation more than has the nascent stress research using the challenge to date. As such, those wishing to draw conclusions about the psychological factors influencing reactivity to the carbon dioxide challenge have a bevy of psychological findings on which to lean. Several such psychological factors are discussed below.

Trait anxiety. Intuitively, it makes sense that those who are characteristically more anxious in general (e.g., trait anxiety) than others would react with more anxiety to the 35% CO_2 challenge (which generates mild anxiety in the typical participant). Some empirical findings have supported this notion generally, and other findings have substantially clarified and refined it.

For example, Schmidt, Richey, and colleagues (2007) determined that the correlation between trait anxiety and self-reported fear post-challenge was a small effect size ($r = .24$; Cohen, 1988) that was in fact not significant ($p > .05$) in their study's participants (both men and women). Further investigating this idea, Monkul et al. (2010) reported that trait anxiety predicted panic after the challenge only in female panic disorder patients. These researchers therefore recommended ongoing study that considers gender in the possible relationship between emotional responding induced by the 35% CO_2 challenge and trait anxiety. Further investigation will undoubtedly clarify matters.

Discomfort intolerance. People vary in the extent to which they tolerate unpleasant sensations they are experiencing. This construct, termed discomfort intolerance by Schmidt and colleagues (2006), appears substantially linked to one's emotional reactivity to the CO_2 stressor, albeit in limited research. Specifically, Schmidt, Richey, and colleagues (2007) reported a nearly large effect size (Cohen, 1988) between discomfort intolerance and fear after the challenge ($r = .46$, $p < .01$). Indeed, even after statistically controlling for trait anxiety (as well as other measures), one's level of discomfort intolerance still predicted significant variance in emotional response to the challenge. Refining their findings, the researchers explored the specific aspects of discomfort intolerance most strongly linked to emotional response post-challenge, finding that discomfort avoidance specifically (e.g., items such as "I take extreme measures to avoid feeling physically uncomfortable") predicted greater fearful responding to the challenge (Schmidt, Richey, et al., 2007). Interestingly, other research as well has illuminated the potentially detrimental effect of avoidance.

For example, a greater tendency to use avoidance coping predicted more emotional response to the 35% CO_2 challenge (Schmidt et al., 2005) and to a 10% CO_2 inhalation (Spira et al., 2004). These findings, along with many others (e.g., Pennebaker and Beall, 1986), suggest that attempts to avoid experiencing one's reaction to a stressor, be it the CO_2 challenge or a trauma, may backfire (Spira et al., 2004).

Anxiety sensitivity. The most established psychological variable affecting emotional response to the CO_2 stressor is anxiety sensitivity. Conceptualized by Reiss and colleagues (1986), anxiety sensitivity denotes fear of one's own symptoms of anxiety. Importantly, despite the similar terminology, anxiety sensitivity and trait anxiety are distinct constructs (McNally, 1989, 2002). Indeed, anxiety sensitivity has consistently outperformed trait anxiety in predicting emotional response to the CO_2 stressor (e.g., a significant correlation of $r = .51$ between anxiety sensitivity and anxious response in Schmidt, Richey, et al., 2007).

Recent research has confirmed the importance of anxiety sensitivity to the prediction of post-CO_2 stressor response, particularly in context with other parameters (e.g., Telch et al., 2011). For example, participants with high anxiety sensitivity reported augmented anxious responding after the CO_2 challenge, relative to those with low anxiety sensitivity; furthermore, high anxiety sensitivity participants who were (misleadingly) instructed that CO_2

would produce relaxation were significantly more likely to respond with intense fear to the CO_2 stressor, compared to high anxiety sensitivity participants told to expect arousal symptoms post-challenge. In contrast, instructional manipulation did not affect the response of low anxiety sensitivity participants.

Explaining this pattern of results, Telch and colleagues (2011, p. 651) suggested that the "under-prediction" of perceived danger likely engendered by the relaxation instructions may have potentiated high sensitivity participants' dispositional tendency to fear anxiety-related symptoms. Indeed, according to danger expectancy theory (Reiss et al., 1986), beliefs about danger garner strength particularly when the danger surpasses expectation. Applied more generally to stress reactivity, this line of reasoning suggests that those high in anxiety sensitivity are likely to respond especially intensely to a stressor that affects them more than was anticipated. Although this idea has yet to receive empirical scrutiny, there is emerging evidence connecting anxiety sensitivity to stress reactivity (see Vickers et al., 2012, p. 161). For example, the joint presence of high anxiety sensitivity and a looming cognitive style (in which the perceived threat dynamically increases as the threat approaches) has potent stress generation effects (Riskind et al., 2010).

Additional psychological factors. Other dispositional variables likely also influence CO_2 reactivity. Some, such as a heightened fear of suffocation (e.g., Shipherd et al., 2001) are potentially most relevant to particular stressors that specifically aggravate respiration (as does the CO_2 stressor) and as such are not considered further here. Others (e.g., a looming cognitive style; Riskind et al., 2012) have yet to be tested in the CO_2 challenge but would be welcome additions to this literature when that research is conducted.

More generally, ongoing investigation into the dispositional variables affecting CO_2 reactivity potentially will identify additional psychological factors that influence response to the CO_2 stressor and by extension to other stressors.

PRACTICAL IMPLICATIONS OF THESE PSYCHOLOGICAL FINDINGS TO STRESS RESEARCH

Ample evidence indicates that it is possible to alter the characteristic way in which one tends to react to stressors, thereby reducing reactivity to stressors and potentially promoting health. To be sure, some factors influencing how one responds to stress (e.g., one's genotype; Schmidt et al., 2000; Schruers et al., 2011) are less easily altered, but psychological factors appear somewhat malleable after appropriate intervention. Reactivity to the 35% CO_2 stressor in particular lessens for numerous reasons, including medication addressing serotonergic functioning for those suffering from extreme emotional distress and under a doctor's care (e.g., Pols et al., 1996). Repeated inhalations of 35% CO_2 may also be beneficial in clinical contexts as a method of generating physiological symptoms of anxiety for interoceptive exposure exercises (e.g., Beck et al., 1997; Griez and van den Hout, 1986; Schmidt and Trakowski, 2004; van den Hout et al., 1987; for a review, see Forsyth and Karekla, 2001; Vickers et al., 2012). In other circumstances, psychotherapy has shown promise in decreasing reactivity to the CO_2 stressor. More specifically, cognitive-behavioral therapy (CBT) interventions reduce anxiety sensitivity (for a review, see Smits et al., 2008), resulting in a reduction in stress reactivity to the CO_2 stressor (Schmidt et al., 1997). Whether similar reductions in discomfort intolerance or the associated more general avoidance coping will also reduce CO_2 reactivity in those undergoing CBT has yet to be tested. Along these lines, Schmidt et al (2005) advocate specifically targeting maladaptive coping in CBT. As such, therapeutic results could improve potentially if dismantling studies reveal benefits of reducing discomfort intolerance and/or avoidance coping in CBT (possibly along with a looming cognitive style; Riskind et al., 2012).

The typical person experiencing daily stressors, however, is not undergoing either CBT or taking medication. With that in mind, it is important to point out that several investigations have shown that anxiety sensitivity in nonclinical participants can be reduced via brief and economically feasible interventions (reviewed in Smits et al., 2008). For example, a 30 minute educational video (Anxiety Sensitivity Amelioration Training; ASAT) delineating the harmless nature of stress symptoms decreased anxiety sensitivity in youth (19 years old on average; Schmidt, Eggleston, et al., 2007). Similarly, a 60-minute psychoeducational presentation (based on panic control treatment; Barlow and Craske, 1994) that included cognitive restructuring about physical sensations reduced anxiety sensitivity in cardiac patients (Esler et al., 2003).

Lifestyle changes also have the potential to reduce one's reactivity to the CO_2 stressor. Appropriate physical exercise in particular has shown promise in several studies (reviewed in Smits et al., 2009, p. 447). For example, participants who vigorously exercised on a stationary bicycle (for 12 minutes or until high blood lactate levels occurred) had fewer panic symptoms and (nonsignificantly) less anxiety after a subsequent CO_2 challenge, compared to participants who bicycled at a relaxed pace for 12 minutes (Esquivel et al., 2002). In a much larger study, 20 minutes of exercise (at 70% of the maximal heart rate) resulted in less fear post-challenge, relative to 20 minutes of sitting quietly (Smits et al., 2009). Exercise therefore may be "an underused wonder," as Esquivel and colleagues (2002, p. 396) suggest, that reduces anxious responding to the CO_2 stressor. Furthermore, exercise itself (six 20-minute sessions over two weeks) may reduce anxiety sensitivity (Broman-Fulks and Storey, 2008), an intriguing finding with important implications if replicated.

CONCLUSION

This chapter overviewed psychological variables influencing reactivity to a particular laboratory stress provocation, the 35% CO_2 stressor. Of these dispositional traits, anxiety sensitivity currently has substantial empirical support as a factor influencing response to the CO_2 challenge. Increasing research indicates that anxiety sensitivity can be reduced via therapeutic and/or psychoeducational interventions (Smits et al., 2008). Potentially, then, beneficial reductions in general responsivity to stressors may ensue following attenuation of anxiety sensitivity. Forthcoming empirical investigations will assuredly answer this question and another question that arguably warrants study, namely, the factors promoting resilience in the face of the CO_2 stressor. Of course, these factors may often be relatively low levels of those psychological variables (e.g., discomfort intolerance) known to aggravate CO_2 reactivity at their higher values. That noted, possibly, reconceptualizing the CO_2 stressor paradigm as a way to study resilience, rather than risk, may enhance the study of resilience in the face of stressors. This research trajectory will make an important contribution by advancing understanding of "individual differences" (Juster et al., 2010, p. 13) in stress reactivity.

Underlying the previous discussion is the assumption that one's reactivity to the CO_2 stressor is a valid probe of the acute stress response (e.g., Wetherell et al., 2006). However, administration of CO_2 is decidedly different than what happens in a real-world stressful situation, such as a traffic jam. The extent to which the CO_2 stressor does indeed faithfully reproduce the stress associated with daily stressors can—and should—be questioned. Nevertheless, arguably, research using the CO_2 stressor provides a useful starting point for thinking about further more refined ways of testing reactivity to stressors in controlled laboratory environments. Other limitations of this chapter include that it is a non-exhaustive overview emphasizing findings from psychological investigations rather than from stress research; additionally, some psychological studies noted (e.g., Monkul et al., 2010; Schmidt et al., 2005) used patients with panic disorder, a condition with only a 4.7% lifetime prevalence rate (Kessler et al., 2005). The extent to which these findings can be generalized is thus questionable. Of course, further investigation will clarify and extend this research.

REFERENCES

American Psychiatric Association. (1994). *Diagnostic and statistical manual of mental disorders* (4th ed.). American Psychiatric Association Press, Washington, DC: Author.

Barlow, D. H., and Craske, M. G. (1994). *Mastery of your anxiety and panic.* San Antonio, TX: Psychological Corporation/Graywind Publications.

Battaglia, M., Ogliari, A., Harris, J., Spatola, C. A. M., Pesenti-Gritti, P., and Reichborn-Kjennerud, T., et al. (2007). A genetic study of the acute anxious response to carbon dioxide stimulation in man. *Journal of Psychiatric Research, 41,* 906-917.

Beck, J.G., Shiperd, J.C., and Zebb, B.J. (1997). How does interoceptive exposure for panic disorder work? An uncontrolled case study. *Journal of Anxiety Disorders, 11,* 541-556.

Blonna, R. (2007). *Coping with stress in a changing world* (4th ed.) Toronto, ON: McGraw-Hill.

Bouton, M. E., Mineka, S., and Barlow, D. H. (2001). A modern learning theory perspective on the etiology of panic disorder. *Psychological Review, 108,* 4-32.

Brewin, C.R., Andrews, B., and Valentine, J.D. (2000). Meta-analysis of risk factors for posttraumatic stress disorder in trauma-exposed adults. *Journal of Consulting and Clinical Psychology, 68,* 748-766.

Broman-Fulks, J., and Storey, K. M. (2008). Evaluation of a brief aerobic exercise intervention for high anxiety sensitivity. *Anxiety, Stress and Coping: An International Journal, 21*(2), 117-128.

Cohen, J. (1988). *Statistical power analysis for the behavioral sciences* (2nd ed.). Hillsdale, NJ: Lawrence Erlbaum Associates.

Cook, M., and Mineka, S. (1989). Observational conditioning of fear to fear-relevant versus fear-irrelevant stimuli in rhesus monkeys. *Journal of Abnormal Psychology, 98,* 448-459.

Davison, G. C., Williams, M. E., Nezami, E., Bice, T. L., and Dequattro, V. (1991). Relaxation, reduction in angry articulated thoughts, and improvements in borderline essential hypertension and heart rate. *Journal of Behavioral Medicine, 14, 453-468.*

Esler, J. L., Barlow, D. H., Woolard, R. H., Nicholson, R. A., Nash, J. M., and Erogul, M. H. (2003). A brief-cognitive behavioral intervention for patients with noncardiac chest pain. *Behavior Therapy, 34*, 129-148.

Esquivel, G., Schruers, K., Kuipers, H., and Griez, E. (2002). The effects of acute exercise and high lactate levels on 35% CO_2 challenge in healthy volunteers. *Acta Psychiatrica Scandinavica, 106*, 394-397.

Foa, E. D., and Riggs, D. S. (1995). Posttraumatic stress disorder following assault: Theoretical considerations and empirical findings. *Current Directions in Psychological Science, 4*, 61-65.

Forsyth, J. P., and Karekla, M. (2001). Biological challenge in the assessment of anxiety disorders. In M.M. Antony, S.M. Orsillo, and L. Roemer L. (Eds.), *Practitioner's guide to empirically based measures of anxiety* (pp. 31-36). Dordrecht, Netherlands: Kluwer Academic Publishers.

Friedman, M., and Rosenman, R. (1974). *Type A behavior and your heart.* Greenwich, CT: Fawcett.

Griez, E. J., and van den Hout, M. A. (1986). CO_2 inhalation in the treatment of panic attacks. *Behaviour Research and Therapy, 24*, 145-150.

Juster, R.-P., McEwen, B.S., and Lupien, S.J. (2010). Allostatic load biomarkers of chronic stress and impact on health and cognition. *Neuroscience and Biobehavioral Reviews, 35*, 2-16.

Kaye, J., Buchanan, F., Kendrick, A., Johnson, P., Lowry, C., Bailey, J., et al. (2004). Acute carbon dioxide exposure in healthy adults: Evaluation of a novel means of investigating the stress response. *Journal of Neuroendocrinology, 16, 256-264.*

Kessler, R. C., Berglund, P., Demler, O., Jin, R., Merikangas, K. R., and Walters, E. E. (2005). Lifetime prevalence and age-of-onset distributions of DSM-IV disorders in the National Comorbidity Survey Replication. *Archives of General Psychiatry, 62*, 593-602.

Lazarus, R.S. (1966). *Psychological stress and the coping process.* New York: McGraw-Hill.

Loft, P., Thomas, M. G., Petrie, K. J., Booth, R. J., Miles, J., and Vedhara, K. (2007). Examination stress results in altered cardiovascular responses to acute challenge and lower cortisol. *Psychoneuroendocrinology, 32*, 367-375.

Lyness, S. (1993) Predictors of difference between Type A and Type B individuals in heart rate and blood pressure reactivity. *Psychological Bulletin, 114*, 266-295.

Margiotta, E., Davilla, D., and Hicks, R. (1990). Type A-B behavior and the self-report of daily hassles and uplifts. *Perceptual and Motor Skills, 70*, 777-778.

McNally, R. J. (1989). Is anxiety sensitivity distinguishable from trait anxiety? Reply to Lilienfeld, Jacob, and Turner (1989). *Journal of Abnormal Psychology, 98*(2), 193-194.

McNally, R. J. (2002). Anxiety sensitivity and panic disorder. *Biological Psychiatry, 52*, 938-946.

McNally, R. J., and Lukach, B. M. (1992). Are panic attacks traumatic stressors? *The American Journal of Psychiatry, 149*, 824-826.

Millon, T. (1996). *Disorders of personality* (2nd ed.) New York: Wiley.

Monkul, E. S., Onur, E., Tural, U., Hatch, J. P., Alkin, T., Yucel, B., and Fidaner, H. (2010). History of suffocation, state-trait anxiety, and anxiety sensitivity in predicting 35% carbon dioxide-induced panic. *Psychiatry Research, 179*, 194-197.

Nolen-Hoeksema, S., and Rector, N.A. (2011). *Abnormal psychology.* (2nd Canadian ed.). Toronto: McGraw-Hill Ryerson.

Ogliari, A., Tambs, K., Harris, J. R., Scaini, S., Maffei, C., Reichborn-Kjennerud, T., et al. (2010). The relationships between adverse events, early antecedents, and carbon dioxide reactivity as an intermediate phenotype of panic disorder. *Psychotherapy and Psychosomatics, 79*, 48-55.

Ohman, A., Erixon, G., and Loftberg, I. (1975). Phobias and preparedness: Phobic versus neutral pictures as conditioned stimuli for human autonomic responses. *Journal of Abnormal Psychology, 84*, 41-45.

Pennebaker, J. W., and Beall, S. K. (1986). Confronting a traumatic event: Toward an understanding of inhibition and disease. *Journal of Abnormal Psychology, 95*, 274–281.

Perna, G., Gabriele, A., Caldirola, D., and Bellodi, L. (1995). Hypersensitivity to inhalation of carbon dioxide and panic attacks. *Psychiatry Research, 57*, 267-273.

Pols, H.J., Hauzer, R.C., Meijer, J.A., Verburg, K., and Griez, E.J. (1996). Fluvoxamine attenuates panic induced by 35% CO_2 challenge. *Journal of Clinical Psychiatry, 57*, 539-542.

Reiss, S., Peterson, R. A., Gursky, D. M., and McNally, R. J. (1986). Anxiety sensitivity, anxiety frequency, and the prediction of fearfulness. *Behaviour Research and Therapy, 24*, 1–8.

Riskind, J.H., Black, D., and Shahar, G. (2010). Cognitive vulnerability to anxiety in the stress generation process: Interaction between the looming cognitive style and anxiety sensitivity. *Journal of Anxiety Disorders, 24*, 124-128.

Riskind, J. H., Rector, N. A., and Taylor, S. (2012). Looming cognitive vulnerability to anxiety and its reduction in psychotherapy. *Journal of Psychotherapy Integration, 22*(2), 137-162.

Rosenberg, R. S., and Kosslyn, S. M. (2011). *Abnormal psychology*. New York: Worth.

Sandstrom, G. M., and Russo, F. A. (2010). Music hath charms: The effects of valence and arousal on recovery following an acute stressor. *Music and Medicine, 2*(3), 137-143.

Schmidt, N.B., Eggleston, A.M., Trakowski, J.H., and Smith, J.D. (2005). Does coping predict CO_2-induced panic in patients with panic disorder? *Behaviour Research and Therapy, 43*, 1311-1319.

Schmidt, N. B., Eggleston, A. M., Woolaway-Bickel, K., Fitzpatrick, K. K., Vasey, M. W., and Richey, J. A. (2007). Anxiety Sensitivity Amelioration Training (ASAT): A longitudinal primary prevention program targeting cognitive vulnerability. *Journal of Anxiety Disorders, 21*, 302-319.

Schmidt, N.B., Richey, J. A., Cromer, K. R., and Buckner, J. D. (2007). Discomfort intolerance: Evaluation of a potential risk factor for anxiety psychopathology. *Behavior Therapy, 38*, 247-255.

Schmidt, N. B., Richey, J. A., and Fitzpatrick, K. K. (2006). Discomfort intolerance: Development of a construct and measure relevant to panic disorder. *Journal of Anxiety Disorders, 20*, 263–280.

Schmidt, N. B., Storey, J., Greenberg, B. D., Santiago, H. T., Li, Q., and Murphy, D. L. (2000). Evaluating gene x psychological risk factor effects in the pathogenesis of anxiety: A new model approach. *Journal of Abnormal Psychology, 109*, 308-320.

Schmidt, N.B., and Trakowski, J. (2004). Interoceptive assessment and exposure in panic disorder: A descriptive study. *Cognitive and Behavioral Practice, 11*, 81-92.

Schmidt, N. B., Trakowski, J. H., and Staab, J. P. (1997). Extinction of panicogenic effects of a 35% CO_2 challenge in patients with panic disorder. *Journal of Abnormal Psychology, 106*, 630–638.

Schruers, K., Esquivel, G., van Duinen, M., Wichers, M., Kenis, G., Colasanti, A., et al. (2011). Genetic moderation of CO_2-induced fear by 5-HTTLPR genotype. *Journal of Psychopharmacology, 25*, 37–42.

Shipherd, J. C., Beck, J. G., and Ohtake, P. J. (2001). Relationships between the anxiety sensitivity index, the suffocation fear scale, and responses to CO_2 inhalation. *Journal of Anxiety Disorders, 15*, 247-258.

Shufflebotham, J., Wetherell, M. A., Hince, D., Hood, S., Lightman, S., Nutt, D., et al. (2009). Women with diarrhoea-predominant irritable bowel syndrome show an increased pressure response to 35% carbon dioxide stress challenge. *Stress, 12*, 30-36.

Smits, J. A. J., Berry, A. C., Tart, C. D., and Powers, M. B. (2008). The efficacy of cognitive-behavioral interventions for reducing anxiety sensitivity: A meta-analytic review. *Behaviour Research and Therapy, 46*, 1047-1054.

Smits, J. A. J., Meuret, A. E., Zvolensky, M. J., Rosenfield, D., and Seidel, A. (2009). The effects of acute exercise on CO_2 challenge reactivity. *Journal of Psychiatric Research, 43*, 446-454.

Spira, A. P., Zvolensky, M. J., Eifert, G. H., and Feldner, M. T. (2004). Avoidance-oriented coping as a predictor of panic-related distress: A test using biological challenge. *Journal of Anxiety Disorders, 18*, 309-323.

Telch, M. J., Harrington, P.J., Smits, J.A.J., and Powers, M.B. (2011). Unexpected arousal, anxiety sensitivity, and their interaction on CO_2-induced panic: Further evidence for the context-sensitivity vulnerability model. *Journal of Anxiety Disorders, 25*, 645–653.

van den Hout, M.A., van der Molen, G.M., Griez, E., Lousberg, H., and Nansen, A. (1987). Reduction of CO_2-induced anxiety in patients with panic attacks after repeated CO_2 exposure. *American Journal of Psychiatry, 144*, 788-791.

Vickers, K., Jafarpour, S., Mofidi, A., Rafat, B., and Woznica, A. (2012). The 35% carbon dioxide test in stress and panic research: Overview of effects and integration of findings. *Clinical Psychology Review, 32*, 153-164.

Wetherell, M. A., Crown, A. L., Lightman, S. L., Miles, J. N. V., Kaye, J., and Vedhara, K. (2006). The four-dimensional stress test: Psychological, sympathetic–adrenal–medullary, parasympathetic and hypothalamic–pituitary–adrenal responses following inhalation of 35% CO_2. *Psychoneuroendocrinology, 31,* 736–747.

Zvolensky, M. J., and Eifert, G. H. (2001). A review of psychological factors/processes affecting anxious responding during voluntary hyperventilation and inhalations of carbon dioxide-enriched air. *Clinical Psychology Review, 21*, 375–400.

Chapter 7

CHRONIC PSYCHOSOCIAL WORK STRESS IN TEACHERS: AN UPDATE ON EMPIRICAL PSYCHOBIOLOGICAL FINDINGS

*Silja Bellingrath[1], Maren Wolfram[2] and Brigitte M. Kudielka[3]**
[1]Institute of Psychology, University Duisburg-Essen, Essen, Germany
[2]Jacobs Center on Lifelong Learning and Institutional Development,
Jacobs University Bremen, Campus, Bremen, Germany
[3]Department of Medical Psychology, Psychological Diagnostics and Research
Methodology, University of Regensburg, Regensburg, Germany

ABSTRACT

Recent evidence from epidemiological and prospective studies suggests that chronic work stress is a relevant risk factor for the progression and development of manifest disease such as cardiovascular disease, type 2 diabetes as well as psychiatric and psychosomatic conditions. Especially teaching has often been described as a highly demanding occupation, leaving many teachers with a general perception of being stressed and overworked. Here, we present an up-date on findings from the second part of our Teacher Stress Study, in which we investigated associations between work-related psychosocial stress in two independent samples of healthy school teachers and alterations in the regulation of different physiological systems. The goal of this project was to investigate the psychobiological pathways which link job stress to an increased risk for disease outcomes in order to increase the knowledge, which is necessary for the development of diagnostic tools that allow the early identification of potential risk factors. Our recent empirical results suggest an impact of chronic work stress in terms of effort-reward-imbalance and overcommitment on hypothalamus-pituitary-adrenal (HPA) axis stress responses and HPA axis feedback regulation, on stress responses of the blood coagulation system as well as on the regulation of the immune system. Furthermore, we found associations between exhaustion as a consequence of chronic work stress and stress reactivity of the blood coagulation system as well as HPA axis feedback regulation.

---

* Corresponding author: Brigitte M. Kudielka. Department of Medical Psychology,Psychological Diagnostics and Research Methodology.University of Regensburg, Universitätsstr. 31, 93053 Regensburg, Germany.

To sum up, we observed subtle dysregulations in multiple stress sensitive, physiological systems even in apparently healthy, working school teachers. Our findings point to the need to protect employees from negative health outcomes. which are potentially associated with chronic work stress in the long run.

INTRODUCTION

During the last decade, a number of epidemiological studies have reported a prospective association between unfavorable psychosocial work conditions and different adverse health outcomes, especially an increased vulnerability for coronary artery disease (CAD) and major depression (Bosma et al., 1998; Hemingway & Marmot, 1999; Rozanski et al., 1999; Kivimäki et al., 2006; Melamed et al., 2006). Especially the teaching profession has been repeatedly described as a potentially stressful occupation (Kyriacou, 1987; Guglielmi & Tatrow, 1998). Increased stress levels in school teachers are reflected in absenteeism and alarmingly high rates of early retirement among German school teachers (Weber et al., 2001; Lehr et al., 2009). The psychophysiological mechanisms however explaining the link between work-related stress and its consequences for health are not yet fully understood. The aim of our teacher stress study is therefore to investigate possible associations between chronic work stress and alterations in different physiological systems, namely the neuroendocrine system, the immune system and the blood coagulation system.

The neuroendocrine system enables the organism to maintain homeostasis under acute stress by regulating the adaptation to increased demands. This originally adaptive response can have numerous deleterious consequences when stress becomes a chronic condition. Disturbances of the neuroendocrine system, especially the hypothalamus-pituitary-adrenal (HPA) axis have been associated with several stress-related diseases and psychopathologies (Heim et al., 2000; Pariante & Miller, 2001; Parker et al., 2003; Raison & Miller, 2003) and could be one potential psychobiological mechanism explaining the link between work-related stress and disease outcomes. Furthermore, states of chronic stress have been shown to induce alterations in immune system activity and one can assume that an increase in inflammatory markers contributes to the increased risk for cardiovascular disease and depressive symptomatology in individuals with high levels of chronic work stress (Miller et al., 2002; Glaser & Kiecolt-Glaser, 2005; Miller et al., 2009). Finally, a hypercoagulable state, characterized by activated coagulation and/or impaired fibrinolysis, in response to acute psychosocial stress has been shown to contribute to atherothrombotic events (von Känel et al., 2001a; von Känel et al., 2001b). Therefore we were also interested whether hyper-coagulability after acute stress is associated with chronic work stress and its consequences, as it might link job stress with atherosclerosis. In the first part of our teacher project we focused on basal measurements of HPA axis, immune and coagulation parameters, whereas the second part concentrates on the response of the systems to psychosocial and pharmacological challenge.

METHODS

In a first step we confronted 62 middle-aged healthy school teachers with the Trier Social Stress Test (TSST) in order to test whether chronic work stress is accompanied by alterations in 1) HPA axis regulation 2) immune functioning and 3) the blood coagulation system. The TSST is a standardized laboratory protocol to induce mild to moderate psychosocial stress and has become a widely used tool in research on stress reactivity (Kirschbaum et al., 1993; Kudielka et al., 2007a; Kudielka et al., 2007b). A recent meta-analysis showed that the components of social evaluative threat and uncontrollability render the TSST a reliable tool to elicit robust physiological stress responses (Dickerson & Kemeny, 2004). The TSST consists of a three min preparation phase followed by a five min free speech phase (mock job interview) and a five min mental arithmetic task in front of a panel. The panel members were graduate students well trained for this task and the panel always comprised one female and one male member.

In a second, independent sample of 53 healthy, middle-aged school teachers, two pharmacological challenge paradigms were implemented to examine the influence of work-related stress on HPA axis functioning in more detail. The combined Dexamethasone/CRH (DEX/CRH) test allows the investigation of HPA axis regulation, examining the stimulating effects of CRH under the suppressive action of DEX (Heuser et al., 1994), while the low-dose $ACTH_{1-24}$ (Synacthen) test is a tool to measure adrenal cortex sensitivity, as it triggers cortisol release from the adrenal cortex directly.

In a third sample of healthy student teachers cortisol responses to a demonstration lesson were assessed and compared to a control day. To further compare stress responses to a real life stressor with responses to a standardized stressor, participants were also exposed to a laboratory stressor, namely the TSST. Additionally, the cortisol awakening response (CAR) was assessed on both days (Kudielka & Wüst, 2008; Kudielka & Wüst, 2010).

Chronic work stress was measured in terms of the effort-reward-imbalance (ERI) model (Siegrist, 1996, 2002). This work stress model provides a conceptual framework for possible associations between adverse psychosocial workplace characteristics and long-term negative health outcomes. Siegrist and co-workers postulate that a lack of reciprocity between personal costs (effort) and personal gains (reward) at the workplace elicits stress, which in the long run may result in the development of stress-related disorders (Siegrist, 2005). Overcommitment (OC), the intrinsic component of the ERI model, reflects a cognitive-motivational pattern of coping with demands that is characterized by an extreme ambition in combination with a special need for control and approval (van Vegchel et al., 2005). Potential consequences of chronic work stress were assessed in terms of exhaustion and depressive symptomatology. Vital exhaustion (VE) has been conceptualized as a state of undue fatigue, loss of energy, increased irritability, and demoralization reflecting a breakdown of the adaptation to chronic stress. VE originates from clinical work with cardiovascular patients, is closely related to the burnout syndrome and was originally identified as an independent risk factor for coronary artery disease (Kop, 1999; Appels, 2004). Emotional exhaustion is closely related to VE and represents the core symptom of the burnout syndrome. It also captures feelings or symptoms of distress resulting from the perception of work related stress (Maslach & Jackson, 1986; Maslach, 2007).

RESULTS

A sample of 53 teachers (mean age 50 ± 9 years; 33 females, 20 males) had complete data for the analysis of cortisol and ACTH responses to acute laboratory stress. ACTH was measured five times, total plasma cortisol six times and free salivary cortisol eight times before and after the TSST. In the total group, ERI and OC were only marginally associated with HPA axis responses to acute stress. However, looking only at those subjects who responded to the TSST with an increase in cortisol > 2.5 nmol/l (subgroup of responders: N = 30) we observed a significant association between high levels of OC and lower ACTH as well as plasma and salivary cortisol responses. These results remained significant controlling for depressive symptoms. The additional control for acute perceived stressfulness of the TSST rendered significant associations between OC and HPA axis responses in responders as well as in the total study sample. With regard to ERI, higher stress levels were solely related to stronger plasma cortisol increases after TSST exposure, this effect however missed statistical significance when controlling for depressive symptomatology. The association between OC and a blunted HPA axis response to acute psychosocial stress may reflect an adaptation of the neuroendocrine system to prolonged or repeated stimulation due to chronic work stress (Bellingrath & Kudielka, 2008).

Immune system responses to acute stress were assessed in a final study sample of 55 healthy teachers (mean age 50 ± 8 years; 34 females, 21 males). We measured lymphocyte subset counts and lymphocyte production of tumor-necrosis-factor (TNF)-a, interferon (IFN)-γ, interleukin (IL)-2, IL-4, IL-6 and IL-10 -45 min before and immediately after the TSST. High levels of ERI and OC were associated with lower numbers of natural killer (NK) cells (CD16+/56+) whereas only high levels of OC were related to a lower increase in T-helper cells (CD4+) after stress. Furthermore, subjects with high levels of ERI showed an overall increase in pro-inflammatory activity, with higher TNF-a production at both time points and elevated pre-stress IL-6 production. Additionally, the production of IL-10 decreased after stress in subjects with levels of ERI. The ratios of TNF-a/IL-10 and IL-6/IL-10 were also significantly increased in subjects high on ERI. Finally, OC was associated with higher IL-2 production post-stress. To conclude, we observed signs of low-grade systemic inflammation and a dampened innate immune defense in relation to work stress in a sample of middle aged otherwise healthy teachers; a finding that has important implications for the prevention and treatment of work-related ill health (Bellingrath et al., 2010).

Among these subjects, a sample of 52 school teachers (mean age 49 ± 8 years, 63% women) was available for the analyses of the coagulation measures fibrinogen and D-dimer in plasma, measured at five time points before and after the TSST. High levels of OC were associated with a stronger D-dimer increase and a smaller fibrinogen decrease during recovery from stress. In contrast, OC was not associated with changes in coagulation measures from pre-stress to immediately post-stress. ERI was not related to stress-induced changes in coagulation measures (von Känel et al., 2009b). In a second set of analyses, a subgroup of 38 (mean age 50 ± 8 years, 55% women) teachers underwent the TSST twice. Again coagulation measures were determined at five time points during the protocol each day. We observed exhaustion in terms of VE as well as depressive symptoms to be related to stress-induced changes in D-dimer levels over time. More specifically, elevated levels of VE and depression were associated with reduced D-dimer increase from pre-stress to immediately post-stress on the one hand and to an attenuated recovery of D-dimer levels between 20 and 45 min post-stress on the other hand. Our results remained stable when controlling for stress hormone and blood pressure reactivity (von Känel et al., 2009a). One can speculate that a prolonged hypercoagulability after an acute stressor might contribute to the atherothrombotic risk previously observed in individuals suffering from exhaustion or depression, even at subclinical levels.

A completely independent sample of 53 healthy, middle-aged (mean age 49 years ± 9 years; 31 female, 22 male) school teachers was recruited for the pharmacological challenge study. ACTH, plasma cortisol and salivary cortisol were measured before as well as six times after stimulation. Emotional exhaustion (EE) was related to higher plasma cortisol profiles after Synacthen injection, pointing to a heightened sensitivity of the adrenal cortex in emotionally exhausted teachers. OC on the other hand, was significantly associated with attenuated ACTH, plasma cortisol and salivary cortisol concentrations following the DEX/CRH test, suggesting hyporeactive pituitary as well as adrenal cortex responses in teachers with high levels of OC (Wolfram et al., 2012). We assume that the observed attenuated HPA axis response is not purely of pituitary and adrenal but also of central origin, which is in line with our findings of a reduced HPA axis reaction to psychosocial stress reported above.

Finally, cortisol responses to a demonstration lesson compared to a control day under naturalistic conditions as well as to the cortisol responses to the TSST in a laboratory setting were assessed in third sample of 21 healthy student teachers (mean age 31 ± 6 years; 9 females, 11 males). Cortisol levels were found to decline after the demonstration lesson. However, when comparing post-stress cortisol levels to the time-matched cortisol levels on the control day, cortisol levels after the lesson were significantly higher. Also for the TSST, higher cortisol responses were found when using the control day as reference baseline. These results indicate that it is important to include a control day in laboratory, and especially in ambulatory stress research. Furthermore, there were no significant correlations in terms of either response magnitude or response height between the demonstration lesson and the TSST, suggesting that responses to the laboratory stressor do not simply mirror natural stress responses. Finally, associations between the CAR and chronic stress measures were observed, however only on the control day. Higher levels of ERI as well as higher levels of exhaustion in terms of EE were related to a lower CAR. Thus, one can speculate that associations between chronic stress measures and the CAR might be obscured by acute stress exposure (Wolfram et al., in press).

DISCUSSION

To conclude, our results show that associations between chronic psychosocial work stress and disturbances in stress-related physiological systems can already be observed in healthy working school teachers and as early as in student teachers. Our findings support the claim for suitable preventive measures that are targeted specifically to the strains of the teaching profession. An improved understanding of the psychobiological mechanisms that lead to health impairments in reaction to chronic work stress can help to develop such measures.

Finally, our society would benefit from a more understanding attitude towards people who suffer from stressful work conditions by putting a greater emphasis on a work-life balance and fairness at work in order to ameliorate the consequences of chronic work stress.

ACKNOWLEDGMENTS

This work was supported by Emmy Noether research grant KU 1401/4-1, KU 1401/4-2 and KU 1401/4-3 of the German Research Foundation (DFG) awarded to Brigitte M. Kudielka.

REFERENCES

Appels, A., 2004. Exhaustion and coronary heart disease: the history of a scientific quest. *Patient Educ Couns* 55, 223-229.

Bellingrath, S., Kudielka, B. M., 2008. Effort-reward-imbalance and overcommitment are associated with hypothalamus-pituitary-adrenal (HPA) axis responses to acute psychosocial stress in healthy working schoolteachers. *Psychoneuroendocrinology* 33, 1335-1343.

Bellingrath, S., Rohleder, N., Kudielka, B. M., 2010. Healthy working school teachers with high effort-reward-imbalance and overcommitment show increased pro-inflammatory immune activity and a dampened innate immune defence. *Brain Behav Immun* 24, 1332-1339.

Bosma, H., Peter, R., Siegrist, J., Marmot, M., 1998. Two alternative job stress models and the risk of coronary heart disease. *Am J Public Health* 88, 68-74.

Dickerson, S. S., Kemeny, M. E., 2004. Acute stressors and cortisol responses: a theoretical integration and synthesis of laboratory research. *Psychol Bull* 130, 355-391.

Glaser, R., Kiecolt-Glaser, J. K., 2005. Stress-induced immune dysfunction: implications for health. *Nat Rev Immunol* 5, 243-251.

Guglielmi, R. S., Tatrow, K., 1998. Occupational stress, burnout, and health in teachers: A methodological and theoretical analysis. *Rev Educ Res* 68, 61-99.

Heim, C., Ehlert, U., Hellhammer, D. H., 2000. The potential role of hypocortisolism in the pathophysiology of stress-related bodily disorders. *Psychoneuroendocrinology* 25, 1-35.

Hemingway, H., Marmot, M., 1999. Evidence based cardiology: psychosocial factors in the aetiology and prognosis of coronary heart disease. Systematic review of prospective cohort studies. *Bmj* 318, 1460-1467.

Heuser, I., Yassouridis, A., Holsboer, F., 1994. The combined dexamethasone/CRH test: a refined laboratory test for psychiatric disorders. *J Psychiatr Res* 28, 341-356.

Kirschbaum, C., Pirke, K. M., Hellhammer, D. H., 1993. The 'Trier Social Stress Test' - a tool for investigating psychobiology stress responses in a laboratory setting. *Neuropsychobiology* 28, 76-81.

Kivimäki, M., Leino-Arjas, P., Kaila-Kangas, L., Luukkonen, R., Vahtera, J., Elovainio, M., Harma, M., Kirjonen, J., 2006. Is incomplete recovery from work a risk marker of cardiovascular death? Prospective evidence from industrial employees. *Psychosom Med* 68, 402-407.

Kop, W. J., 1999. Chronic and acute psychological risk factors for clinical manifestations of coronary artery disease. *Psychosom Med* 61, 476-487.

Kudielka, B. M., Hellhammer, D. H., Kirschbaum, C., 2007a. Ten years of research with the Trier Social Stress Test (TSST) - revisited. In: Harmon-Jones, E. & Winkielman, P. (Eds.), Social Neuroscience. New York, Guilford Press, pp. 56-83.

Kudielka, B. M., Wüst, S., 2010. Human models in acute and chronic stress: assessing determinants of individual hypothalamus-pituitary-adrenal axis activity and reactivity. *Stress* 13, 1-14.

Kudielka, B. M., Wüst, S., 2008. The cortisol awakening response (CAR): A useful tool for ambulant assessment of hypothalamus-pituitary-adrenal (HPA) axis activity. In: Columbus, F. (Ed.), *Progress in circadian rhythm research*. New York, Nova Science Publishers Inc., pp. in press.

Kudielka, B. M., Wüst, S., Kirschbaum, C., Hellhammer, D. H., 2007b. Trier Social Stress Test. In: Fink, G., Chrousos, G., Craig, I., de Kloet, E. R., Feuerstein, G., McEwen, B. S., Rose, N. R., Rubin, R. T., & Steptoe, A. (Eds.), *Encyclopedia of stress*. 2nd ed. Oxford, Elsevier, pp. 767-781.

Kyriacou, C., 1987. Teacher Stress and burnout: an international review. Educational Research 29, 146-152.

Lehr, D., Hillert, A., Keller, S., 2009. What can balance the effort? Associations between effort-reward imbalance, overcommitment, and affective disorders in German teachers. *Int J Occup Environ Health* 15, 374-384.

Maslach, C., 2007. Burnout. In: Fink, G., Chrousos, G., Craig, I., de Kloet, E. R., Feuerstein, G., McEwen, B. S., Rose, N. R., Rubin, R. T., & Steptoe, A. (Eds.), *Encyclopedia of stress*. 2nd revised edition ed. Oxford, Elsevier, pp. 368-371.

Maslach, C., Jackson, S., 1986. Maslach Burnout Inventory Manual (2nd ed.). Palo Alto, CA: Consulting Psychologists Press.

Melamed, S., Shirom, A., Toker, S., Berliner, S., Shapira, I., 2006. Burnout and risk of cardiovascular disease: evidence, possible causal paths, and promising research directions. *Psychol Bull* 132, 327-353.

Miller, G. E., Chen, E., Fok, A. K., Walker, H., Lim, A., Nicholls, E. F., Cole, S., Kobor, M. S., 2009. Low early-life social class leaves a biological residue manifested by decreased glucocorticoid and increased proinflammatory signaling. *Proc Natl Acad Sci U S A* 106, 14716-14721.

Miller, G. E., Stetler, C. A., Carney, R. M., Freedland, K. E., Banks, W. A., 2002. Clinical depression and inflammatory risk markers for coronary heart disease. *Am J Cardiol* 90, 1279-1283.

Pariante, C. M., Miller, A. H., 2001. Glucocorticoid receptors in major depression: relevance to pathophysiology and treatment. *Biol Psychiatry* 49, 391-404.

Parker, K. J., Schatzberg, A. F., Lyons, D. M., 2003. Neuroendocrine aspects of hypercortisolism in major depression. *Horm Behav* 43, 60-66.

Raison, C. L., Miller, A. H., 2003. When not enough is too much: the role of insufficient glucocorticoid signaling in the pathophysiology of stress-related disorders. *Am J Psychiatry* 160, 1554-1565.

Rozanski, A., Blumenthal, J. A., Kaplan, J., 1999. Impact of psychological factors on the pathogenesis of cardiovascular disease and implications for therapy. *Circulation* 99, 2192-2217.

Siegrist, J., 1996. Adverse health effects of high-effort/low-reward conditions. *J Occup Health Psychol* 1, 27-41.

Siegrist, J., 2002. Effort-reward imbalance at work and health. In: Perrewé, P. L. & Ganster, D. C. (Eds.), *Historical and Current Perspectives on Stress and Health*. Amsterdam, JAI, pp. 261-291.

Siegrist, J., 2005. Social reciprocity and health: new scientific evidence and policy implications. *Psychoneuroendocrinology* 30, 1033-1038.

van Vegchel, N., de Jonge, J., Bosma, H., Schaufeli, W., 2005. Reviewing the effort-reward imbalance model: drawing up the balance of 45 empirical studies. *Soc Sci Med* 60, 1117-1131.

von Känel, R., Bellingrath, S., Kudielka, B. M., 2009a. Association of vital exhaustion and depressive symptoms with changes in fibrin D-dimer to acute psychosocial stress. *J Psychosom Res* 67, 93-101.

von Känel, R., Bellingrath, S., Kudielka, B. M., 2009b. Overcommitment but not effort-reward imbalance relates to stress-induced coagulation changes in teachers. *Ann Behav Med* 37, 20-28.

von Känel, R., Dimsdale, J. E., Ziegler, M. G., Mills, P. J., Patterson, T. L., Lee, S. K., Grant, I., 2001. Effect of acute psychological stress on the hypercoagulable state in subjects (spousal caregivers of patients with Alzheimer's disease) with coronary or cerebrovascular disease and/or systemic hypertension. *Am J Cardiol* 87, 1405-1408.

von Känel, R., Mills, P. J., Fainman, C., Dimsdale, J. E., 2001. Effects of psychological stress and psychiatric disorders on blood coagulation and fibrinolysis: a biobehavioral pathway to coronary artery disease? *Psychosom Med* 63, 531-544.

Weber, A., Weltle, D., Lederer, P., 2001. "Macht Schule krank?" Zur Problematik krankheitsbedingter Frühpensionierung von Lehrkräften. *Bayerische Schule* 6, 214-215.

Wolfram, M., Bellingrath, S., Feuerhahn, N., Kudielka B.M. in press. Cortisol responses to naturalistic and laboratory stress in student teachers: Comparison with a non-stress control day. *Stress and Health*. doi: 10.1002/smi.2439.

Wolfram, M., Bellingrath, S., Feuerhahn, N., Kudielka, B. M., 2012. Emotional exhaustion and overcommitment to work are differentially associated with hypothalamus-pituitary-adrenal (HPA) axis responses to a low-dose ACTH(1-24) (Synacthen) and dexamethasone-CRH test in healthy school teachers. *Stress*. doi: 10.3109/ 10253890. 2012.683465.

INDEX

B

C

F

G

K

L

M

RNA, 33, 43

RNA processing, 33, 43

Romania, 123

room temperature, 135

root, 4, 16, 27, 28

routes, 21, 30, 94

routines, 125

rules, 98

S